Topics in Spine Imaging

Editor

LUBDHA M. SHAH

RADIOLOGIC CLINICS
OF NORTH AMERICA

www.radiologic.theclinics.com

Consulting Editor
FRANK H. MILLER

March 2019 • Volume 57 • Number 2

ELSEVIER

1600 John F. Kennedy Boulevard • Suite 1800 • Philadelphia, Pennsylvania, 19103-2899

http://www.theclinics.com

RADIOLOGIC CLINICS OF NORTH AMERICA Volume 57, Number 2
March 2019 ISSN 0033-8389, ISBN 13: 978-0-323-65532-3

Editor: John Vassallo (j.vassallo@elsevier.com)
Developmental Editor: Donald Mumford

Radiologic Clinics of North America (ISSN 0033-8389) is published bimonthly by Elsevier Inc., 360 Park Avenue South, New York, NY 10010-1710. Months of issue are January, March, May, July, September, and November. Periodicals postage paid at New York, NY and additional mailing offices. Subscription prices are USD 508 per year for US individuals, USD 933 per year for US institutions, USD 100 per year for US students and residents, USD 594 per year for Canadian individuals, USD 1193 per year for Canadian institutions, USD 683 per year for international individuals, USD 1193 per year for international institutions, and USD 315 per year for Canadian and international students/residents. To receive student and resident rate, orders must be accompanied by name of affiliated institution, date of term and the signature of program/residency coordinatior on institution letterhead. Orders will be billed at individual rate until proof of status is received. Foreign air speed delivery is included in all *Clinics* subscription prices. All prices are subject to change without notice. **POSTMASTER:** Send address changes to *Radiologic Clinics of North America*, Elsevier Health Sciences Division, Subscription Customer Service, 3251 Riverport Lane, Maryland Heights, MO63043. **Customer Service: Telephone: 1-800-654-2452** (U.S. and Canada); **1-314-447-8871** (outside U.S. and Canada). **Fax: 1-314-447-8029. E-mail: journalscustomerservice-usa@ elsevier.com (for print support); journalsonlinesupport-usa@elsevier.com (for online support)**.

Reprints. For copies of 100 or more of articles in this publication, please contact the Commercial Reprints Department, Elsevier Inc., 360 Park Avenue South, New York, New York 10010-1710. Tel.: +1-212-633-3874; Fax: +1-212-633-3820; E-mail: reprints@elsevier.com.

Radiologic Clinics of North America also published in Greek Paschalidis Medical Publications, Athens, Greece.

Radiologic Clinics of North America is covered in *MEDLINE/PubMed (Index Medicus), EMBASE/Excerpta Medica, Current Contents/Life Sciences, Current Contents/Clinical Medicine, RSNA Index to Imaging Literature, BIOSIS, Science Citation Index,* and *ISI/BIOMED.*

Contributors

CONSULTING EDITOR

FRANK H. MILLER, MD, FACR
Lee F. Rogers MD Professor of Medical
Education, Chief, Body Imaging Section and
Fellowship Program, Medical Director, MRI,
Department of Radiology, Northwestern
Memorial Hospital, Northwestern University
Feinberg School of Medicine, Chicago, Illinois

EDITOR

LUBDHA M. SHAH, MD
Associate Professor of Radiology, Department
of Radiology and Imaging Sciences, University
of Utah, Salt Lake City, Utah

AUTHORS

TIMOTHY J. AMRHEIN, MD
Assistant Professor, Division of Neuroradiology,
Department of Radiology, Duke University
Medical Center, Durham, North Carolina

MICHAEL S. BEATTIE, PhD
Department of Neurological Surgery, University
of California, San Francisco, Brain and Spinal
Injury Center, Zuckerberg San Francisco
General Hospital, San Francisco, California

JACQUELINE C. BRESNAHAN, PhD
Department of Neurological Surgery, University
of California, San Francisco, Brain and Spinal
Injury Center, Zuckerberg San Francisco
General Hospital, San Francisco, California

AARON J. CLARK, MD, PhD
Assistant Professor of Neurological Surgery,
University of California, San Francisco, San
Francisco, California

SANJAY S. DHALL, MD
Department of Neurological Surgery, University
of California, San Francisco, Brain and Spinal
Injury Center, Zuckerberg San Francisco
General Hospital, San Francisco, California

SEAN C. DODSON, MD
Radiology Specialists of Florida, Maitland,
Florida

AMISH H. DOSHI, MD
Associate Professor, Department of
Radiology, Icahn School of Medicine at
Mount Sinai, New York, New York

LAURA EISENMENGER, MD
Assistant Professor, Department of Radiology,
University of Wisconsin-Madison School of
Medicine and Public Health, Madison,
Wisconsin

ADAM R. FERGUSON, PhD
Department of Neurological Surgery,
University of California, San Francisco, Brain
and Spinal Injury Center, Zuckerberg San
Francisco General Hospital, San Francisco,
California

WENDE N. GIBBS, MD, MA
Assistant Professor, Department of
Radiology, Keck School of Medicine at
the University of Southern California,
Los Angeles, California

CHRISTOPHER J. HANRAHAN, MD, PhD
Associate Professor, Department of Radiology and Imaging Sciences, University of Utah, Salt Lake City, Utah

JOHN RUSSELL HUIE, PhD
Department of Neurological Surgery, University of California, San Francisco, Brain and Spinal Injury Center, Zuckerberg San Francisco General Hospital, San Francisco, California

TROY A. HUTCHINS, MD
Assistant Professor, Neuroradiology Division, Department of Radiology and Imaging Sciences, University of Utah, Salt Lake City, Utah

SCOTT M. JOHNSON, MD
Neuroradiology Fellow, Department of Radiology and Imaging Sciences, University of Utah, Salt Lake City, Utah

NICHOLAS A. KOONTZ, MD
Director of Fellowship Programs, Dean D.T. Maglinte Scholar in Radiology Education, Assistant Professor of Radiology and Otolaryngology–Head and Neck Surgery, Indiana University School of Medicine, Indianapolis, Indiana

PETER G. KRANZ, MD
Associate Professor, Director of Spine Intervention, Division of Neuroradiology, Department of Radiology, Duke University Medical Center, Durham, North Carolina

RICHARD L. LEAKE, MD
Assistant Professor, Department of Radiology and Imaging Sciences, University of Utah, Salt Lake City, Utah

LUKE N. LEDBETTER, MD
Department of Radiology, University of Kansas Health System, Kansas City, Kansas

JOHN D. LEEVER, MD
Department of Radiology, University of Kansas Health System, Kansas City, Kansas

MEGAN K. MILLS, MD
Assistant Professor, Department of Radiology and Imaging Sciences, University of Utah, Salt Lake City, Utah

KAMBIZ NAEL, MD
Associate Professor, Department of Radiology, Icahn School of Medicine at Mount Sinai, New York, New York

MIRIAM E. PECKHAM, MD
Assistant Professor, Neuroradiology Division, Department of Radiology and Imaging Sciences, University of Utah, Salt Lake City, Utah

PRASHANT RAGHAVAN, MBBS
Associate Professor, Department of Diagnostic Radiology and Nuclear Medicine, University of Maryland School of Medicine, Baltimore, Maryland

ULRICH RASSNER, MD
Department of Radiology and Imaging Sciences, University of Utah, Salt Lake City, Utah

JESSICA RECORD, MD
Neuroradiology Fellow, Department of Diagnostic Radiology and Nuclear Medicine, University of Maryland School of Medicine, Baltimore, Maryland

LUBDHA M. SHAH, MD
Associate Professor of Radiology, Department of Radiology and Imaging Sciences, University of Utah, Salt Lake City, Utah

VINIL N. SHAH, MD
Assistant Professor of Radiology, University of California, San Francisco, San Francisco, California

JASON F. TALBOTT, MD, PhD
Department of Radiology and Biomedical Imaging, Zuckerberg San Francisco General Hospital, Department of Neurological Surgery, University of California, San Francisco, San Francisco, California

LAWRENCE N. TANENBAUM, MD, FACR
Director of MRI, CT, and Advanced Imaging, Vice President, Medical Director of RadNet, Eastern Division, New York, New York

LORENNA VIDAL, MD
Assistant Professor, Department of Diagnostic Radiology and Nuclear Medicine, University of Maryland School of Medicine, Baltimore, Maryland

Contents

T2-weighted (T2W) imaging is the most important sequence for detection of acute traumatic spinal cord pathology in clinical practice. Intramedullary hemorrhage on T2W imaging is associated with some component of irreversible injury and arguably the most robust MR imaging predictor of injury severity. The MR imaging appearance of the injured spinal cord in the early stages of injury is highly dynamic, and the time delay from injury to imaging must be considered in image interpretation. Diffusion imaging offers promise as specific tool for interrogating spinal cord integrity, although well-designed, prospective clinical studies validating its application remain limited.

Nonosseous spinal tumors are rare and encompass a wide range of benign and malignant masses. Compartmental localization of the mass to the intramedullary, intradural extramedullary, or extradural spaces can narrow the differential of possibilities. Ependymomas and astrocytomas are the most common intramedullary masses. Nerve sheath tumors and meningiomas are the most common intradural extramedullary tumors, and nerve sheath tumors dominate the nonosseous extradural tumors. These tumors and other less common masses are described in this article through a space-based approach.

Benign and malignant as well as focal and diffuse disease processes can involve the spinal marrow. This is a review of the commonly encountered spinal marrow abnormalities and the distinguishing magnetic resonance features that may provide clues to disease.

Osseous metastases are the most common spine tumor and increasingly prevalent as advances in cancer treatments allow patients to live longer with their disease. Evidence-based algorithms derive the majority of their data from imaging studies and reports; the radiologist should understand the most current treatments and report in the language of the treatment team for efficient and effective communication and patient care. Advanced imaging techniques such as diffusion-weighted imaging and dynamic contrast-enhanced MRI are increasingly used for diagnosis and problem solving. Radiologists have a growing role in treatment of patients with metastatic disease, performing cement augmentation and tumor ablation.

Acute low back pain, defined as less than 6 weeks in duration, does not require imaging in the absence of "red flags" that may indicate a cause, such as fracture, infection, or malignancy. When imaging is indicated, it is important to rule out a host of abnormalities that may be responsible for the pain and any associated symptoms. A common mnemonic VINDICATE can help ensure a thorough consideration of the possible causes.

Imaging of the postoperative spine is commonly obtained but is often challenging to interpret. Accurate and clinically relevant interpretation requires a strong understanding of the preoperative spinal pathologic condition, the surgical procedure performed, and the expected imaging appearance of postoperative changes. This article reviews common surgical approaches to the degenerative spine, the most appropriate imaging modalities to use, how to optimize imaging protocols, and how to interpret those images. The reader will therefore possess the tools required to effectively assess postoperative spine imaging, identify early and late complications, and provide the surgeon with relevant information to guide patient management.

This article reviews the role of imaging in the diagnosis, management, and treatment of spontaneous intracranial hypotension (SIH). SIH is a debilitating and often misdiagnosed condition caused by either a spinal cerebrospinal fluid (CSF) leak or a CSF to venous fistula. This pathologic condition is identified and localized via spinal imaging, including computed tomographic (CT) myelography, dynamic myelography, dynamic (ultrafast) CT myelography, MR imaging, or MR myelography with intrathecal gadolinium. Treatment of SIH involves conservative measures, surgery, or imaging-guided epidural blood patching.

Cross-sectional spinal imaging is common, and extraspinal findings are often incidentally identified during interpretation. Although some of these findings may cause symptoms that mimic a spinal disorder, the majority are entirely asymptomatic and incidental. It is essential that the radiologist not only identify those abnormalities that may have clinical significance but also recognize those that are clinically irrelevant and thereby prevent patients from being subjected to further unnecessary, expensive and potentially harmful interventions. This article focuses on those abnormalities that are commonly encountered and provides practical guidance for follow-up and management based on current recommendations.

PROGRAM OBJECTIVE

The objective of the *Radiologic Clinics of North America* is to keep practicing radiologists and radiology residents up to date with current clinical practice in radiology by providing timely articles reviewing the state of the art in patient care.

TARGET AUDIENCE

Practicing radiologists, radiology residents, and other healthcare professionals who provide patient care utilizing radiologic findings.

LEARNING OBJECTIVES

Upon completion of this activity, participants will be able to:
1. Review imaging highlights of spinal pathologies and their clinical importance.
2. Discuss postoperative spine imaging and patient management.
3. Recognize the role of advanced imaging techniques in improved diagnoses and post treatment problem solving.

ACCREDITATION

The Elsevier Office of Continuing Medical Education (EOCME) is accredited by the Accreditation Council for Continuing Medical Education (ACCME) to provide continuing medical education for physicians.

The EOCME designates this enduring material for a maximum of 15 *AMA PRA Category 1 Credit*(s)™. Physicians should claim only the credit commensurate with the extent of their participation in the activity.

All other healthcare professionals requesting continuing education credit for this enduring material will be issued a certificate of participation.

DISCLOSURE OF CONFLICTS OF INTEREST

The EOCME assesses conflict of interest with its instructors, faculty, planners, and other individuals who are in a position to control the content of CME activities. All relevant conflicts of interest that are identified are thoroughly vetted by EOCME for fair balance, scientific objectivity, and patient care recommendations. EOCME is committed to providing its learners with CME activities that promote improvements or quality in healthcare and not a specific proprietary business or a commercial interest.

The planning committee, staff, authors and editors listed below have identified no financial relationships or relationships to products or devices they or their spouse/life partner have with commercial interest related to the content of this CME activity:

Timothy J. Amrhein, MD; Michael S. Beattie, PhD; Jacqueline C. Bresnahan, PhD; Sean C. Dodson, MD; Laura Eisenmenger, MD; Adam R. Ferguson, PhD; Wende N. Gibbs, MD, MA; Christopher J. Hanrahan, MD, PhD; John Russell Huie, PhD; Troy A. Hutchins, MD; Scott M. Johnson, MD; Alison Kemp; Nicholas A. Koontz, MD; Peter G. Kranz, MD; Pradeep Kuttysankaran; Richard L. Leake, MD; Luke N. Ledbetter, MD; John D. Leever, MD; Frank H. Miller, MD, FACR; Megan K. Mills, MD; Miriam E. Peckham, MD; Prashant Raghavan, MBBS; Ulrich Rassner, MD; Jessica Record, MD; Lubdha M. Shah, MD; Vinil N. Shah, MD; Jason F. Talbott, MD, PhD; Lawrence N. Tanenbaum, MD, FACR; John Vassallo; Lorenna Vidal, MD.

The planning committee, staff, authors and editors listed below have identified financial relationships or relationships to products or devices they or their spouse/life partner have with commercial interest related to the content of this CME activity:

Aaron J. Clark, MD, PhD: is a consultant/advisor for NuVasive, Inc.
Sanjay S. Dhall, MD: participates in a speakers burea for Globus Medical Inc. and DePuy Synthes.
Amish H. Doshi, MD: participates in a speakers burea for Merit Medical Systems.
Kambiz Nael, MD: is a consultant/advisor for Olea Medical and Siemens Corporation.

UNAPPROVED/OFF-LABEL USE DISCLOSURE

The EOCME requires CME faculty to disclose to the participants:
1. When products or procedures being discussed are off-label, unlabelled, experimental, and/or investigational (not US Food and Drug Administration [FDA] approved); and
2. Any limitations on the information presented, such as data that are preliminary or that represent ongoing research, interim analyses, and/or unsupported opinions. Faculty may discuss information about pharmaceutical agents that is outside of FDA-approved labelling. This information is intended solely for CME and is not intended to promote off-label use of these medications. If you have any questions, contact the medical affairs department of the manufacturer for the most recent prescribing information.

TO ENROLL

To enroll in the *Radiologic Clinics of North America* Continuing Medical Education program, call customer service at 1-800-654-2452 or sign up online at http://www.theclinics.com/home/cme. The CME program is available to subscribers for an additional annual fee of USD 327.60.

METHOD OF PARTICIPATION

In order to claim credit, participants must complete the following:

1. Complete enrolment as indicated above.
2. Read the activity.
3. Complete the CME Test and Evaluation. Participants must achieve a score of 70% on the test. All CME Tests and Evaluations must be completed online.

CME INQUIRIES/SPECIAL NEEDS

For all CME inquiries or special needs, please contact elsevierCME@elsevier.com.

RADIOLOGIC CLINICS OF NORTH AMERICA

RELATED SERIES

Magnetic Resonance Imaging Clinics
Neuroimaging Clinics
PET Clinics

THE CLINICS ARE AVAILABLE ONLINE!
Access your subscription at:
www.theclinics.com

Preface
New View of Spine Imaging

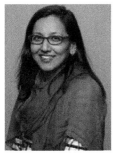

Lubdha M. Shah, MD
Editor

Imaging of the spine is exciting as advances in imaging techniques improve our diagnoses from the vague categories of previous years (eg, extradural mass, intramedullary abnormality, and intradural extramedullary lesion) to more specific diagnoses (eg, cavernous malformation, arachnoid adhesion with presyrinx state). The spine is particularly challenging to image because of several factors, including the osseous cerebrospinal fluid (CSF)-spinal cord interfaces, the small size of the spinal cord, the CSF pulsation artifact, and the poor signal-to-noise with conventional MR imaging sequences. Newer techniques are enabling us to overcome these limitations. Strides have also been made in imaging of the postoperative spine, which will be adroitly reviewed by two authors in this issue.

The topics in this issue cover spine diagnoses that we encounter routinely in a fresh, new perspective, integrating conventional imaging findings with those on advanced techniques. Lesions involving the spine may not be isolated to spinal disease but may be a manifestation of systemic disease. It is also important to understand the treatment implications of imaging features of various spinal pathologies. There are some lesions for which it is important to employ judicious follow-up rather than immediate biopsy at the acute presentation. The authors review not only the imaging highlights of spinal pathologies but also their clinical importance. Algorithms of imaging underscore the importance of appropriate diagnostic imaging and reporting, which is increasingly important in this era of value-based imaging and meaningful use.

The esteemed authors are experts in the field of neuroradiology, particularly in spine imaging, and bring expertise to their respective articles. They represent various institutions and have contributed a rich case selection. I am very grateful to each of the authors for their efforts and dedication in preparing this issue of *Radiologic Clinics of North America*. Their outstanding efforts illustrate how thrilling current spine imaging is and the even more exciting diagnostic discoveries that are on the horizon.

Lubdha M. Shah, MD
Department of Radiology
University of Utah
University of Utah Health Sciences Center
30N 1900, Room 1A071
Salt Lake City, UT 84132, USA

E-mail address:
lubdha.shah@hsc.utah.edu

Radiol Clin N Am 57 (2019) xi
https://doi.org/10.1016/j.rcl.2018.11.002
0033-8389/19/© 2018 Published by Elsevier Inc.

Pearls and Pitfalls of Spine Imaging

Ulrich Rassner, MD

KEYWORDS

- Artifact • Tissue suppression • Hardware • MR sequences • Protocol optimization

KEY POINTS

- Metal artifact on computed tomography is a combination of different artifacts; each can be addressed by different parameter changes.
- Volumetric T2 sequences (CUBE, SPACE, VISTA) have lower whereas T2* GRE have higher T2 contrast for spinal cord lesions.
- Gradient echo (GRE) sequences tend to have less pulsation but are more affected by spinal hardware.
- Fat saturation can saturate water, in which case enhancement will also be nulled.
- Remedies for metal artifact on MR imaging depend on the sequence. Some changes beneficial on one sequence can be ineffective or detrimental on other sequences.

COMPUTED TOMOGRAPHY

Although computed tomography (CT) imaging of the spine is quite routine, slight variations in slice thickness and used imaging kernels are common. A challenge when imaging the spine with CT is the presence of hardware. Although bone attenuates X rays 2 to 3 times as much as water, metals used for spinal hardware can have more than 30 times the attenuation of water resulting in a variety of effects, including beam hardening, photon starvation, and data inconsistencies. The problem is 2-fold: how to evaluate the hardware and how to minimize artifact in the tissues surrounding the hardware.

Hardware evaluation is hampered by the much higher attenuation of metal compared with soft tissues. With exception of dental enamel, CT numbers of biological tissues range from −1000 HU to ≈ 2300 HU, whereas spinal hardware can have CT numbers exceeding 30,000. For most scanners, the standard CT image is a 12-bit image with a CT number range of −1024 to 3071. The hardware and the directly adjacent soft tissues with artifactual elevation of CT numbers are in excess of 3071 HU and thus will appear as the same attenuation (3071). The artifact directly adjacent to the hardware, which also is in excess of 3071 HU will be indistinguishable from the hardware, leading to blooming. Some scanners allow for an extended CT scale reconstruction, where CT numbers change in increments of 10, covering a range exceeding 30,000, whereas some vendors allow 16-bit CT image reconstruction with an inherently larger dynamic range.[1] Both methods allow windowing away the blooming artifact with improved visualization of hardware (Fig. 1).

The degree of artifact surrounding the hardware depends on the material used. While stainless steel and vitallium hardware causes striking artifact, titanium less so due to the decreased attenuation coefficient (1 cm of steel attenuate 99% of 80 keV photons, whereas 1 cm of titanium only attenuates 83%). The variety of different artifacts caused by metal are jointly referred to as "streak artifact" (Figs. 2 and 3); however it is helpful to consider them separately[2,3] (Table 1):

Disclosures: None.
Department of Radiology and Imaging Sciences, University of Utah, 30 North 1900 East #1A071, Salt Lake City, UT 84132-2140, USA
E-mail address: Ulrich.rassner@hsc.utah.edu

Radiol Clin N Am 57 (2019) 233–255
https://doi.org/10.1016/j.rcl.2018.09.003

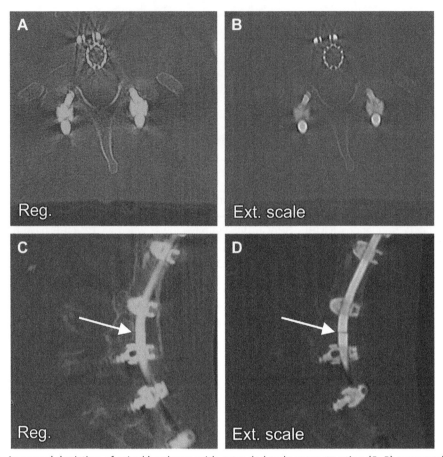

Fig. 1. The improved depiction of spinal hardware with extended scale reconstruction (*B, D*) compared with regular reconstruction (*A, C*). The CT-number scale of routine reconstructions ranges from −1024 to 3071 HU. Extending the scale to more than 30,000 (*D*) allows a window wide enough to minimize blooming; see more detail within the hardware and demonstrate better conspicuity of hardware fracture (*arrow*).

1. Beam hardening: due to preferential attenuation of low-energy photons the average energy of the x-ray photons increases as the beam traverses materials, more pronounced with high-attenuation materials. This leads to decreased attenuation of the hardened beam and therefore artificial decrease of CT numbers and is improved with increased kV and dual-energy scanning calculating virtual monoenergetic images.

2. Aliasing: due to insufficient data points to accurately represent high spatial frequencies. This leads to fine streaks arising either directly adjacent to the hardware or at some distance. It is improved by increasing number of sample (in some scanners accomplished by increasing rotation time).

3. Windmill artifact: due to interpolation errors of data between 2 detector rows. In helical scanning a thin reconstructed slice alternatingly lines up with a detector row and lies between 2 detector rows. When in between detector rows, data from both rows are interpolated for reconstruction. Interpolation can be incorrect at high-contrast interfaces, with resulting alternating brighter and darker streaks that rotate when scrolling through the images. It is improved by increasing slice thickness, which leads to volume averaging of the streaks. Non-integer pitch values can also slightly reduce artifact.[2]

4. Photon starvation: due to attenuation of large number of photons. As the number of photons decreases quantum mottle increases, resulting in noisier data. It is improved with increased kV and mAs at the expense of dose and decreased contrast resolution, most conspicuously with iodine.

5. Reconstruction error: due to data inconsistencies in part due to bream hardening, scatter and photon starvation is improved with specialized metal artifact reduction algorithms that use data segmentation and iterative reconstruction approaches.[3]

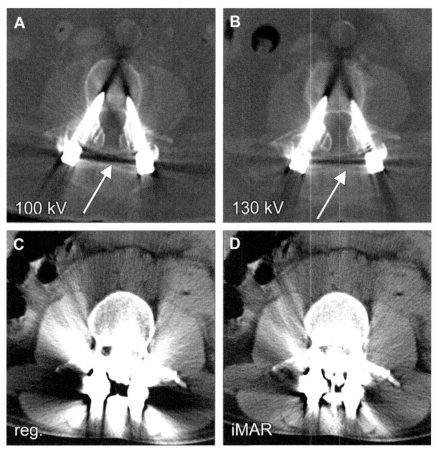

Fig. 2. Change in metal artifact with changes in kV (*A, B*) and with specialized metal artifact reduction reconstruction (*C, D*). Beam hardening is slightly reduced with a kV of 130 (*B*) compared with 100 kV (*A*). Streak artifact (*arrow*) is slightly reduced due to less photon starvation. Specialized metal artifact reduction reconstruction (*D*) shows a noticeable improvement in artifact adjacent to the metal hardware compared with a standard reconstruction (*C*).

MR IMAGING
Standard Sequences

T1

Although a conventional T1 spin echo (SE) or fast spin echo (FSE) is the most commonly used sequence, some people favor inversion recovery (IR) prepared T1 FSE (IR-FSE, T1- fluid ttenuation inversion recovery [FLAIR]). The preference for one or the other may also be influenced by the field strength of the used scanner. T1 IR-FSE and T1 SE/FSE have many similarities and the difference between them is much more pronounced on 3 Tesla (T) scans (**Fig. 4**) than 1.5 T scans, owing to the poor T1 contrast on 3 T T1 SE/FSE. Improvement in contrast and decrease in signal-to-noise ratio (SNR) have been demonstrated.[4,5] However, some feel that the improvement in contrast has the disadvantage of making the marrow seem more heterogeneous. Lastly, the

choice of imaging parameters can vary quite greatly for different IR-T1 sequences. The sharpness of the image and the exact contrast behavior depends on the TE and number of refocused echoes (turbo factor/echo train length). The larger the number of refocused echoes and the shorter the TE, the more the unsharpness that will result. When the repetition time (TR) and the inversion time (TI) are not matched, fluid signal increases. Furthermore, if TI is relatively too short for a given TR, water will maintain antiparallel magnetization, whereas all other tissues will have parallel longitudinal magnetization. After the excitation pulse, water and all other tissues will be 180° out of phase (OOP), resulting in bounce point artifact (signal cancellation at the water/tissue interface).[6] Bounce point artifact can simulate superficial siderosis (see **Fig. 4**).

Flow effects in cerebrospinal fluid (CSF), and also vessels, can be prominent in T1 sequences,

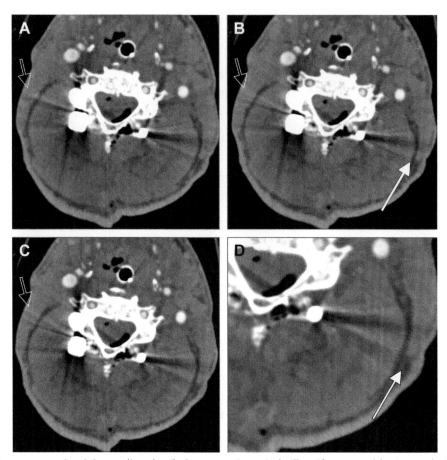

Fig. 3. Three consecutive 0.6 mm slices (*A–C*) demonstrating windmill artifact caused by interpolation errors. When scrolling (*A–C*) the artifact moves clockwise in this example (*open arrow*). Also visible is aliasing artifact starting at a distance from the responsible metal hardware (*arrow*). Higher magnification (*D*) shows the artifact more clearly.

leading to artificially elevated T1 signal, particularly in the axial plane. This is seen due to flow-related enhancement, with inflow of fully magnetized spins into the image plane, further discussed later.[7]

Pulsation/phase artifact from mediastinal structures and lungs can cause image degradation more pronounced on T1 SE/FSE or IR-T1 FSE, particularly on postcontrast sequences due to the high signal in the vasculature, and can make evaluation of potential spinal cord enhancement challenging. In general, gradient echo (GRE) sequences are less susceptible to pulsation artifact (**Fig. 5**). Three-dimensional (3D) T1 GRE images greatly reduce pulsation artifact; however, these sequences have their own drawbacks, such as increased artifact from spinal hardware. Depending on the hardware, artifact can render T1 GRE sequences nondiagnostic (see **Fig. 5**). The contrast behavior of T1 GRE and SE/FSE is different and thus obtaining the GRE sequence pre- and

postcontrast is advisable. Pulsation artifact maybe reduced with gated (respiratory and/or electrocardiogram [ECG]) sequences; however, this increases imaging time and shows variable improvement.[8] Non-Cartesian k-space readout has also shown to offer improved image quality[9] but is not widely available and can cause unique artifacts.

T2/T2*

Although conventional 2D T2-FSE is the most commonly used techniques, 3D sequences have the appeal of only acquiring one sequence (commonly in the sagittal plane) and reconstructing the other planes. Although 2D T2-FSE sequences are a good routine sequence, there are certain drawbacks: flow artifact can be quite pronounced,[7] particularly in areas of disc disease, where the narrowed area of the thecal sac results in increased CSF flow velocities and increases flow-related signal loss. The signal loss can be so pronounced that it blends together with

Table 1
Computed tomography metal artifact

Artifact	Remedy	Drawback of Remedy
Beam hardening	↑ kV	↑Dose unless mAs is adjusted ↓ Contrast
Aliasing	↑ Rotation time	↑ Scan time ↑ Chance of motion
Windmill	↑ Slice thickness Noninteger pitch values	↓ Spatial resolution
Photon starvation	↑kV ↑mAs	↓ Contrast ↑ Dose
Reconstruction error	Specialized reconstruction	Availability

herniated disc and creates the appearance of even more severe narrowing (**Fig. 6**).

Pulsation artifact can also be present from lung and mediastinum, particularly in the thoracic spine, where swapping phase- and frequency-encoding direction often does not improve the situation; rather it replaces pulsation artifact from the mediastinum with motion artifact from the lungs. Furthermore, in larger patients, wraparound from the arms can cause additional image degradation.

3D T2 sequences can be used. Often the variety with variable flip angles (SPACE, CUBE, VISTA) is used. These sequences allow for high-quality multiplanar reformats and at TEs used in regular 2D T2 FSE sequences, with often, but not invariably, reduced CSF flow artifact[10] (see **Fig. 6**). However, there can be certain drawbacks. For time reasons, the coverage of the reformatted images is often less than a native acquisition.

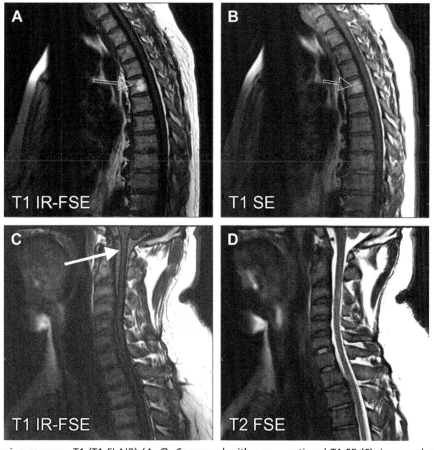

Fig. 4. Inversion recovery T1 (T1 FLAIR) (*A, C*). Compared with a conventional T1 SE (*B*), increased contrast between spinal cord and CSF is noticeable, as well as the higher contrast within the bone marrow (*arrow* indicates incidental hemangioma). (*C*) The effect of mismatched inversion time (TI) and TR. CSF signal is too high and an artificial black line (bounce point artifact) is seen on the surface of the spinal cord (*arrow*). Although any mismatch of TI and TR results in incomplete CSF signal suppression, only when TI is relatively too short for a given TR, will bounce point artifact occur. (*D*) T2 FSE on the same patient as (*C*) demonstrating lack of superficial siderosis, which bounce point artifact could be confused with.

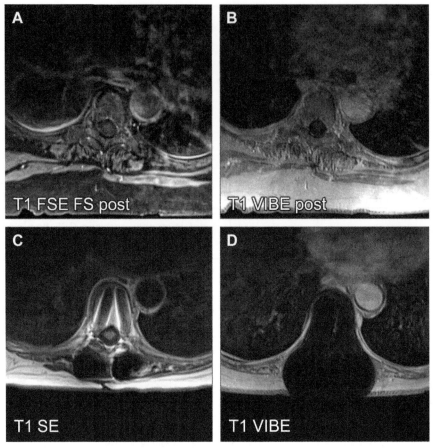

Fig. 5. 3D T1 VIBE sequence (*B, D*) compared with T1 SE (*A, C*). (*A, B*) Both sequence types postcontrast with noticeably more pulsation/breathing artifact in the SE sequence. (*C, D*) Axial precontrast T1 SE and 3D T1 VIBE. Clearly noticeable is the large artifact surrounding spinal fusion hardware on the VIBE sequence due to absence of a refocusing pulse.

Similarly, the spatial resolution of reformatted images from a 3D acquisition is often inferior (**Fig. 7**)[11] unless very high spatial resolution images are used, which require longer acquisition times and therefore increase chance of motion artifact. The contrast behavior is somewhat different than conventional 2D-T2 FSE.[12] With TE values used in conventional T2 FSE, cord lesion contrast is poor and subtle T2 lesion in the cord may not be seen or seen less well (see **Fig. 7**). To achieve good T2 contrast for subtle cord lesions and gray/white matter differentiation, TE values need to be longer than for conventional T2 sequences, which can lead to more pronounced CSF flow artifact and even complete loss of CSF signal (see **Fig. 6**), depending on individual CSF dynamics. Thus, when using these types of T2 sequences, the study needs to be optimized for either spinal cord lesion contrast or visibility of thecal sac encroachment/nerve root lesions (bright CSF).

T2* GRE-based sequences have been used predominantly not only in the evaluation of demyelinating spinal cord lesions[13] but also in the setting of traumatic spinal cord injury.[14] These maybe conventional T2* GRE images or variants that combine multiple echoes (eg, multiple echo recombined gradient echo and multi-echo data image combination). Although these sequences exhibit higher sensitivity for subtle spinal cord lesions, some studies demonstrate decreased specificity[13,15] (**Fig. 8**). In the setting of trauma, GRE sequences and susceptibility weighted imaging are useful for detection of spinal cord hemorrhage.[14,16] Because of the lack of a refocusing pulse, these sequences will be more negatively affected by susceptibility effects from hardware than SE or FSE sequences.

SHORT TAU INVERSION RECOVERY

This widely used fat suppressed sequence is valuable in the evaluation of osseous and ligamentous

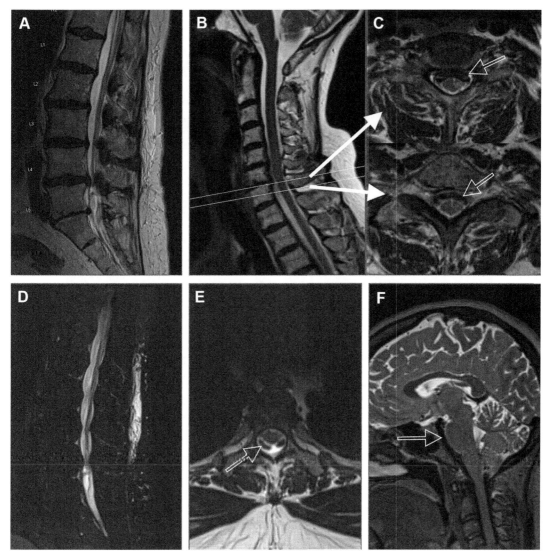

Fig. 6. CSF flow artifact on sagittal T2 FSE with TE 100 ms (A) and T2 SPACE with TE of 120 (D) show mild and similar flow effects anterior to conus and cauda equina. Axial T2 FSE (E) shows very pronounced flow artifact (*open arrow*). (F) Sagittal T2 SPACE with TE 265 ms shows good grey-white contrast in cerebellum and occipital lobes, however demonstrates complete loss of CSF signal in the cervical spine (*open arrow*). (B, C) Cervical spine T2 FSE sagittal image (B) shows narrowing of the thecal sac, with some CSF maintained anterior to the cord. Two axial images from the same study (C) shows how flow artifact blends together with the disc disease on the upper slice giving the appearance of no residual CSF between disc and cord (solid arrows indicate the 2 slice locations shown in [C]). Flow artifact extends below level of disc disease, as seen on the lower slice.

injury but is also characterized by its high sensitivity for spinal cord lesions.[17] Although it does seem to have the same image weighting as a T2 FSE image with fat saturation, the contrast is influenced by different features. The main cause of the high fluid signal on STIR is a T1, more precisely an inverse T1, effect. After the inversion pulse, fat, owing to its short T1 time (300–400 ms), quickly loses antiparallel magnetization, whereas all the other tissues lose antiparallel magnetization at a much slower rate, in particular water, due to the very long T1 time (4–5 seconds). When fat has recovered to the null point, all other tissues (particularly water) will still have antiparallel magnetization, which will be flipped into the transverse plane by the excitation pulse.[18,19] Fluid is bright because of inverse T1 rather than T2 effects, although the often slightly longer TE (30–60 ms) used with STIR superimposes some T2 weighting, emphasizing the bright fluid signal.

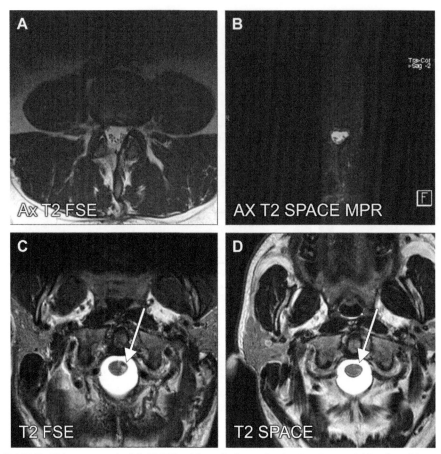

Fig. 7. T2 SPACE (*B, D*) is compared with T2 FSE. Although the native 3D SPACE acquisition has thinner slices than a comparable 2D T2 FSE, multiplanar reformats (*B*) often suffer from lower in-plane resolution and less coverage than a natively acquired 2D FSE (*A*). With a TE of 120 ms, flow artifact is minimal on T2 SPACE (*D*); however, sensitivity for subtle cord lesions is diminished compared with a 2D T2 FSE with a TE of 100 ms. Cord lesion in this patient with multiple sclerosis (MS) is much better seen on the T2 FSE, than on the SPACE sequence.

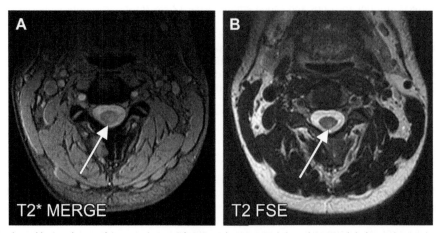

Fig. 8. Spinal cord lesion (*arrows*) in a patient with MS with T2* GRE (*A*) and T2 FSE (*B*) shows better lesion conspicuity on the GRE sequence. Central gray matter in the cord is also brighter and maybe misinterpreted as a lesion, explaining higher sensitivity but lower specificity described for T2* GRE sequences in evaluation of cord lesions.

The preference for how completely fat signal is suppressed varies. The inversion time can be used to control how complete fat suppression will be. Typical inversion times for STIR are 150 to 200 ms, with 150 ms resulting in partial and 180 to 200 ms resulting in more complete fat suppression (**Fig. 9**). Care should be taken that TI is not set too high, to avoid bounce point artifact, which typically is thought of in the context of water-suppressed sequences (T1 and T2 FLAIR) but can be seen with STIR at fat/water interfaces, giving a similar appearance to an OOP GRE. In contrast, on T1 and T2 FLAIR sequences, the artifact is seen at brain/water interfaces.

It is important to remember that not only fat can be suppressed on STIR, but also other T1 bright lesions, as STIR targets fat by its T1 time (see **Fig. 9**).

SPECIALTY SEQUENCES
In- and Out-of-Phase

In-phase (IP) and OOP images are often used to distinguish malignant from nonmalignant lesions. These sequences use chemical shift artifact of the second kind (signal loss due to signal cancellation from out of phase fat and water hydrogen spins).[20] They are typically GRE sequences and as such sensitive to susceptibility artifact (the

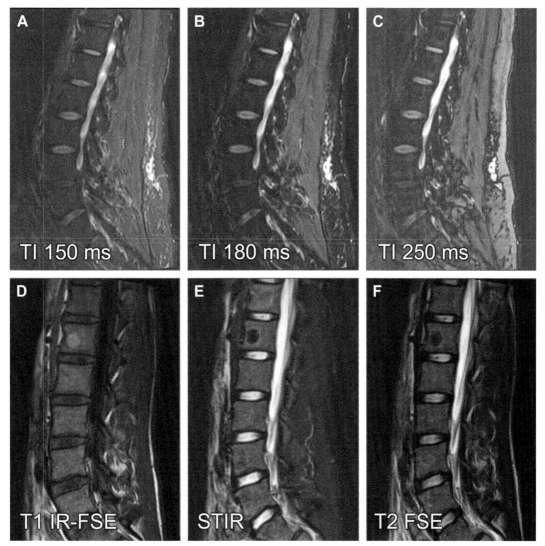

Fig. 9. (*A–C*) The effect of changes in TI on STIR image. Although a TI of 180 ms (*B*) gives the most complete fat suppression, some prefer slightly less fat suppression, which can be achieved by shortening TI to 150 ms (*A*). Although increasing TI more than 180 ms also results in decreased fat suppression, it now shows signal cancellation at fat/water interfaces due to bounce point artifact, giving an appearance akin to chemical shift artifact of the second kind (OOP). (*D–F*) shows a melanoma metastasis that is bright on T1 (*D*) and dark on STIR (*E*), mimicking a hemangioma. T2 FSE (*F*) shows low signal, not typical for hemangioma.

longer TE sequence more so than the shorter TE sequence). Of note, it is important to acquire OOP images with a shorter TE than the IP images, to ensure that when lower signal is present in a lesion on OOP images, it is due to chemical shift of the second kind and not due to T2* decay. This effect is well known to affect IP and OOP imaging in iron storage disease[21] but could similarly occur in hemorrhagic spinal lesions. Signal loss will occur when fat and water are present in the same voxel, whereas no signal loss will be seen when it is a watery lesion devoid of fat. However, no signal loss will be present in a purely fatty lesion either and thus lack of signal loss does not necessarily indicate a malignant lesion.

Diffusion

Routine diffusion-weighted imaging (DWI) is done with echoplanar imaging (EPI) sequences. This proves challenging in the spine imaging due to more heterogeneous anatomy and susceptibility effects, which are more pronounced at higher-field strengths and even more problematic with spinal hardware.[22,23] Echoplanar sequences use only gradients to refocus signal during readout and are typically done as single-shot sequences (sampling all of k-space in one shot). Changes that reduce the number of gradient refocusing steps are helpful, such as narrow field of view (FOV), parallel imaging, and multi-shot EPI sequences. Some vendors also have FSE-based diffusion-weighted sequences, which inherently are much more robust in respect to susceptibility effects (PROPELLER DWI). It is important to remember that EPI-based diffusion images will always be fat suppressed because of the large chemical shift artifact of the first kind (see the later discussion), whereas FSE-based DWI (eg, PROPELLER DWI) does not require fat suppression. However, the suppression of fat will change absolute apparent diffusion coefficient (ADC) values, as has been demonstrated in liver imaging.[24] It is also important to recognize that there is no accepted standard of b-values used in spine imaging. Although in brain imaging most commonly b-values of 1000 and 2000 s/mm^2, in spine imaging the b-values range from 400 to 1000 s/mm^2, with some using 2 b-values, but others 3 or even 6 different b-values.[22,25,26] These differences can affect the appearance of pathology and will certainly affect measured ADC values.

ARTIFACTS
Flow-Related Enhancement

Although loss of signal in CSF due to flow is well known, it maybe overlooked that flow-related enhancement can also occur.[7] Because of short TR, spins in the image plane are not allowed to fully recover and thus will have lower signal than inflowing fully recovered spins. This effect is typically seen at the first and last slice, called entry-slice phenomenon. Because of the typically larger number of slices required during axial imaging, they are often acquired in multiple blocks (acquisitions, concatenations), particularly for T1 sequences. Because the scanner typically interleaves these, entry slice phenomenon can occur on every single slice (imagine we are imaging with 3 concatenations: first block will contain slice 1,4,7,10..., the second block slice 2,5,8,11...., and the last block slice 3.6,9,12.... Thus, while acquiring the slices in block 1, fully recovered spins from slice 2 and 3 can flow into slice 1 or 4 to cause flow-related enhancement). This can lead to artificially high CSF signal. Although more commonly observed on T1-weighted sequences, the same effect maybe seen on T2-weighted sequences. Given the typically used TR (3000–6000 ms), water is not completely recovered (it takes water about 20–25 s to fully recover longitudinal magnetization) and inflow of fully recovered water leads to increased signal. In 3D sequences this will only occur at the top and/or bottom slice. Flow-related enhancement is also seen in vessels (Fig. 10). The latter can be helpful if an enhancing nerve root is suspected. If there is flow-related enhancement in the structure on precontrast images, it represents a vessel, not a nerve root.

Chemical Shift

Chemical shift artifact is a group of artifacts caused by the difference in resonance frequency between fat and water, and also silicone when present. This causes problems whenever frequency is used as a marker of location (frequency encoding and slice selection)[27] and when spins are not refocused by a refocusing pulse, causing signal loss when fat and water spins are OOP at TE (chemical shift artifact of the second kind). Although spatial misregistration artifacts are often grouped together as chemical shift artifacts, some also describe them as separate entities: chemical shift artifact of the first kind = misregistration in frequency encoding direction and chemical misexcitation = misregistration in slice select direction (through-plane). The benefit of separating them is that they are affected by different scan parameters.

Chemical shift of the first kind: during frequency encoding, a gradient causes differences in precession frequency along the gradient. Akin to a piano,

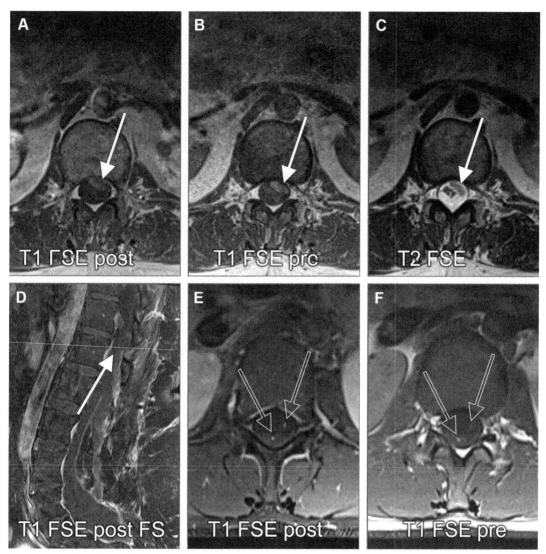

Fig. 10. Examples of CSF flow artifact, with artificially elevated T1 signal in CSF (*arrows, A–D*), which could be confused with a mass. Artificial high T1 signal is present on axial post- (*A*) and precontrast (*B*) images. T2 (*C*) shows prominent signal loss. Sagittal postcontrast fat saturated T1 (*D*) shows no corresponding lesion. (*E, F*) Two apparent enhancing nerve roots (*open arrows*) on T1 postcontrast sequence (*E*). Flow-related enhancement on the precontrast T1 (*F*) indicates that these represent vessels.

where the frequency of a note corresponds to the location of the key that was struck, location information is encoded into the frequency of the signal. Since fat always precesses at a lower frequency than water (3.5 ppm), it always gets assigned to the incorrect location and is shifted in the direction of lower frequency. The severity of this effect depends on the chosen receive bandwidth (rBW). At 1.5 T the difference in resonance frequency between fat and water is about 210 Hz. Thus if an rBW of 210 Hz/px (pixel) is chosen, the spatial misregistration will be 1 pixel. If rBW is decreased to 105 Hz/px, misregistration increases to 2 pixels.

Note that different vendors use different nomenclatures to describe rBW: Hz/px, kHz over FOV or chemical shift in pixels between fat and water. Increasing rBW to reduce chemical shift artifact of the first kind comes at the expense of the SNR, with doubling rBW reducing SNR 1.4 fold. Chemical shift artifact can be helpful in the identification of fatty lesions such as filum lipomas but can also cause artificial narrowing of the spinal canal when frequency encoding direction is chosen in anterior-posterior direction (posterior epidural fat can be shifted anteriorly) (**Fig. 11**). The direction of the shift depends on the gradient slope

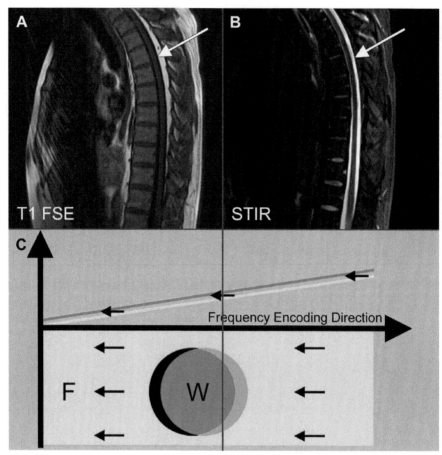

Fig. 11. Effects of chemical shift (resonance frequency difference between fat and water). (*A*) The appearance of a narrowed thecal sac (*arrow*) with minimal CSF dorsal to the cord due to epidural fat on the sagittal T1 SE; however, the sagittal STIR (*B*) shows that this is due to chemical shift of the first kind with anterior misregistration of epidural fat in frequency encoding direction. (*C*) The mechanism of chemical shift of the first kind. Fat always precesses at a lower frequency than water. Because frequency is used as a marker of location with frequency encoding gradient turned on, fat in the image is shifted toward the lower frequency (*arrows*).

direction, and while it can be shifted anteriorly in some scanners, it can also be shifted posteriorly in other scanners.

Chemical misexcitation: frequency is also used as a marker of location when slices are selected with a slice select gradient and a radiofrequency pulse with a certain transmit bandwidth (tBW). The resonance frequency difference between fat and water results in a slightly different slice plane for fat and water—fat is shifted through-plane. This artifact is much less conspicuous than chemical shift artifact, but it is almost always visible. It can lead to neuroforaminal fat being shifted into the thecal sac, simulating perineural cysts. Epidural fat can also be shifted into the thecal sac, sometimes even superimposing on the spinal cord simulating cord lesions or obscuring cord lesions (**Fig. 12**). As is the case with chemical shift of the first kind, the direction of shift depends on the

gradient slope direction and can be different from scanner to scanner. Chemical misexcitation is reduced by increasing tBW at the expense of increasing energy deposition (SAR—Specific Absorption Rate) and typically a less ideal slice profile with more potential for crosstalk. Not all scanners allow for adjustment of tBW, or it may not be obvious as such and may be labeled as a different type of rf-pulse, such as a fast pulse (increasing tBW shortens rf-pulse duration)

Pulsation/Breathing Artifact

Artifact from pulsation and breathing is a common problem and most bothersome in thoracic spine imaging. The artifact projects in phase encoding direction, and although choosing phase encoding direction in left-right direction reduces artifact from mediastinum, motion from the lungs can still

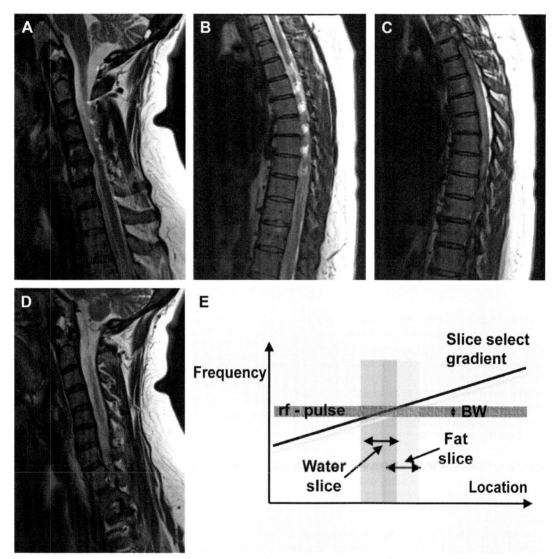

Fig. 12. Effects of chemical misexcitation. Because of resonance frequency difference of fat and water, fat and water slices are not identical. This through-plane shift of fat relative to water is seen on a left paramedian slice (*A*) with interspinous fat shifted into the thecal sac partially superimposing on the cord. The right paramedian slice (*D*) does not show this effect, because the fat is shifted away from the thecal sac. (*B*) and (*C*) show the same effect in the thoracic spine, with neuroforaminal fat shifted into the thecal sac on the right paramedian slice (*B*), giving the appearance of cysts, while no such effect is seen on the left paramedian slice (*D*). The direction of shift depends on the direction of gradient slope and can be different from scanner to scanner, as is seen in the first 2 examples. (*E*) The cause of chemical misexcitation, with the excitation rf-pulse selecting slightly different slice planes for fat and water due to the lower resonance frequency of fat (*yellow line*) compared with water (*blue line*).

produce prominent artifact and wraparound can pose additional problems in larger patients. In general terms, artifact is more pronounced on SE and FSE sequences, sequences with Cartesian k-space acquisition, and with contrast-enhanced T1 sequences. Artifacts are less pronounced on GRE sequences, non-Cartesian readouts (radial or PROPELLER/BLADE), and in the absence of intravenous contrast on T1 sequences.

Respiratory and/or ECG gating[28] can be performed, but results are variable and can carry a noticeable time penalty.

Fat Suppression

Fat suppression is a vital part of spine imaging.[19] Four different techniques are used (**Table 2**), with the first 2 available on most scanners: chemical

Table 2
Fat suppression techniques

Techniques	Mechanism Targets Fat by	Advantage	Drawback
Fat saturation	Resonance frequency	Specific for fat Can be added to virtually any other sequence	Sensitive to B_0 inhomogeneity (can saturate water) Time penalty
STIR	T1 time	Insensitive to B_0 inhomogeneity	Not specific for fat (can suppress other T1 bright tissues)
Dixon	Resonance frequency difference from fat	Insensitive to B_0 inhomogeneity Acquires IP/OOP images Can calculate fat, water, and nonfat suppressed images	Swap artifact Availability
Water excitation	Resonance frequency difference from fat	Fairly specific for fat	Sensitive to B_0 inhomogeneity Only with SE and GRE

saturation (Fat-Sat), inversion recovery (STIR), water excitation (binomial pulses), and dixon (**Fig. 13**). Although the scope of this article does not allow a detailed review of these different techniques, the basic principles and important characteristics will be discussed. Familiarity with these techniques will not only allow fine tuning of protocols but will also enable effective trouble shooting.

In order to suppress fat, it needs to be targeted by a property that distinguishes it from nonfatty tissues. Only 2 properties are commonly used: precession frequency (fat saturation, water excitation, and Dixon) and T1 time (inversion recovery).

Fat Saturation

This technique targets fat by its resonance frequency. Because of chemical shift, hydrogen in fat resonate at a slightly lower frequency than water (3.5 ppm). A fat-specific narrow bandwidth saturation pulse is given, turning the magnetization of fat into the transverse plane, where it is spoiled (saturation). Before fat can recover significant longitudinal magnetization, the regular sequence is started (excitation pulse given). Because fat has recovered virtually no longitudinal magnetization at the time of the excitation pulse, it will have no

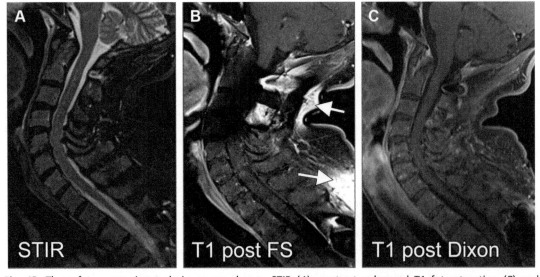

Fig. 13. Three fat suppression techniques are shown: STIR (*A*), contrast enhanced T1 fat saturation (*B*) and contrast enhanced T1 Dixon (*C*). Clearly visible are areas of fat saturation failure (*arrows* on [*B*]), with robust fat suppression with Dixon and inversion recovery.

transverse magnetization and hence no signal. As the fat saturation pulse should only null fat, a narrow bandwidth saturation pulse is required. Because the duration of a radio frequency pulse increases with decreasing bandwidth, a fat saturation pulse can incur a substantial time penalty (1–2 minutes at 1.5 T, but less at 3 T because the greater frequency difference between fat and water allows for a larger bandwidth saturation pulse and thus less time penalty).

SPIR (Spectral Presaturation with Inversion Recovery) and SPAIR (SPectral Attenuated Inversion Recovery) are similar; however they use a fat-specific inversion pulse (adiabatic pulse for SPAIR, which is less sensitive to rf-pulse inhomogeneities) to null fat signal. Like fat saturation, these pulses are preparation pulses that can be added on to a variety of sequences.

Advantages:
- Because the chemical shift property of fat is unique to fat, saturation pulse will only target fat (specific for fat).
- Can be added to virtually any sequence.

Drawbacks:
- Time penalty
- With field inhomogeneities, the saturation pulse may miss the actual fat frequency in some areas (fat saturation failure) and even saturate water (if the field is slightly weaker than expected, water can have the same resonance frequency that fat is supposed to have). Remember that in enhancing soft tissues the enhancement occurs in the water component; if water saturation occurs, enhancement will be saturated (**Fig. 14**)!!

Short Tau Inversion Recovery

This technique targets fat by its T1 time.[29,30] Magnetization of all tissues is inverted by a $180°$ inversion pulse resulting in net magnetization antiparallel to the main magnetic field of the scanner (B_0). Immediately after the inversion pulse, tissue will recover toward its equilibrium state with parallel magnetization. First it will lose antiparallel magnetization, then it will regain parallel magnetization. How quickly this recovery process occurs depends on the T1 property of a particular tissue (fast for fat, slow for water). At no point will there be transverse magnetization and signal during this process. At some point, the tissue will have no longitudinal magnetization. The time when this occurs depends on the T1 time of the particular tissue. Tissues can be targeted by giving the excitation pulse at the time point when the target tissue

has no longitudinal magnetization. The time between the inversion and excitation pulse is called TI (inversion time—also Tau). Because fat has a short T1 time, the inversion time needed to target fat must also be short (around 180 ms), hence the name "short tau inversion recovery".

Advantages:
- As T1 changes little with changes of the main magnetic field caused by metal or air, STIR is very robust even in the presence of hardware.

Disadvantages:
- Because inversion recovery targets tissues by their T1 times, it is not specific for certain tissues, but for a particular T1 time. Tissues other than fat (proteinaceous fluid, subacute blood products, or occasionally even melanin) can have the similar T1 time as fat and then will also be suppressed by STIR (see **Fig. 9**).
- STIR is its own sequence, unlike fat saturation, which can be added on to virtually any sequence.

Dixon

This method also uses the frequency difference between fat and water to target fat, but rather than targeting fat directly it acquires IP and OOP images (**Fig. 15**).[31] In simplified terms, the IP image signal is the sum of water and fat signal (water + fat), whereas OOP image signal is the difference of the fat and water signal (water − fat). When IP and OOP images are added ([water + fat]+[water − fat]), fat cancels out and a fat-suppressed image results. If the OOP image is subtracted from the IP image ([water + fat]−[water − fat]), water cancels out and a fat image is generated (see **Fig. 15**). This technique is very robust, even in the setting of field inhomogeneity from head and neck anatomy or field distortion from surgical hardware.

Advantage:
- Good fat suppression even in the setting of surgical hardware (in most cases)
- Can be added to a variety of different sequences

Disadvantage:
- In order to generate fat and water images, the location of fat and water need to be mapped. This is in part done by the resonance frequency. Because of field inhomogeneities, fat and water may be misidentified. Fatty

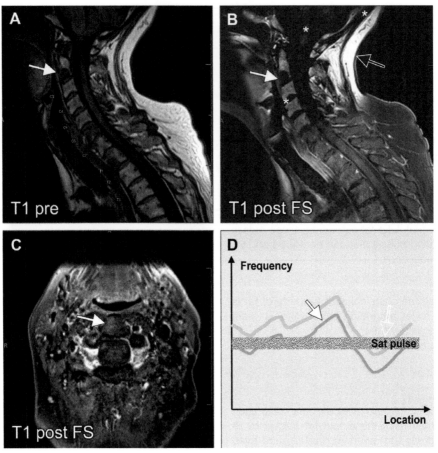

Fig. 14. Example of fat saturation failure with water saturation. A marrow replacing lesion (*arrow*) is seen on pre-contrast T1 (*A*), with apparent lack of enhancement on sagittal fat saturated postcontrast T1 (*B*). Note the failure of fat saturation (*open arrow*) with complete signal void in water tissues (*asterisks*), such as brain, muscle, and cervical disks. Enhancement in the lesion is seen on the fat saturated axial postcontrast T1 (*C*). (*D*) The cause of fat saturation failure and water saturation. In the presence of field inhomogeneities (from metal or other causes, such as air), the resonance frequencies change proportional to the field strength. The narrow bandwidth saturation pulse can miss fat (*green line, arrow*) and in areas of slightly decreased field strength even saturate water (*blue line, open arrow*).

tissues are assigned to the water image and watery tissues to the fat image (swap artifact) (**Fig. 16**). For this reason, the fat image should always be reconstructed (may not be possible retrospectively), so that if swap artifact occurs, complete evaluation is still possible.

- Even though it is more commonly seen nowadays, availability maybe limited.

Water Excitation

This technique also targets fat by its resonance frequency difference from water by using the IP and OOP phenomenon.[30] In its simplest form, the 90° excitation pulse is divided into 2 successive 45° pulses (adding up to 90°). A short time interval between the two 45° pulses allows fat and water to go 180° OOP. The second 45° pulse will

flip water into the transverse plane, whereas the OOP fat will be flipped back into the longitudinal direction, thus suppressing fat signal.

Advantage:
- Very similar appearance to fat saturation (**Fig. 17**)
- Faster than fat saturation

Drawbacks:
- Availability
- Not available with fast spin echo sequences
- Although it looks indistinguishable from fat saturation in most cases, it is not identical, and certain materials (such as silicone) may have a different imaging appearance than with fat saturation.

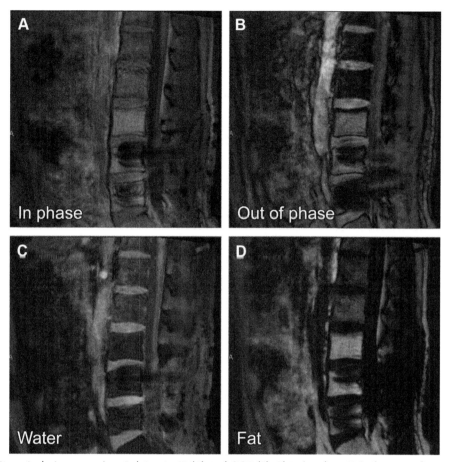

Fig. 15. Dixon technique acquires 2 datasets: IP (*A*) and OOP (*B*). The signal on IP is the sum of water and fat signal (W + F), whereas the OOP image is the subtraction of fat from water signal (W − F). When IP and OOP images are added ([W + F]+[W − F] = 2xW) a water image is generated (*C*). Subtraction of OOP image from IP image ([W + F]−[W − F] = 2xF) results in a fat image (*D*).

METAL ARTIFACT

The presence of metal causes distortion of the magnetic field due to the difference of the magnetic susceptibility of metal compared with soft tissues. The resulting change in the magnetic field strength changes the Larmor frequency of tissues and hence interferes when we use frequency as a marker of location (geometric distortion) or to target tissues (fat saturation, water excitation, as discussed earlier). The amount of artifact greatly depends on the type and volume of offending metal, with stainless steel hardware producing less severe and titanium much less severe artifact (see **Fig. 17**). However, the radiographic appearance is not necessarily predictive of the magnetic properties. Although titanium produces less artifact on computed tomography (CT) and MR imaging compared with stainless steel, vitallium has the radiographic appearance of stainless steel but creates MR imaging artifact similar to titanium.[32] Thus, pronounced artifact on CT should not discourage MR imaging evaluation when the actual composition of the hardware is unknown (**Fig. 18**).

Generally, susceptibility effects increase with field strength, and therefore lower-field scanners should be preferred over high-field scanners when a patient with hardware is to be scanned. Because field distortion changes with distance from the offending metallic objects, there will be inhomogeneity of B_0 even within a single voxel, resulting in loss of phase coherence. This is largely corrected for by the refocusing pulse used in SE and FSE sequences, but GRE sequences lacking a refocusing pulse are unable to correct, resulting in signal loss. Because the area of signal loss is typically much larger than and obscures geometric distortion, parameter changes aiming at reducing geometric distortion are not warranted with GRE

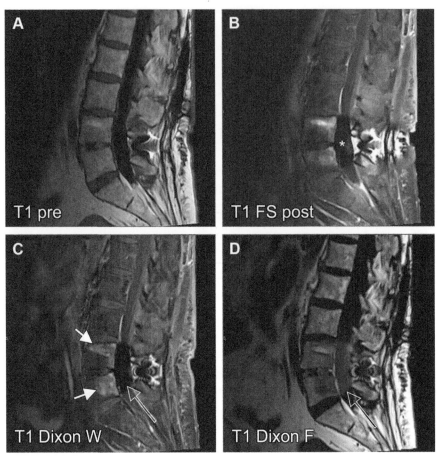

Fig. 16. The appearance of SWAP artifact. T1 precontrast image (*A*) with L4/L5 fusion hardware shows no suspicious marrow lesion. Postcontrast T1 with fat saturation (*B*) suffers from fat saturation failure (*asterisks*) with water saturation. Dixon technique shows swap artifact of the same area with mismapping of some of the water data into the fat image and vice versa; areas are swapped (*open arrow*; *C*, *D*). This gives the appearance of marrow replacing lesions in L4 and L5 (*arrow*) on the water image (*C*). (*Courtesy of* Dr Edward Quigley, MD, PhD, Salt Lake city, UT.)

sequences. For that reason, protocol changes should largely focus on reduction of geometric distortion in SE/FSE and reduction of signal loss with GRE sequences (Table 3). Although there are specialized sequences reducing geometric distortion, such as view angle tilting and slice encoding for metal artifact correction for example, there are easily performed changes that can improve image quality even on scanners that lack these techniques.

Spin Echo/Fast Spin Echo

Because metallic susceptibility effects change the precession frequency of spins, it interferes with frequency encoding and distortion occurs in frequency encoding direction. The amount of distortion depends on our rBW. Let us assume that metal causes an error of 1000 Hz. If we have an rBW of 100 Hz/px, this will translate to a distortion of 10 pixels. Increasing rBW to 500 Hz/px reduces the error to 2 pixels (Fig. 19). The drawback of increasing rBW is decreased SNR (doubling rBW reduces SNR to 70%) (Fig. 20). Because increased rBW shortens readout duration, it allows for shorter minimum TE, shorter echo spacing, and reduces chemical shift artifact of the first kind.

Equally present is through-plane distortion (warping of the slice plane) during slice selection. The distortion effects are quite similar to what is seen in frequency encoding direction but is less noticeable unless multiplanar reformats are done. Some scanners allow increasing tBW, which reduces this through plane distortion at the expense of increasing SAR and less ideal slice profiles (increased chance of crosstalk).

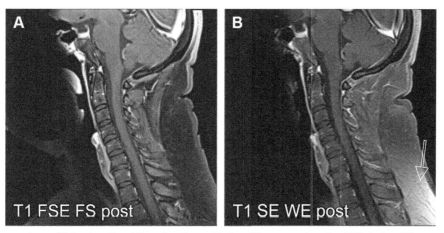

Fig. 17. Comparison of fat saturation (A) and water excitation (B) on a postcontrast T1 study of the cervical spine. In most cases the appearance is very similar and both are sensitive to B_0 inhomogeneities. In this case, some loss of fat suppression is seen in an area on the water excitation image (open arrow).

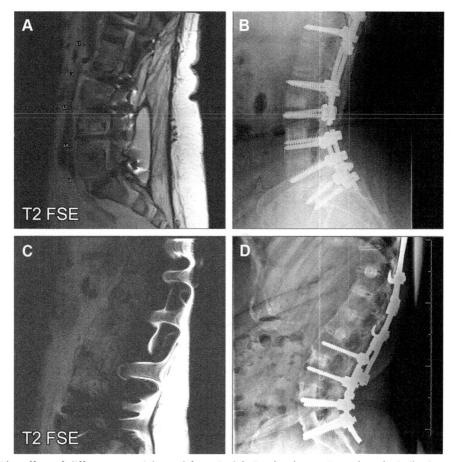

Fig. 18. The effect of different materials used for spinal fusion hardware. Even though similar in appearance radiographically, materials used in patient 1 (A, B) cause much less susceptibility effects than in patient 2 (C, D).

Table 3
MR imaging metal artifact remedies

Sequence	Adjustment	Advantage	Drawback
GRE	↓ TE	↓Signal void	Can change image weighting ↓ Sensitivity for microscopic hemorrhage on T2*
SE/FSE	↑ rBW	↓In plane distortion ↓ Min. TE ↓ Echo spacing on FSE ↓ Chemical shift first kind	↓ SNR
	↑ tBW	↓Through plane distortion ↓ min. TE ↓ Echo spacing on FSE ↓ Chemical misexcitation	↑ SAR ↑ Crosstalk
	Swap phase/frequency	Project artifact in less offensive direction	Changes direction of other artifacts (chemical shift, pulsation, wraparound) Can affect quality of parallel imaging

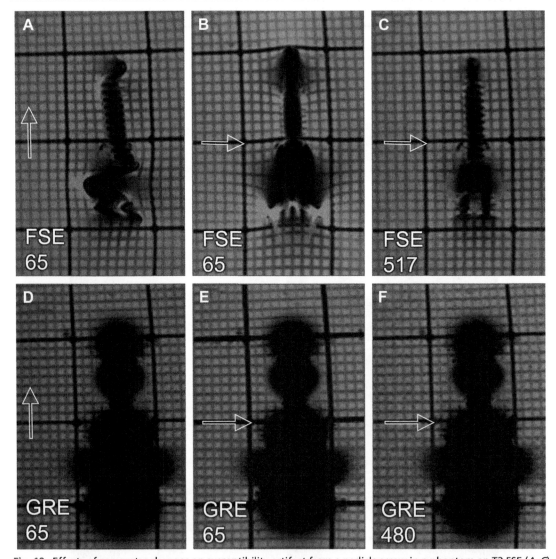

Fig. 19. Effects of parameter changes on susceptibility artifact from a pedicle screw in a phantom on T2 FSE (*A–C*) and T2* GRE sequences (*D–F*). On FSE distortion occurs in frequency encoding direction (*open arrow* indicates phase encoding direction). Increasing rBW (65 Hz/px on (*B*), 517 Hz/px on [*C*]) reduces distortion. On T2* GRE (*D, E*), neither phase encoding direction nor rBW (65 Hz/px on [*C, D*]; 480 Hz/px on [*F*]) has an effect, because signal loss from the absent refocusing pulse overwhelms any underlying distortion.

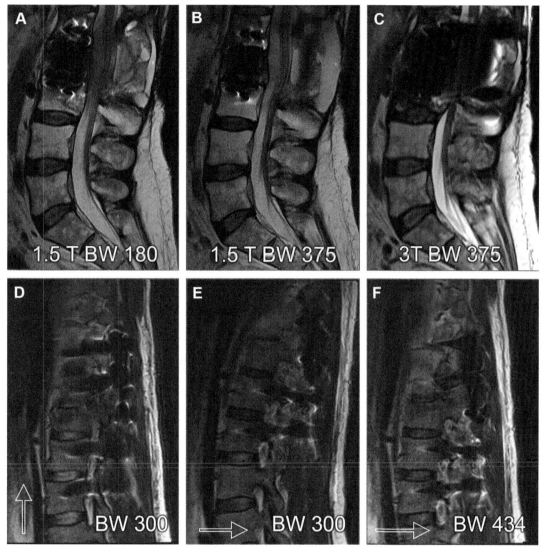

Fig. 20. (A–C) The effects of rBW and field strength on artifact from pedicle screws. 1.5 T and higher rBW–375 Hz/ px (B) provide the best image quality. 3T has inherently more susceptibility artifact (C). (D–F) The effects of rBW and phase encoding direction (*open arrow*) on artifact. For pedicle screws, choosing frequency encoding direction AP results in the artifact projecting onto the screws (E, F). Increasing rBW further improves image quality, at the expense of SNR.

Swapping Phase- and Frequency-Encoding Direction

This can project the artifact into a different, potentially less offensive direction (see **Fig. 20**).

View Angle Tilting

By tilting the plane of frequency encoding, through-plane distortion corrects for in-plane distortion. In simplified terms, it is akin to having a round disk that has been distorted into an oval and tilted relative to the imaging plane due to metal distortion. By tilting light source (frequency encoding), the shadow projected by it onto a flat plane will again be a round. TE and turbofactor/echotrain length have minor effects on the amount of artifacts.

Gradient Echo

The lack of a refocusing pulse causes loss of phase coherence and signal loss in an area much greater than the geometric distortion. The less time spins are given to lose phase coherence, the smaller the area of signal loss/void

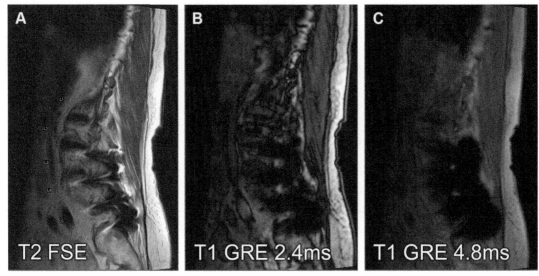

Fig. 21. The lesser amount of susceptibility artifact on FSE (*A*) compared with GRE (*B, C*). On GRE, TE has the most influence on susceptibility artifact, with shorter TE (*B*) being clearly better than longer TE (*C*).

will be. Hence, reducing TE reduces the artifact, easily seen on IP and OOP GRE sequences (**Fig. 21**). If parameter changes are done to reduce geometric distortion (as described for SE/FSE sequences), the drawbacks will occur in terms of SNR and SAR, without any improvement of artifact.

SUMMARY

There is not one optimal protocol that can fulfill the needs of all diagnostic questions or meet the preferences of the interpreting physician. Familiarity with the different sequence options and their advantages and drawbacks allows to build better protocols and better modifications of routine protocols when problems arise. Familiarity with different fat suppression strategies as well as common artifacts and their mechanisms can aid in building better MR imaging protocol and reducing artifacts or in some case even use artifacts for better image interpretation.

REFERENCES

1. Lee MJ, Kim S, Lee SA, et al. Overcoming artifacts from metallic orthopedic implants at high-field-strength MR imaging and multi-detector CT. Radiographics 2007;27(3):791–803.
2. Barrett JF, Keat N. Artifacts in CT: recognition and avoidance. Radiographics 2004;24(6):1679–91.
3. Boas FE, Fleischmann D. Evaluation of two iterative techniques for reducing metal artifacts in computed tomography. Radiology 2011;259(3):894–902.
4. Erdem LO, Erdem CZ, Acikgoz B, et al. Degenerative disc disease of the lumbar spine: a prospective comparison of fast T1-weighted fluid-attenuated inversion recovery and T1-weighted turbo spin echo MR imaging. Eur J Radiol 2005;55(2):277–82.
5. Lavdas E, Vlychou M, Arikidis N, et al. Comparison of T1-weighted fast spin-echo and T1-weighted fluid-attenuated inversion recovery images of the lumbar spine at 3.0 Tesla. Acta Radiol 2010;51(3):290–5.
6. Pusey E, Lufkin RB, Brown RK, et al. Magnetic resonance imaging artifacts: mechanism and clinical significance. Radiographics 1986;6(5):891–911.
7. Lisanti C, Carlin C, Banks KP, et al. Normal MRI appearance and motion-related phenomena of CSF. AJR Am J Roentgenol 2007;188(3):716–25.
8. Ehman RL, McNamara MT, Pallack M, et al. Magnetic resonance imaging with respiratory gating: techniques and advantages. AJR Am J Roentgenol 1984;143(6):1175–82.
9. Bamrungchart S, Tantaway EM, Midia EC, et al. Free breathing three-dimensional gradient echo-sequence with radial data sampling (radial 3D-GRE) examination of the pancreas: Comparison with standard 3D-GRE volumetric interpolated breathhold examination (VIBE). J Magn Reson Imaging 2013;38(6):1572–7.
10. Chokshi FH, Sadigh G, Carpenter W, et al. Diagnostic quality of 3D T2-SPACE compared with T2-FSE in the evaluation of cervical spine MRI anatomy. AJNR Am J Neuroradiol 2017;38(4):846–50.
11. Sayah A, Jay AK, Toaff JS, et al. Effectiveness of a rapid lumbar spine MRI protocol using 3D T2-weighted SPACE imaging versus a standard

protocol for evaluation of degenerative changes of the lumbar spine. AJR Am J Roentgenol 2016; 207(3):614–20.

12. Mugler JP 3rd. Optimized three-dimensional fast-spin-echo MRI. J Magn Reson Imaging 2014;39(4): 745–67.

13. Martin N, Malfair D, Zhao Y, et al. Comparison of MERGE and axial T2-weighted fast spin-echo sequences for detection of multiple sclerosis lesions in the cervical spinal cord. AJR Am J Roentgenol 2012;199(1):157–62.

14. Kumar Y, Hayashi D. Role of magnetic resonance imaging in acute spinal trauma: a pictorial review. BMC Musculoskelet Disord 2016;17:310.

15. Held P, Dorenbeck U, Seitz J, et al. MRI of the abnormal cervical spinal cord using 2D spoiled gradient echo multiecho sequence (MEDIC) with magnetization transfer saturation pulse. A T2* weighted feasibility study. J Neuroradiol 2003; 30(2):83–90.

16. Wang M, Dai Y, Han Y, et al. Susceptibility weighted imaging in detecting hemorrhage in acute cervical spinal cord injury. Magn Reson Imaging 2011; 29(3):365–73.

17. Philpott C, Brotchie P. Comparison of MRI sequences for evaluation of multiple sclerosis of the cervical spinal cord at 3 T. Eur J Radiol 2011; 80(3):780–5.

18. Pooley RA. AAPM/RSNA physics tutorial for residents: fundamental physics of MR imaging. Radiographics 2005;25(4):1087–99.

19. Delfaut EM, Beltran J, Johnson G, et al. Fat suppression in MR imaging: techniques and pitfalls. Radiographics 1999;19(2):373–82.

20. Erly WK, Oh ES, Outwater EK. The utility of in-phase/opposed-phase imaging in differentiating malignancy from acute benign compression fractures of the spine. AJNR Am J Neuroradiol 2006;27(6): 1183–8.

21. Merkle EM, Nelson RC. Dual gradient-echo in-phase and opposed-phase hepatic MR imaging: a useful tool for evaluating more than fatty infiltration or fatty sparing. Radiographics 2006;26(5):1409–18.

22. Andre JB, Bammer R. Advanced diffusion-weighted magnetic resonance imaging techniques of the human spinal cord. Top Magn Reson Imaging 2010; 21(6):367–78.

23. Stroman PW, Wheeler-Kingshott C, Bacon M, et al. The current state-of-the-art of spinal cord imaging: methods. Neuroimage 2014;84:1070–81.

24. Poyraz AK, Onur MR, Kocakoc E, et al. Diffusion-weighted MRI of fatty liver. J Magn Reson Imaging 2012;35(5):1108–11.

25. Chen P, Wu C, Huang M, et al. Apparent diffusion coefficient of diffusion-weighted imaging in evaluation of cervical intervertebral disc degeneration: an observational study with 3.0 T magnetic resonance imaging. Biomed Res Int 2018;2018:6843053.

26. Holder CA, Muthupillai R, Mukundan S Jr, et al. Diffusion-weighted MR imaging of the normal human spinal cord in vivo. AJNR Am J Neuroradiol 2000; 21(10):1799–806.

27. Smith RC, Lange RC, McCarthy SM. Chemical shift artifact: dependence on shape and orientation of the lipid-water interface. Radiology 1991;181(1): 225–9.

28. Enzmann DR, Rubin JB, Wright A. Use of cerebrospinal fluid gating to improve T2-weighted images. Part I. The spinal cord. Radiology 1987;162(3): 763–7.

29. Bydder GM, Young IR. MR imaging: clinical use of the inversion recovery sequence. J Comput Assist Tomogr 1985;9(4):659–75.

30. Thomasson D, Purdy D, Finn JP. Phase-modulated binomial RF pulses for fast spectrally-selective musculoskeletal imaging. Magn Reson Med 1996; 35(4):563–8.

31. Ma J. Dixon techniques for water and fat imaging. J Magn Reson Imaging 2008;28(3):543–58.

32. Knott PT, Mardjetko SM, Kim RH, et al. A comparison of magnetic and radiographic imaging artifact after using three types of metal rods: stainless steel, titanium, and vitallium. Spine J 2010;10(9):789–94.

Imaging Approach to Myelopathy
Acute, Subacute, and Chronic

Peter G. Kranz, MD*, Timothy J. Amrhein, MD

KEYWORDS

- Myelopathy • Transverse myelitis • MR imaging • Spinal imaging • Neuromyelitis optica

KEY POINTS

- MR imaging is the imaging test of choice in the evaluation of patients presenting with myelopathy.
- Compression is the most frequent etiology of myelopathy, and must be excluded first.
- Determining of the acuity of presentation can help narrow the differential diagnosis.
- The cross-sectional distribution and longitudinal extent of lesions of the spinal cord may further narrow the diagnostic possibilities and, in some cases, suggest a specific diagnosis.

INTRODUCTION

Myelopathy is a commonly encountered neurologic scenario, and one in which imaging plays a vitally important role. The first step in diagnosis is the clinical attribution of neurologic deficits to the spinal cord, rather than peripheral nerves, the brain, or other conditions that may mimic myelopathy.[1] Signs that strongly suggest myelopathy include a defined sensory level on the torso, unilateral corticospinal tract signs with contralateral spinothalamic tract signs, and urinary retention.[2] Once spinal cord pathology is suspected clinically, imaging is usually the next and most important step as it can help to narrow the differential diagnosis or suggest a specific diagnosis. In this article, we discuss the imaging approach to patients who present with acute, subacute, or chronic myelopathy, focusing on primary disorders of the spinal cord.

TERMINOLOGY

The term *myelopathy* refers to any pathologic process affecting the spinal cord and encompasses both primary disorders of the spinal cord itself, as well as conditions that secondarily affect the cord, such as compression. Myelopathy is considered acute when the symptoms progress to their nadir within 21 days of onset.[3] Myelopathy that exhibits a more progressive time course can be considered subacute (weeks to months) or chronic (months to years).

Acute myelopathy can be subdivided into noninflammatory causes (such as compression or ischemia) and inflammatory causes; the condition is given the more specific term *myelitis* when inflammation is demonstrated.[4]

Acute transverse myelitis (ATM) is a clinical presentation of acute myelitis in which the spinal cord is affected in a bilateral fashion, resulting in sensory or motor changes on both sides of the body.[3] ATM refers to the clinical syndrome that may be caused by a variety of diagnoses, rather than a specific diagnosis itself. It can be classified as either disease-associated, when the causative demyelinating or inflammatory condition is known, or idiopathic. In contrast to transverse myelitis, *partial myelitis* denotes a process limited to one

Disclosures: All authors report no conflicts of interest or of financial relationships relevant to this work.
Division of Neuroradiology, Department of Radiology, Duke University Medical Center, Box 3808, Durham, NC 27710, USA
* Corresponding author.
E-mail address: peter.kranz@duke.edu

Radiol Clin N Am 57 (2019) 257–279
https://doi.org/10.1016/j.rcl.2018.09.006

side of the spinal cord or a particular tract and is seen more commonly in certain conditions such as multiple sclerosis.

APPROACH TO THE PATIENT WITH MYELOPATHY

Causes of myelopathy are manifold, and many conditions will have overlapping clinical signs, symptoms, and imaging findings. Because the conditions that cause acute myelopathy are generally different from those that cause sub-acute to chronic presentations, acuity of clinical presentation is a useful first discriminator. This review subdivides diseases of the spinal cord into those that cause acute myelopathy (**Fig. 1**) and those that cause subacute to chronic myelopathy (**Fig. 2**). This approach carries the

Compression   *Rule out first*

Ischemia

Demyelinating
- *Multiple Sclerosis*
- *NMOSD*
- *ADEM*

Systemic Inflammatory
- *Lupus*
- *Sjögrens*
- *Other connective tissue disorders*
- *Sarcoidosis*

Infectious
- *Viral*
- *Bacterial*
- *Other – fungal, parasitic*

Idiopathic

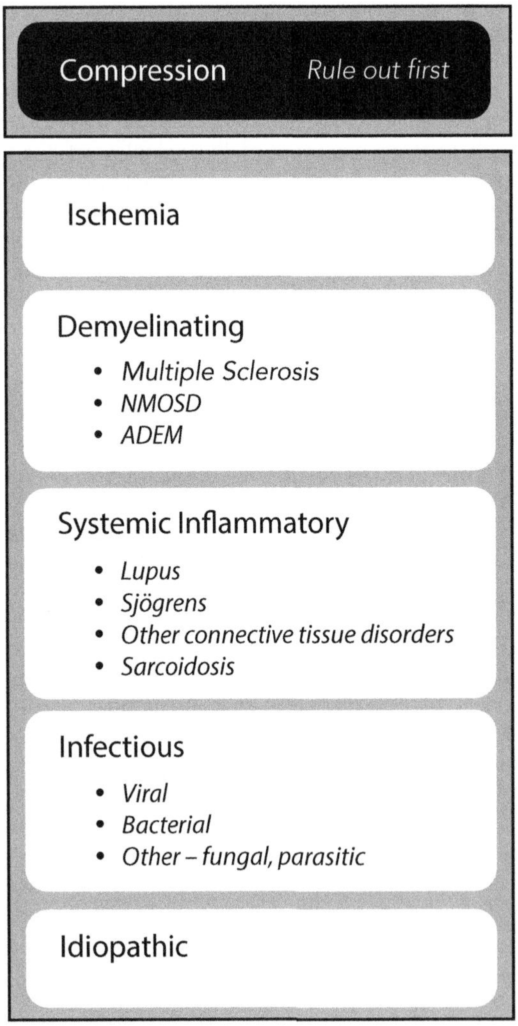

Fig. 1. Differential diagnosis (Ddx) of acute myelopathy.

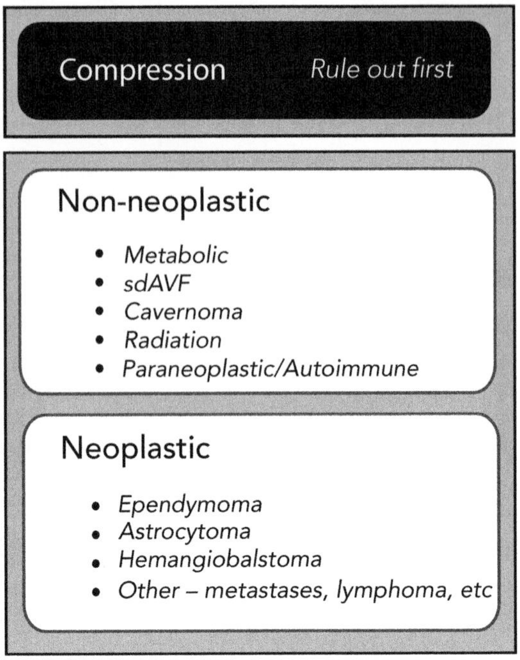

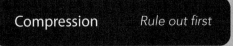

Compression   *Rule out first*

Non-neoplastic
- *Metabolic*
- *sdAVF*
- *Cavernoma*
- *Radiation*
- *Paraneoplastic/Autoimmune*

Neoplastic
- *Ependymoma*
- *Astrocytoma*
- *Hemangioblastoma*
- *Other – metastases, lymphoma, etc*

Fig. 2. Ddx of subacute-chronic myelopathy.

caveat that chronic causes of myelopathy may uncommonly present in a more acute fashion, sometimes after an event that causes abrupt deterioration, thereby mimicking an acute myelopathy. In general, however, determination of acuity provides a very good place to start refining an otherwise broad differential diagnosis.

Extrinsic causes of spinal cord compression must be excluded before considering intrinsic spinal cord pathology. This may include causes of compression that present acutely as well as those that chronically compress the spinal cord. In all cases of myelopathy, MR imaging is the imaging test of choice, both to evaluate for compression and abnormalities of the spinal cord itself. The pattern of spinal cord involvement seen on MR imaging may help to narrow the differential diagnosis (**Fig. 3**).

If MR imaging is not immediately available or contraindicated, computed tomography (CT) myelography can be used to exclude cord compression, but will be limited in its evaluation of intrinsic spinal cord diseases. Nonmyelographic CT evaluation is not sensitive in detecting many causes of compression, such as that caused by epidural hematoma or abscess, for example, and should not be considered to be a replacement for MR imaging. This review, therefore, focuses on the MR imaging appearance of myelopathic conditions.

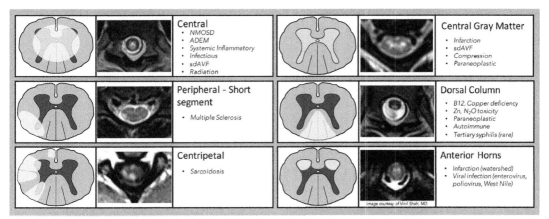

Fig. 3. Cross-sectional patterns of spinal cord involvement in various causes of myelopathy.

COMPRESSION

Extrinsic compression of the spinal cord is the most common cause of myelopathy, and the cervical spine is the most commonly affected spinal segment (**Fig. 4**). It may manifest with hand numbness, arm paresthesia, ataxic gait, Lhermitte phenomenon, and weakness.[5] Degenerative spondylosis is the most common cause and may be caused by a combination of disk protrusions, osteophytes, ligament flavum infolding, and ossification of the posterior longitudinal ligament. Other important causes of spinal cord compression include trauma, epidural pathology (such as metastases, hematoma, or abscess), and intradural tumors.

On MR imaging, the compressed spinal cord can show normal signal, elevated T2 signal, or in the most severe cases, evidence of cavitation with T1 hypointensity accompanying the T2 hyperintensity. The presence of T1 hypointensity usually indicates more severe clinical deficits and worse postoperative prognosis.[6] The presence of T2 hyperintensity may indicate reversible edema and/or permanent gliosis. In isolation, T2 hyperintensity does not necessarily predict a worse postoperative outcome in degenerative cervical myelopathy.[6,7]

Other imaging changes of the spinal cord can be associated with chronic compression. These include *myelomalacia*, a term referring to permanent spinal cord damage with volume loss, although assessing the caliber of a compressed segment of the spinal cord is not typically possible until after the cord is decompressed. Ischemia due to vascular compression may cause central gray matter T2 hyperintensity. Syringohydromyelia may occur in the spinal cord either above or below the level of compression due to altered cerebrospinal fluid flow dynamics. After decompression, contrast enhancement can be seen in the spinal cord on T1 postcontrast images for weeks to months.

ACUTE MYELOPATHY

After compression has been excluded, causes of acute myelopathy can be generally subdivided into broad 4 categories: ischemic, demyelinating, systemic inflammatory, and infectious. A fifth category, idiopathic, is reserved for cases of acute myelopathy in which no clear etiology can be determined.

Pearls: acute myelopathy

- Asymmetric short-segment (<2 vertebral segments) lesions in the dorsal/lateral spinal cord are characteristic of multiple sclerosis.

- Longitudinally extensive lesions (3 or more vertebral segments in length) have many causes, but neuromyelitis optica spectrum disorder is common in adult patients.

- Hyperacute onset (<4 hours) suggests arterial ischemia.

- Brain imaging is often useful in refining the differential diagnosis, especially in demyelinating diseases.

- Chest imaging to look for hilar lymphadenopathy or pulmonary disease can be helpful in diagnosing sarcoidosis, although spinal involvement may occur without thoracic involvement.

- Cerebrospinal fluid analysis to look for markers of inflammation and specific antibodies (such as AQP4-IgG) is very helpful establishing a diagnosis of acute myelopathies.

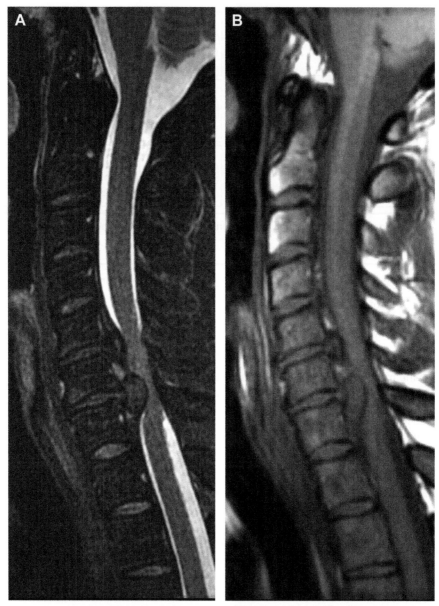

Fig. 4. Compressive myelopathy. (*A*) Sagittal STIR and (*B*) sagittal T1-weighted images demonstrate spinal cord compression due to large disk extrusions in a patient presenting with pain and subacute myelopathic complaints.

Ischemia

Spinal cord ischemia is the result of abrupt occlusion of one of the arteries that supply the spinal cord parenchyma. One of the most notable clinical features of ischemia is the hyperacute progression to symptom nadir, often within 4 hours or less. This rapid onset and the profound deficits that accompany ischemia frequently prompt very early clinical presentation.

Ischemia most commonly affects the territory of anterior spinal artery (ASA), which irrigates a large portion of the central gray matter of the spinal cord. Anterior radiculomedullary arteries enter the neural foramen to supply the ASA, but are present at an average of only 6 spinal levels, and are most numerous in the cervical spine.[8,9] This results in a system of vascular supply that is dependent on a relatively small number of vessels, particularly in the lower thoracic spinal cord, where infarction is most common.[10]

The most common identified etiology of ischemia is atherosclerosis, although no definite cause is identified in a substantial number of cases. Other causes include aortic dissection or aortic surgery/stenting, vertebral artery occlusion, hypotension, and fibrocartilaginous embolism.[11] Hyperextension of the thoracic spine among novice surfers has also been found to induce ischemia in rare cases and has been termed "surfer's myelopathy."[12]

On MR imaging, characteristic findings include T2 hyperintense signal within the central gray matter, producing an "H-shaped" or "butterfly-shaped" region of abnormality (**Fig. 5**). If diffusion-weighted imaging is performed, diffusion restriction will be seen (**Fig. 6**). Patients most commonly present and are imaged early in the course of ischemia, at which point the process is typically nonexpansile, resulting in a thin "pencil-like" stripe of T2 hyperintense signal on sagittal images. These 2 imaging features, central gray matter predominance and absence of expansion, together with the hyperacute onset of symptoms, are highly suggestive of ischemia, and help to discriminate it from many of the other causes of acute myelopathy.

Similar to cerebral infarction, swelling of the spinal cord may be seen if imaging is delayed. Contrast enhancement is absent early on but may develop after several days.

The pattern of central gray matter involvement is typical in acute ischemia, but other variants may be seen. Posterior spinal artery infarction may cause dorsal column involvement, and watershed territory infarction may cause abnormalities in the anterior horns of the gray matter only, producing a "snake-eyes" or "owl's-eyes" appearance.[11]

Demyelinating Disease

Multiple sclerosis

Multiple sclerosis (MS) is a demyelinating disorder that affects the brain and spinal cord, and is characterized by lesions (and their corresponding clinical defects) that are disseminated in both space and time. The spinal cord is involved in 80% to 90% of patients with MS,[13] with lesions most common in the cervical cord.[14] Patients with primary progressive MS tend to have more spinal cord lesions than patients with relapsing-remitting MS. Although transverse myelitis is a possible clinical presentation of MS, partial myelitis is much more common, resulting in asymmetric clinical deficits.

MS lesions are typically *short-segment* lesions, meaning that they are less than 2 vertebral bodies in craniocaudal extent.[15] This notable feature separates them from many of the other acute

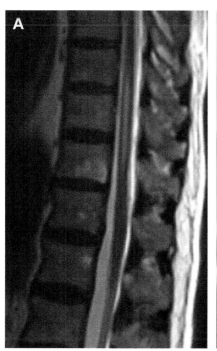
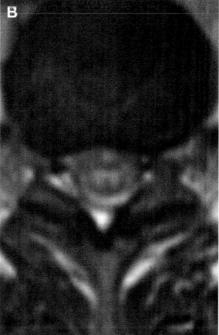

Fig. 5. Acute spinal cord ischemia. (*A*) Sagittal and (*B*) axial T2-weighted images demonstrate abnormal signal in the central spinal cord that preferentially affects the central gray matter. Expansion of the cord is typically absent or mild in cases of ischemia.

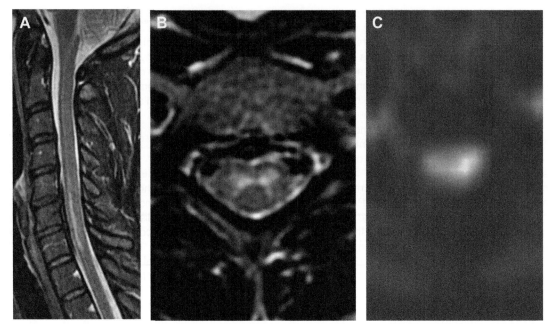

Fig. 6. Acute spinal cord ischemia. (*A*) Sagittal STIR and (*B*) axial T2-weighted images demonstrate increased T2 signal in the central gray matter in a patient who presented with hyperacute onset of sensory and motor dysfunction. Axial diffusion-weighted image (*C*) shows restricted diffusion in the central gray matter due to acute ischemia.

myelopathies, which take the form of *longitudinally extensive transverse myelitis (LETM)*, meaning that they extend over 3 or more vertebral segments in length.

The cross-sectional distribution of MS lesions is also typically characteristic (**Fig. 7**). Lesions occur with greatest frequency in the dorsal and lateral portions of the spinal cord, often extending to the periphery of the cord where white matter predominates. Asymmetric lesion distribution is common, accounting for the frequent presentation with partial myelitis.

On MR imaging, MS lesions are T2 hyperintense. Acute lesions may be expansile, a feature that decreases over time. Chronic lesions often remain visible on T2-weighted images. Numerous investigators have found lesions to be more conspicuous on short tau inversion recovery (STIR) imaging compared with fast spin echo T2-weighted imaging.[16–18]

Contrast enhancement is seen in active demyelinating lesions, and persists for 6 to 8 weeks after onset. There may be a peripheral rim of enhancement, or an "open ring" of c-shaped enhancement (which is highly suggestive of demyelinating disease when present).[19] Small lesions may show nodular or ill-defined enhancement. Enhancement usually does not persist beyond 3 months, which can be a useful way of discriminating MS from other diseases such

as tumors (in addition to the acuity of presentation and brain imaging).

Neuromyelitis optica

Neuromyelitis optica (NMO) is a condition characterized by spinal cord involvement, most commonly resulting in ATM, and optic neuritis. Clinical deficits in NMO are typically more severe than those seen with MS.[20] Recurrent attacks are common.[21]

Most patients with NMO have elevated levels of serum antibodies to aquaporin-4 (AQP4), a water transport channel found in the ependymal cells that line the ventricles within the central nervous system.[22] This antibody (AQP4-IgG) is highly specific for the diagnosis of NMO.[23] More recently, the term "NMO-spectrum disorders" (NMOSDs) has been introduced to encompass patients with clinical NMO who are AQP4-IgG negative; some of these patients demonstrate immunoreactivity to another antibody against myelin oligodendrocyte glycoprotein (MOG).[24]

On imaging, NMO characteristically demonstrates a longitudinally extensive (3 more vertebral levels in length), T2 hyperintense, expansile lesion (**Fig. 8**). On axial imaging, the central portions of the spinal cord are involved, but the process in not confined to gray or white matter alone. The presence of small foci of very hyperintense T2 signal within the cord, so-called "bright

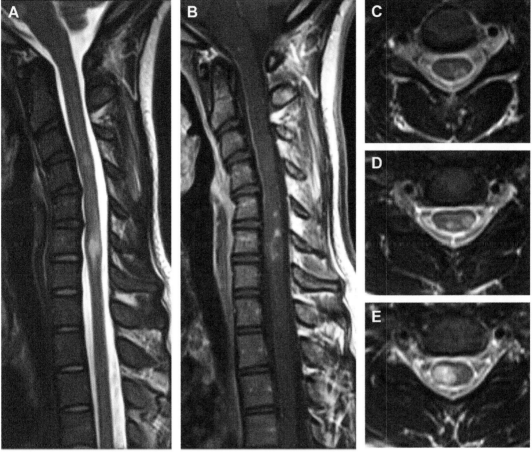

Fig. 7. MS. Numerous short-segment lesions are visible on (A) sagittal T2-weighted and (B) sagittal postcontrast T1-weighted images. Note that there is enhancement of some, but not all, lesions, indicating that some are active and others are chronic. Axial T2-weighted images (C–E) show the typical peripheral, dorsolateral distribution of MS lesions.

spotty lesions," is relatively specific for NMO.[25] Ill-defined or patchy contrast enhancement is very common.

Although brain lesions were initially thought to be absent in NMO, it is now recognized that brain lesions are not uncommon. They tend to predominate in the regions around the third and fourth ventricles,[26,27] regions where AQP4 is expressed in greatest concentration.[22] This distribution is in contrast to the ovoid "Dawson's fingers" lesions seen at the margin of the lateral ventricle and in the corpus callosum in patients with MS.[28]

Acute disseminated encephalomyelitis

Acute disseminated encephalomyelitis (ADEM) is a demyelinating disease that affects the brain and spinal cord, but the primary neurologic manifestation is typically encephalopathy. Although ADEM can occur at any age, the overwhelming majority of cases occur in childhood.[29]

It is an autoimmune-mediated disease, and in many cases, there is a history of antecedent upper respiratory or gastrointestinal illness. Classically, ADEM is considered a monophasic illness, with no new disease activity after 3 months from onset. A small proportion of patients may develop a second episode of ADEM and may be classified as multiphasic disseminated encephalomyelitis.[30]

On imaging, the spinal cord is involved in approximately one-quarter of patients,[31] and typically produces an LETM appearance, with T2 hyperintensity, expansion, and variable enhancement (Fig. 9). The appearance on spinal imaging may be difficult to distinguish from other LETMs. Brain imaging, however, is very useful in suggesting the diagnosis of ADEM. Brain lesions are T2 hyperintense and may variably enhance, but are distributed throughout the white matter and

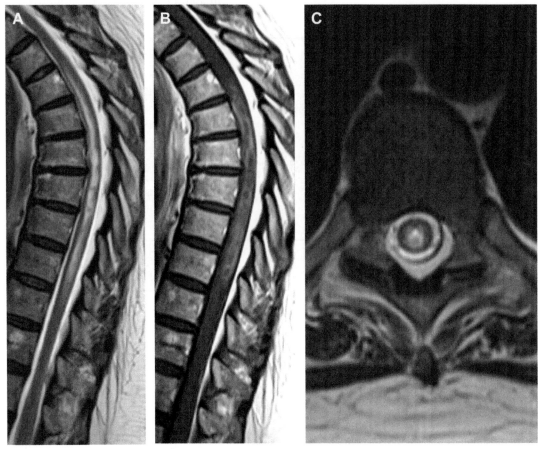

Fig. 8. NMO. (*A*) Sagittal T2-weighted image shows a longitudinally extensive, expansile lesion. There is ill-defined enhancement on (*B*) the sagittal postcontrast T1-weighted image. (*C*) Axial T2-weighted image shows the typical central distribution of NMO in the spinal cord.

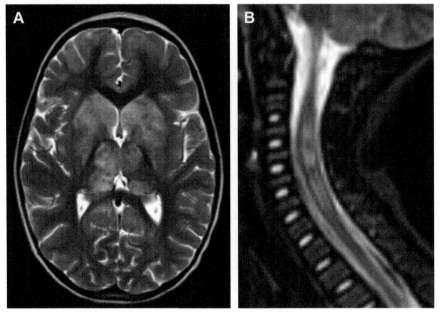

Fig. 9. ADEM. (*A*) Axial T2-weighted image of the brain in a child presenting with encephalopathy and myelopathy after recent viral illness shows T2 hyperintense lesions in the basal ganglia. (*B*) Sagittal T2-weighted image of the cervical spinal cord shows fusiform expansion and T2 hyperintensity.

brainstem (unlike the periventricular predominance seen in MS), may be larger than typical MS lesions, and frequently involve the deep gray nuclei, an imaging feature uncommon in other demyelinating conditions.

Systemic Inflammatory

Acute myelopathy can be a manifestation of multisystem inflammatory disorders, including systemic lupus erythematosus (SLE) (Fig. 10), Sjögren's syndrome (Fig. 11), mixed connective tissue disorder, Behçet disease, and sarcoidosis.

Imaging features in these conditions overlap, generally producing an expansile LETM with variable contrast enhancement. Despite a similar imaging appearance, the pathophysiology of these conditions is different. For example, SLE myelitis has been found to be associated with antiphospholipid antibodies in many cases, leading to the suggestion that SLE myelitis is a thrombotic rather than a truly inflammatory myelopathy.[32] Behçet disease, a condition accompanied by oral and genital aphthous ulcers, is a systemic vasculitis. Some patients with of SLE and Sjögren's syndrome may test positive for AQP4 antibody, indicating that there may be crossover with NMOSD.[33]

Sarcoidosis, on the other hand, is a granulomatous condition. It often shows enhancement along the surface of the spinal cord that can be sheetlike or plaquelike. Centripetal spread of enhancement into the spinal cord in a wedgelike pattern may be seen (Fig. 12), a feature that may help distinguish sarcoidosis from other LETMs. It has been hypothesized that this feature represents involvement of the leptomeninges with granulomatous inflammation that subsequently extends into the spinal cord parenchyma along perivascular

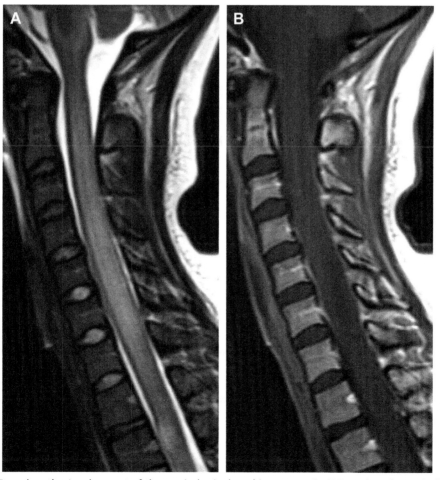

Fig. 10. SLE myelopathy. Involvement of the cervical spinal cord is common in SLE myelopathy, typically producing a longitudinally extensive lesion on T2-weighted images (A). Contrast enhancement is variably present in cases of SLE; this case shows no abnormal enhancement on (B) the sagittal postcontrast T1-weighted image.

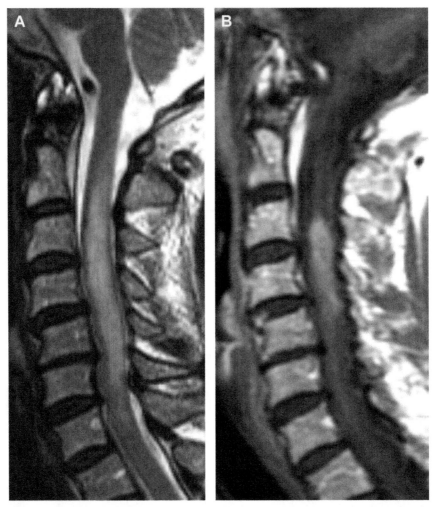

Fig. 11. Sjögren's syndrome. (*A*) Sagittal T2 and (*B*) sagittal postcontrast T1-weighted images demonstrate a longitudinally extensive, T2 hyperintense, enhancing lesion in this patient with Sjögren's syndrome. This appearance is common to several diseases that cause ATM.

spaces.[34] Involvement of the cauda equina or optic nerves can be seen. Chest CT or chest radiographs can be helpful if sarcoidosis is suspected, as roughly half of patients with neurosarcoidosis will have hilar lymphadenopathy.[35] Serum and cerebrospinal fluid (CSF) angiotensin-converting enzyme levels have moderate sensitivity but high specificity for sarcoidosis and may be a useful adjunctive test.[33]

Infection

Infection of the spinal cord and spinal nerve roots can be caused by viruses, bacteria, parasites, or fungi. It is distinct from postinfectious myelopathy, which is an autoimmune-mediated process that occurs after an infection elsewhere in the body (often gastrointestinal or respiratory infections). Compared with other causes of acute myelopathy, direct infection of the spinal cord is relatively uncommon in developed countries. In addition to the motor and sensory changes that may accompany myelopathy, radiculopathy may be present in some cases of infectious myelitis, resulting in lower motor neuron signs.[36]

Among the more common viral causes of myelitis are enteroviruses (including EV-D68, EV-71, and poliovirus), herpesviruses (including varicella zoster virus [VZV], cytomegalovirus [CMV], and herpes simplex), and arboviruses (arthropod-borne viruses, including West Nile virus).

Poliovirus infection affects lower motor neurons, causing acute flaccid paralysis. The incidence of poliomyelitis has decreased dramatically since

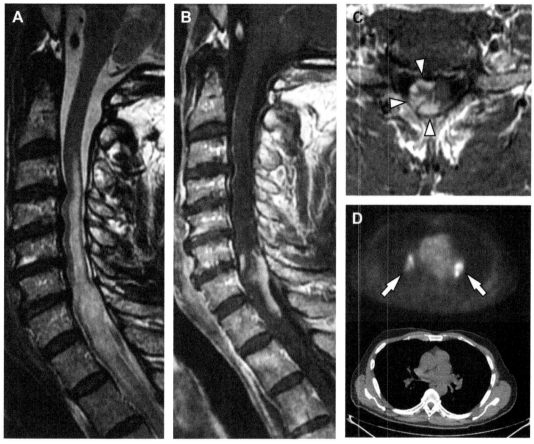

Fig. 12. Sarcoidosis. (A) Sagittal T2 weighted image shows fusiform expansion and longitudinally extensive T2 hyperintense signal abnormality. (D) Sagittal postcontrast T1 weighted image shows plaquelike enhancement along the surface of the spinal cord. (C) Axial postcontrast T1-weighted image shows wedgelike areas of enhancement (arrowheads) spreading in a centripetal pattern into the spinal cord. (D) Axial images from a fluorodeoxyglucose (FDG)- PET-CT shows hypermetabolic hilar lymph nodes (arrows).

the widespread introduction of vaccination, but still persists in parts of the developing world. MR imaging classically shows T2 hyperintensity of the anterior horn cells (**Fig. 13**).[37] Other strains of enterovirus also show a predilection for the anterior horn cells and cause periodic seasonal outbreaks in the late summer–early fall among children.[38]

VZV infection causes chickenpox in pediatric patients, after which it may lie dormant in neurons for decades. Reactivation may cause herpes zoster (also known as shingles), a painful rash in a dermatomal distribution. Extension along the nerve roots into the spinal cord can occur in some cases of herpes zoster, resulting in radiculomyelitis. Imaging can show involvement of the dorsolateral spinal cord at the site of the nerve root entry (**Fig. 14**), and may show enhancement of the affected spinal cord and

affected root.[36] Infection with CMV, another herpesvirus, is typically seen in immunocompromised individuals, often diffusely affecting the lumbar nerve roots, and extending into the spinal cord in some cases.[39]

Bacterial infection of the spinal cord can be associated with bacterial meningitis or adjacent vertebral or disk infection (**Fig. 15**). Rarely, an intramedullary abscess may develop, producing an expansile, ring-enhancing lesion.[39] Other fungal (*Aspergillus*, *Candida*) and atypical organisms (*Nocardia*, *Actinomyces*) may cause an acute necrotizing myelitis,[40] with spinal cord enhancement, expansion, and T2 hyperintensity on MR imaging.

Parasitic infections such as cysticercosis, schistosomiasis, and echinococcus are uncommon outside of endemic areas, but may be encountered due to travel or migration.[41] These

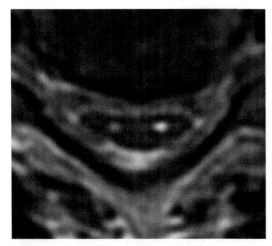

Fig. 13. Poliomyelitis. Axial T2-weighted image shows increased signal in the anterior horn cells of the gray matter, in the classic "snake-eyes" or "owl's-eyes" pattern. Spinal cord atrophy is also present. (*Courtesy of* C. Torres, MD, Ottawa, Canada)

patients may present with either acute or chronic myelopathy, depending on the chronicity of the infection.

Idiopathic

Idiopathic ATM, by definition, lacks an identifiable cause after comprehensive evaluation for demyelinating, vascular, and infectious causes and connective tissue disorders. Arriving at a specific diagnosis, when possible, is important to direct appropriate therapy and to avoid the side effects of long-term immunosuppressive regimens. Idiopathic ATM should be an uncommon diagnosis; previous studies have shown that among patients with initially suspected idiopathic ATM, only 16% to 18% retained this diagnosis after appropriate workup.[3,42]

SUBACUTE-CHRONIC MYELOPATHY

As with acute myelopathies, compression of the spinal cord must be excluded first in cases of subacute to chronic myelopathy. After exclusion of compression, subacute to chronic myelopathies can be broadly divided into nonneoplastic and neoplastic causes. The nonneoplastic myelopathies constitute a diverse spectrum of diseases including metabolic causes, dural arteriovenous fistula (dAVF), radiation-related myelopathy, autoimmune causes, and cavernomas of the spinal cord. Tumors of the spinal cord are a relatively uncommon but important cause of chronic progressive myelopathy.

Pearls: subacute to chronic myelopathy

- Selective involvement of the dorsal columns should prompt evaluation for metabolic myelopathy such as B12 deficiency.
- Carefully examine the dorsal surface of the spinal cord for flow voids in older men who present with myelopathy, as this can indicate a spinal dural arteriovenous fistula.
- Tract-specific abnormalities suggest an autoimmune or paraneoplastic cause.
- Ill-defined, longitudinally extensive lesions in adults are much more common to be demyelinating or inflammatory lesions than tumors. Repeat imaging in 2 to 3 months can be helpful in discriminating these entities.
- Don't jump to a diagnosis of spinal cord tumor too quickly, especially if there is an acute presentation. Spinal cord biopsy carries significant morbidity, and alternative diagnoses can often be established with cerebrospinal fluid analysis and judicious follow-up imaging.

Nonneoplastic Causes of Subacute-Chronic Myelopathy

Metabolic

The best known of the metabolic myelopathies is vitamin B12 (cobalamin) deficiency. Vitamin B12 deficiency causes patchy areas of demyelination of the spinal cord, with a particular predilection for the dorsal columns and, to a lesser extent, the lateral spinal cord.[43] These changes, known as subacute combined degeneration (SCD), result in peripheral neuropathy and gait disturbance due to sensory ataxia.

The classic appearance of SCD on MR imaging is increased T2 signal in the dorsal columns of the cervical and upper thoracic spinal cord bilaterally, resulting in a chevron-shaped appearance on axial images (**Fig. 16**), sometimes referred to as the "inverted-V sign."[44] There is typically no spinal cord expansion or contrast enhancement.

Exposure to nitrous oxide, either as an inhaled anesthetic during dental procedures or as a drug of abuse, causes functional B12 deficiency by oxidizing the cobalt atom needed for proper functioning of cobalamin.[45] Copper deficiency, usually the result of gastric surgery, malabsorption, or prolonged parenteral nutrition, produces clinical findings that are indistinguishable from B12 deficiency.[46] Excessive ingestion of zinc can cause copper deficiency by stimulating the binding of copper ions in the gastrointestinal tract, preventing proper absorption. Toxic levels of zinc have

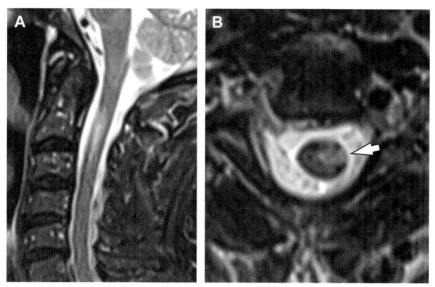

Fig. 14. Varicella zoster myelitis. (A) Sagittal STIR and (B) axial T2-weighted images in a patient with left-sided weakness developing after shingles outbreak, with vesicular skin lesions in the C2-C3 dermatome show T2 hyperintensity and slight expansion of the cervical spinal cord at the location of the left C2 nerve root insertion (arrow). Polymerase chain reaction of the cerebrospinal fluid was positive for VZV.

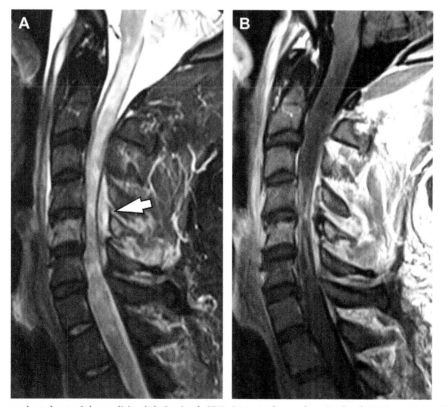

Fig. 15. Secondary bacterial myelitis. (A) Sagittal STIR image shows longitudinal T2 hyperintensity in the spinal cord, with spinal cord compression from an adjacent epidural abscess (arrow). (B) Sagittal postcontrast T1-weighted image shows enhancement of the spinal cord due to spread of bacterial infection from the epidural space. There is abnormal T2 signal and enhancement in the C5 vertebral body due to associated osteomyelitis.

been reported with inadvertent swallowing of zinc-containing denture cream, and with overingestion of zinc-containing dietary supplements.[47,48] All of these entities can show dorsal column T2 hyperintensity on spinal MR imaging in a pattern identical to B12 deficiency.

Spinal dural arteriovenous fistula

Spinal dAVFs (sdAVFs) are a direct connection between an artery and vein, usually adjacent to a spinal nerve root. This abnormal communication of one or more meningeal arteries to an intradural radiculomedullary vein along the inner dural surface results in arterial pressure being transmitted to the veins that drain the spinal cord, leading to progressive venous dilation and tortuosity.[49,50] Increased venous pressure causes vascular congestion in the spinal cord parenchyma, producing cord edema and decreased arterial perfusion. Fistulas most commonly are found at the mid and lower spinal levels, from T4 to L3.[51] Rarely, they may be located intracranially,

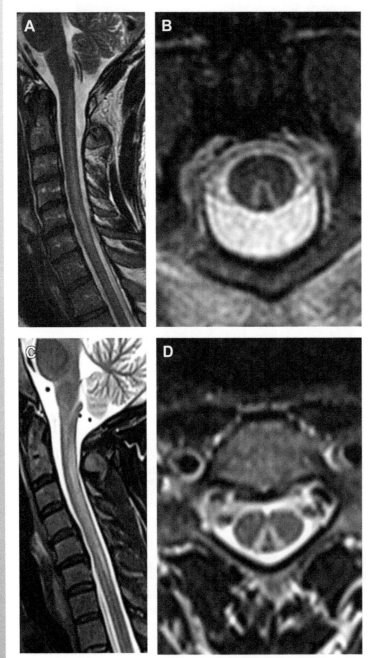

Fig. 16. Metabolic myelopathy. (*A*) Sagittal and (*B*) axial T2-weighted images of the cervical spinal cord in a patient with SCD due to vitamin B12 deficiency shows abnormal T2 hyperintensity confined to the dorsal columns of the spinal cord, in a pattern known as the "inverted-V" sign. (*C*) Sagittal and (*D*) axial T2-weighted images of the cervical spinal cord in a different patient with copper deficiency show a similar distribution of T2 signal abnormality in the dorsal columns.

resulting in involvement of the brainstem and descending cervical symptoms.

Demographically, sdAVFs are overwhelmingly found in male patients in the fifth decade of life and beyond.[51] Gait disturbance is the most common symptom, present in 96% of cases. Lower extremity sensory deficits and urinary dysfunction are also common. Spastic paraplegia may be present initially, eventually progressing to flaccid paralysis. If left untreated, additional spinal levels may become affected in an ascending fashion; this clinical presentation associated with sdAVF is known as Foix-Alajouanine syndrome.[52]

On MR imaging, the most characteristic finding is the presence of enlarged veins along the dorsal surface of the spinal cord (Fig. 17). These will appear as flow voids on T2-weighted images, with intravascular enhancement visible after intravenous contrast administration. The spinal cord itself demonstrates T2 hyperintensity due to edema caused by venous hypertension. Ill-defined parenchymal contrast enhancement of the spinal cord can be seen.

Localization of the fistula is typically performed using catheter angiography, to confirm the level of arterial supply. MR angiography also can be useful in localizing the fistula site, allowing for a more focused catheter angiogram.[53,54] Treatment of sdAVF is with microsurgical obliteration of the fistula or endovascular occlusion. Although some patients may see symptomatic improvement after treatment, some deficits may be irreversible.[55]

Cavernomas

Cavernous malformations (cavernomas) are another form of vascular pathology that can affect the spinal cord. In contrast to high-flow vascular malformations like sdAVFs, cavernomas are low-flow lesions that lack arterial feeding vessels. As a result, they are occult on angiographic imaging. The clinical presentation is nonspecific, and may include progressive sensory deficits, motor deficits, or pain.[56] Acute episodes of deterioration are common due to hemorrhage within the lesion.

Pathologically, spinal cavernomas are identical to cavernomas of the brain. They are circumscribed lesions composed of blood-filled vascular channels separated by single endothelial layers. Gliosis and abundant hemosiderin-containing macrophages are seen at the interface with the

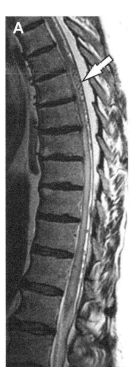 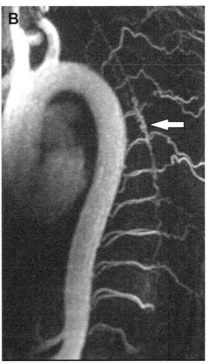 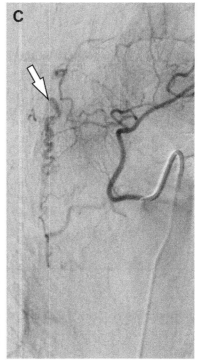

Fig. 17. SdAVF. (A) Sagittal T2-weighted image of the thoracic spine shows T2 hyperintensity in the thoracic spinal cord with tortuous flow voids (*arrow*) over the dorsal aspect of the cord. (B) Sagittal maximum-intensity projection from time-resolved MR angiogram shows enlarged veins filling during arterial phase of imaging (*arrow*) due to shunting in the fistula. (C) Catheter angiogram with selective injection into a spinal segmental artery shows the fistula, with the same enlarged tortuous veins (*arrow*) at the surface of the spinal cord.

spinal cord.[57] MR imaging reveals a multicystic-appearing lesion confining internal locules of blood in various stages of breakdown (**Fig. 18**), often showing T1 hyperintensity due to the presence of methemoglobin. A characteristic feature of cavernomas is a very low signal T2 rim, representing hemosiderin deposition at the margin of the lesion. Contrast enhancement can be seen within the cystic spaces of the lesion, but no flow voids will be present, because cavernomas lack arterial feeding vessels. Similar to cavernomas seen in the brain, techniques that are sensitive to magnetic field inhomogeneity, such as gradient-based MR sequences, will show "blooming" of the lesions due to the paramagnetic effects of hemosiderin.[58]

Radiation

Radiation-induced myelopathy is a rare complication of treatment of primary and metastatic neoplastic disease. The risk of myelopathy is dose-dependent; most centers limit total dose to less than 45 Gy in 1.8-Gy to 2.0-Gy fractions to help reduce this risk.[59] Average time to presentation is 6 months to 2 years, but may develop as soon as 2 months and as late as several years after radiation.[59,60]

Pathologically, radiation myelopathy is characterized by preferential white matter damage and demyelination and vasculopathy.[61] The most common symptoms are motor weakness, pain, and paresthesias.[59,60]

The appearance of the spinal cord on MR imaging in radiation myelopathy has no specific features. T2 hyperintensity is universally present, usually involving the central spinal cord (**Fig. 19**).[59] Spinal cord expansion and contrast enhancement are present in roughly half of cases. However, the key to recognizing radiation-induced myelopathy is the recognition that the changes correlate with a prior radiation port. Examination of adjacent vertebral bodies for T1 hyperintense

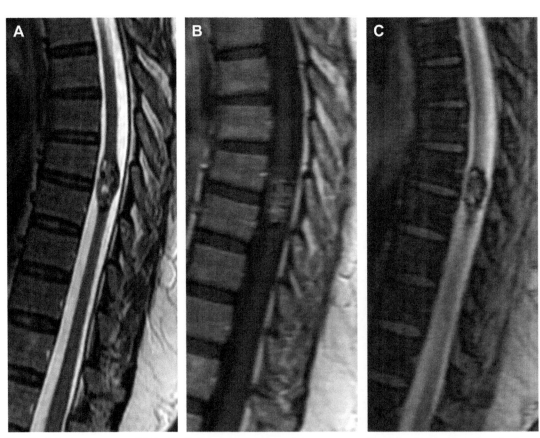

Fig. 18. Spinal cavernoma. (*A*) Sagittal T2-weighted image shows an expansile lesion in the thoracic spinal cord with multiple internal locules. (*B*) Sagittal postcontrast T1-weighted image shows enhancement within the lesion (precontrast T1-weighted image not shown) but no enhancement surrounding the lesion. (*C*) Sagittal gradient recalled echo image shows increased conspicuity of T2 hypointense signal at the margin of the lesion, a phenomenon known as "blooming," due to hemosiderin deposition.

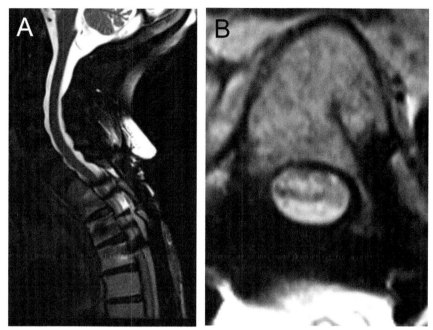

Fig. 19. Chronic radiation myelopathy. (A) Sagittal and (B) axial T2-weighted images in a patient with prior vertebral body metastases treated with radiation and surgery show abnormally increased T2 signal and mild volume loss in the upper thoracic spinal cord. Artifact is seen due to pedicle screws related to the prior surgical intervention. There is increased T2 signal in the bone marrow in the irradiated portion of the vertebral bodies that corresponds with the area or myelopathic change in the spinal cord.

marrow indicating prior radiation can be very helpful in this regard.

Paraneoplastic and autoimmune myelitis

Paraneoplastic myelopathy is the result of cross-reaction of antibodies formed against tumor antigens with antigens present in normal neural tissue. This immune response results in neuronal dysfunction and injury, causing progressive neurologic symptoms that may sometimes precede the diagnosis of the tumor itself. Common tumors associated with paraneoplastic myelopathy include lung (especially small cell lung cancer), breast, thymoma, and ovarian tumors (**Fig. 20**).[62]

Another potential trigger for an autoimmune response against neural elements is viral infection. For example, herpesvirus infection can trigger a reaction to N-methyl-D-aspartate (NMDA) receptors, resulting in encephalitis or myelitis occurring weeks after the incident infection (**Fig. 21**).[63]

The characteristic MR imaging finding that should suggest paraneoplastic or autoimmune myelitis is *tract-specific* distribution of T2 signal abnormality. The lateral columns, dorsal columns, and central gray matter are commonly affected tracts, and contrast enhancement is often present.[64]

Neoplastic Causes of Subacute-Chronic Myelopathy

Spinal cord tumors are a relatively rare cause of myelopathy and are certainly much less common than acute demyelinating and inflammatory

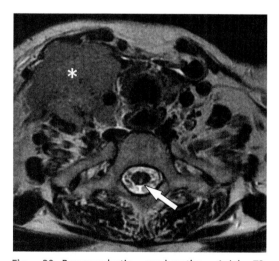

Fig. 20. Paraneoplastic myelopathy. Axial T2-weighted image demonstrates abnormal increased signal in the dorsal columns of the spinal cord (*arrow*) in this patient with metastatic small cell lung cancer. Note the large conglomerate nodal metastasis in the right supraclavicular region (*asterisk*).

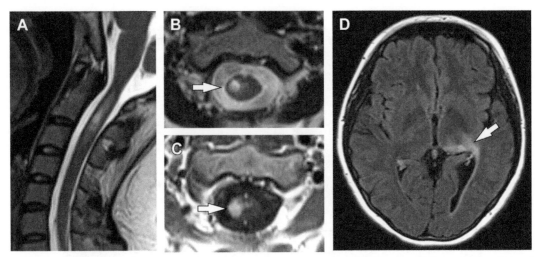

Fig. 21. Anti-NMDA receptor encephalomyelitis. (*A*) Sagittal T2-weighted image shows a hyperintense lesion in the upper cervical spinal cord in this patient presenting with encephalopathy and right-sided motor deficits. (*B*) Axial T2-weighted and (*C*) axial postcontrast T1-weighted images show involvement of the lateral corticospinal tracts (*arrows*). (*D*) Axial fluid attenuated inversion recovery image of the brain showed ill-defined lesions involving the left periatrial white matter and thalamus (*arrow*). CSF analysis revealed the presence of anti-NMDA receptor antibodies.

causes. For example, rates of ATM have been estimated at 3.1 per 100,000 person-years, compared with a rate of 0.17 per 100,000 for ependymomas and 0.03 per 100,000 for pediatric glial/neuronal tumors.[65,66] Establishing the diagnosis of a spinal cord tumor may require biopsy, which can be associated with substantial morbidity and permanent neurologic deficit.

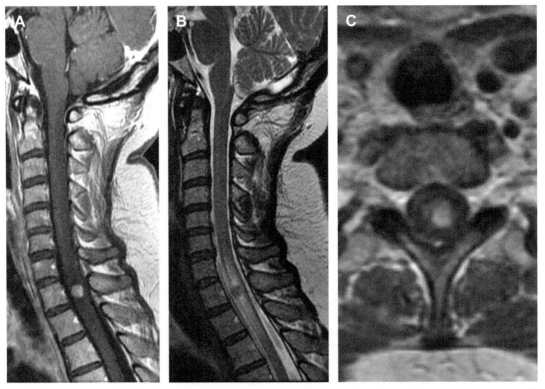

Fig. 22. Ependymoma. (*A*) Sagittal postcontrast T1-weighted and (*B*) sagittal T2-weighted images show a well-defined, homogeneously enhancing nodule in the upper thoracic spinal cord of an adult patient. (*C*) Axial postcontrast T1-weighted image shows the typical central location of an ependymoma.

For these reasons, the diagnosis of a spinal cord tumor should be entertained with caution unless there are clear features on imaging that suggest the presence of a tumor over inflammatory disease. As a general rule, spinal cord tumors will show cord expansion and will enhance on postcontrast imaging in the vast majority of cases.[67] If these features are absent, other diagnoses should be entertained first. Although spinal cord tumors occasionally present acutely, most tumors present with chronic progressive neurologic symptoms, differentiating them from acute myelopathies.

Demyelinating causes of myelopathy, which also show expansion and contrast enhancement, typically stop enhancing after 6 to 8 weeks, whereas spinal cord tumors will show persistent enhancement beyond this time. Because most spinal cord tumors exhibit slow clinical progression, repeating imaging after 2 to 3 months is a useful strategy when initial imaging features are not definitive, to avoid unnecessary biopsy.

Tumors of glial origin comprise 90% of all intramedullary spinal cord tumors, with ependymomas and low-grade astrocytomas constituting the bulk (~95%) of these tumors.[68] Hemangioblastomas are the third most common tumor. Other tumor types, such as lymphoma, metastases, and ganglioglioma, are rare and are not covered in this review.

Ependymoma

In adults, the most common primary spinal cord tumor is ependymoma. Most ependymomas of the spinal cord are World Health Organization (WHO) grade 2 "classic" ependymomas, with higher-grade anaplastic ependymomas (WHO grade 3) much less frequent.[69] Myxopapillary ependymomas, a subtype of ependymomas that arises from the conus medullaris or filum terminale, typically appear as intradural extramedullary

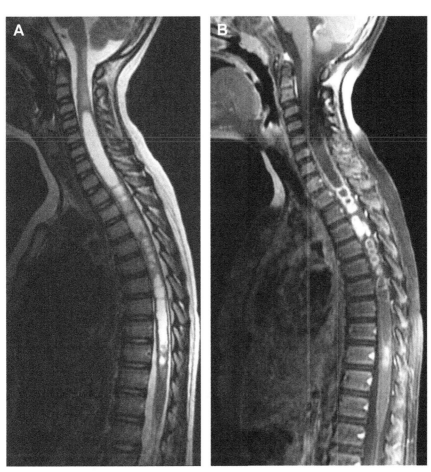

Fig. 23. Spinal cord astrocytoma. (A) Sagittal T2-weighted and (B) sagittal postcontrast T1-weighted images show a holocord enhancing mass expanding the spinal cord in a pediatric patient. The lesion contains internal tumoral cysts surrounded by enhancing tissue.

masses; they are not typically mistaken for other causes of myelopathy on imaging.

Spinal cord ependymomas arise from ependymal cells lining the central canal of the spinal cord, and as a result, are typically located centrally, rather than eccentrically, within the spinal cord. They are not infiltrating tumors histologically and can potentially be cured surgically.[70]

Most ependymomas demonstrate well-circumscribed margins on imaging. A focal, homogeneous, enhancing nodular mass located in the central spinal cord is seen in most cases (**Fig. 22**). The spinal cord is focally expanded at the level of the mass. Because of the location within the central canal, ependymomas are often associated with a syrinx or a "polar cyst," a nontumoral cyst located above or below the tumor nodule.[67] Cysts within the tumor itself are less common, seen more often in astrocytomas

than ependymomas. Further, as a result of the vascularity of the lesion, hemorrhage at the margins of the tumor is not uncommon, resulting in a T2 hypointense rim due to a hemosiderin "cap" in approximately one-third of cases.[71]

Astrocytoma

The most common tumor in pediatric patients and the second most common tumor in adults is the astrocytoma. Spinal cord astrocytomas are low-grade (WHO grade I or II) in 60% to 80% of cases.[72] As opposed to gliomas in the brain, glioblastoma multiforme (WHO grade IV) is uncommonly encountered in the spinal cord.[67,72]

Unlike the circumscribed tumor nodule of ependymomas, astrocytomas are infiltrative histologically, with poorly defined margins both pathologically and radiographically. Whereas the tumor nodules of ependymomas are localized to a short

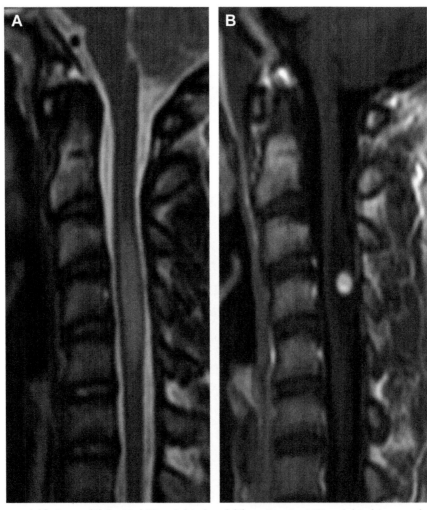

Fig. 24. Hemangioblastoma. (*A*) Sagittal T2-weighted and (*B*) postcontrast T1-weighted images demonstrate a circumscribed nodule of enhancement eccentrically located within the dorsal aspect of the cervical spinal cord, with a relatively large component of surrounding edema.

segment of the spinal cord, astrocytomas are often extensive and may involve nearly all of the spinal cord ("holocord" astrocytomas) at presentation (Fig. 23). Fusiform expansion is the rule, with corresponding T2 hyperintense signal representing a combination of tumor and vasogenic edema. Scoliosis may be present, and there may be remodeling and enlargement of the spinal canal, a reflection of the slow-growing nature of the tumor.[73] Enhancement is usually present and is often ill defined, although may occasionally appear more sharply marginated in pilocytic (WHO grade I) tumors. Commonly, one will note cysts located within the tumor, so-called "tumoral cysts." These are different from the polar cysts located immediately adjacent, but external, to tumors (such as ependymomas). Hemorrhage is not a common feature of astrocytomas.

Hemangioblastoma

Hemangioblastomas are the third most frequent tumor of the spinal cord, accounting for approximately 3% to 4% of intramedullary spinal cord tumors.[68] They are characterized by one or more circumscribed and intensely enhancing nodules that are usually eccentrically located within the spinal cord or are found along the cord surface (Fig. 24). These highly vascular lesions may be occasionally associated with dilated vessels, producing flow voids on imaging. Edema surrounding hemangioblastomas, seen as spinal cord T2 hyperintensity and expansion, is often disproportionately extensive compared with the size of the tumor mass. An associated cyst, producing the "cyst with a mural nodule" appearance, may be present, although in many cases is not. Multiple hemangioblastomas indicate the presence of von Hippel-Lindau syndrome and should prompt a search not only for cerebellar hemangioblastomas, but also for visceral malignancies in organs that may be contained within the scan field-of-view, such as the pancreas, kidneys, and adrenal glands.

SUMMARY

Imaging plays a critical role in the evaluation of the patient with myelopathy, with MR imaging being the preferred modality. Spinal cord compression must be excluded first in both acute and chronic presentations. Although the MR features of many causes of myelopathy overlap, careful attention to the time course of presentation, knowledge of common and uncommon causes of myelopathy, and identification of specific imaging patterns and features can help narrow the differential diagnosis or establish a definitive diagnosis.

REFERENCES

1. Seidenwurm DJ, Expert Panel on Neurologic Imaging. Myelopathy. AJNR Am J Neuroradiol 2008; 29(5):1032–4.
2. Schmalstieg WF, Weinshenker BG. Approach to acute or subacute myelopathy. Neurology 2010; 75(18 Suppl 1):S2–8.
3. Transverse Myelitis Consortium Working Group. Proposed diagnostic criteria and nosology of acute transverse myelitis. Neurology 2002;59:499–505.
4. Ross JS. ATM–OMG! AJNR Am J Neuroradiol 2008; 29(4):618.
5. Kalsi-Ryan S, Karadimas SK, Fehlings MG. Cervical spondylotic myelopathy: the clinical phenomenon and the current pathobiology of an increasingly prevalent and devastating disorder. Neuroscientist 2013;19(4):409–21.
6. Nouri A, Martin AR, Kato S, et al. The relationship between MRI signal intensity changes, clinical presentation, and surgical outcome in degenerative cervical myelopathy: analysis of a global cohort. Spine (Phila Pa 1976) 2017;42(24):1851–8.
7. Tetreault LA, Dettori JR, Wilson JR, et al. Systematic review of magnetic resonance imaging characteristics that affect treatment decision making and predict clinical outcome in patients with cervical spondylotic myelopathy. Spine (Phila Pa 1976) 2013;38(22 Suppl 1):S89–110.
8. Piscol K. Blood supply of the spinal cord and its clinical importance. Schriftenr Neurol 1972;8:1–91 [in German].
9. Santillan A, Nacarino V, Greenberg E, et al. Vascular anatomy of the spinal cord. J Neurointerv Surg 2012; 4(1):67–74.
10. Kister I, Johnson E, Raz E, et al. Specific MRI findings help distinguish acute transverse myelitis of neuromyelitis optica from spinal cord infarction. Mult Scler Relat Disord 2016;9(C):62–7.
11. Weidauer S, Nichtweiß M, Hattingen E, et al. Spinal cord ischemia: aetiology, clinical syndromes and imaging features. Neuroradiology 2014;57(3):241–57.
12. Freedman BA, Malone DG, Rasmussen PA, et al. Surfer's myelopathy. Neurosurgery 2016;78(5): 602–11.
13. Gass A, Rocca MA, Agosta F, et al. MRI monitoring of pathological changes in the spinal cord in patients with multiple sclerosis. Lancet Neurol 2015; 14(4):443–54.
14. Kearney H, Miller DH, Ciccarelli O. Spinal cord MRI in multiple sclerosis–diagnostic, prognostic and clinical value. Nat Rev Neurol 2015;11(6):327–38.
15. Tartaglino LM, Friedman DP, Flanders AE, et al. Multiple sclerosis in the spinal cord: MR appearance

and correlation with clinical parameters. Radiology 1995;195(3):725–32.

16. Rocca MA, Mastronardo G, Horsfield MA, et al. Comparison of three MR sequences for the detection of cervical cord lesions in patients with multiple sclerosis. AJNR Am J Neuroradiol 1999;20(9): 1710–6.

17. Campi A, Pontesilli S, Gerevini S, et al. Comparison of MRI pulse sequences for investigation of lesions of the cervical spinal cord. Neuroradiology 2000; 42(9):669–75.

18. Philpott C, Brotchie P. Comparison of MRI sequences for evaluation of multiple sclerosis of the cervical spinal cord at 3 T. Eur J Radiol 2011; 80(3):780–5.

19. Klawiter EC, Benzinger T, Roy A, et al. Spinal cord ring enhancement in multiple sclerosis. Arch Neurol 2010;67(11):1395–8.

20. Wingerchuk DM. Diagnosis and treatment of neuromyelitis optica. Neurologist 2007;13(1):2–11.

21. Wingerchuk DM, Banwell B, Bennett JL, et al. International consensus diagnostic criteria for neuromyelitis optica spectrum disorders. Neurology 2015; 85(2):177–89.

22. Pittock SJ, Weinshenker BG, Lucchinetti CF, et al. Neuromyelitis optica brain lesions localized at sites of high aquaporin 4 expression. Arch Neurol 2006; 63(7):964–8.

23. Lennon VA, Wingerchuk DM, Kryzer TJ, et al. A serum autoantibody marker of neuromyelitis optica: distinction from multiple sclerosis. Lancet 2004;364(9451):2106–12.

24. Sato DK, Callegaro D, Lana-Peixoto MA, et al. Distinction between MOG antibody-positive and AQP4 antibody-positive NMO spectrum disorders. Neurology 2014;82(6):474–81.

25. Pekcevik Y, Mitchell CH, Mealy MA, et al. Differentiating neuromyelitis optica from other causes of longitudinally extensive transverse myelitis on spinal magnetic resonance imaging. Mult Scler 2016;22(3): 302–11.

26. Kim HJ, Paul F, Lana-Peixoto MA, et al. MRI characteristics of neuromyelitis optica spectrum disorder: an international update. Neurology 2015;84(11): 1165–73.

27. Jurynczyk M, Craner M, Palace J. Overlapping CNS inflammatory diseases: differentiating features of NMO and MS. J Neurol Neurosurg Psychiatry 2015;86(1):20–5.

28. Matthews L, Marasco R, Jenkinson M, et al. Distinction of seropositive NMO spectrum disorder and MS brain lesion distribution. Neurology 2013;80(14): 1330–7.

29. Absoud M, Lim MJ, Chong WK, et al. Paediatric acquired demyelinating syndromes: incidence, clinical and magnetic resonance imaging features. Mult Scler 2013;19(1):76–86.

30. Pohl D, Alper G, Van Haren K, et al. Acute disseminated encephalomyelitis: updates on an inflammatory CNS syndrome. Neurology 2016;87(9 Suppl 2):S38–45.

31. Tenembaum S, Chamoles N, Fejerman N. Acute disseminated encephalomyelitis: a long-term follow-up study of 84 pediatric patients. Neurology 2002;59(8):1224–31.

32. Tellez-Zenteno JF, Remes-Troche JM, Negrete-Pulido RO, et al. Longitudinal myelitis associated with systemic lupus erythematosus: clinical features and magnetic resonance imaging of six cases. Lupus 2001;10(12):851–6.

33. West T, Hess C, Cree B. Acute transverse myelitis: demyelinating, inflammatory, and infectious myelopathies. Semin Neurol 2012;32(02):097–113.

34. Nesbit GM, Miller GM, Baker HL Jr, et al. Spinal cord sarcoidosis: a new finding at MR imaging with Gd-DTPA enhancement. Radiology 1989;173(3): 839–43.

35. Joseph FG, Scolding NJ. Neurosarcoidosis: a study of 30 new cases. J Neurol Neurosurg Psychiatry 2009;80(3):297–304.

36. Yokota H, Yamada K. Viral infection of the spinal cord and roots. Neuroimaging Clin N Am 2015; 25(2):247–58.

37. Malzberg MS, Rogg JM, Tate CA, et al. Poliomyelitis: hyperintensity of the anterior horn cells on MR images of the spinal cord. AJR Am J Roentgenol 1993;161(4):863–5.

38. Maloney JA, Mirsky DM, Messacar K, et al. MRI findings in children with acute flaccid paralysis and cranial nerve dysfunction occurring during the 2014 enterovirus D68 outbreak. AJNR Am J Neuroradiol 2015;36(2):245–50.

39. Thurnher MM, Olatunji RB. Infections of the spine and spinal cord. Handb Clin Neurol 2016;136: 717–31.

40. Tihan T. Pathologic approach to spinal cord infections. Neuroimaging Clin N Am 2015;25(2):163–72.

41. Faria do Amaral LL, Nunes RH, da Rocha AJ. Parasitic and rare spinal infections. Neuroimaging Clin N Am 2015;25(2):259–79.

42. Zalewski NL, Flanagan EP, Keegan BM. Evaluation of idiopathic transverse myelitis revealing specific myelopathy diagnoses. Neurology 2018;90(2): e96–102.

43. Cao J, Su ZY, Xu SB, et al. Subacute combined degeneration: a retrospective study of 68 cases with short-term follow-up. Eur Neurol 2018;79(5–6): 247–55.

44. Sun HY, Lee JW, Park KS, et al. Spine MR imaging features of subacute combined degeneration patients. Eur Spine J 2014;23(5):1052–8.

45. Pema PJ, Horak HA, Wyatt RH. Myelopathy caused by nitrous oxide toxicity. AJNR Am J Neuroradiol 1998;19(5):894–6.

46. Kumar N, Gross JB, Ahlskog JE. Copper deficiency myelopathy produces a clinical picture like subacute combined degeneration. Neurology 2004;63(1):33–9.

47. Nations SP, Boyer PJ, Love LA, et al. Denture cream: an unusual source of excess zinc, leading to hypocupremia and neurologic disease. Neurology 2008;71(9):639–43.

48. Rowin J, Lewis SL. Copper deficiency myeloneuropathy and pancytopenia secondary to overuse of zinc supplementation. J Neurol Neurosurg Psychiatry 2005;76(5):750–1.

49. Takai K, Komori T, Taniguchi M. Microvascular anatomy of spinal dural arteriovenous fistulas: arteriovenous connections and their relationships with the dura mater. J Neurosurg Spine 2015;23(4):526–33.

50. McCutcheon IE, Doppman JL, Oldfield EH. Microvascular anatomy of dural arteriovenous abnormalities of the spine: a microangiographic study. J Neurosurg 1996;84(2):215–20.

51. Flores BC, Klinger DR, White JA, et al. Spinal vascular malformations: treatment strategies and outcome. Neurosurg Rev 2017;40(1):15–28.

52. Marcus J, Schwarz J, Singh IP, et al. Spinal dural arteriovenous fistulas: a review. Curr Atheroscler Rep 2013;15(7):335.

53. Saraf-Lavi E, Bowen BC, Quencer RM, et al. Detection of spinal dural arteriovenous fistulae with MR imaging and contrast-enhanced MR angiography: sensitivity, specificity, and prediction of vertebral level. AJNR Am J Neuroradiol 2002;23(5):858–67.

54. Luetmer PH, Lane JI, Gilbertson JR, et al. Preangiographic evaluation of spinal dural arteriovenous fistulas with elliptic centric contrast-enhanced MR angiography and effect on radiation dose and volume of iodinated contrast material. AJNR Am J Neuroradiol 2005;26(4):711–8.

55. Steinmetz MP, Chow MM, Krishnaney AA, et al. Outcome after the treatment of spinal dural arteriovenous fistulae: a contemporary single-institution series and meta-analysis. Neurosurgery 2004;55(1):77–87 [discussion: 87–8].

56. Gross BA, Du R, Popp AJ, et al. Intramedullary spinal cord cavernous malformations. Neurosurg Focus 2010;29(3):E14.

57. Ogilvy CS, Louis DN, Ojemann RG. Intramedullary cavernous angiomas of the spinal cord: clinical presentation, pathological features, and surgical management. Neurosurgery 1992;31(2):219–29 [discussion: 229–30].

58. Koennecke HC. Cerebral microbleeds on MRI: prevalence, associations, and potential clinical implications. Neurology 2006;66(2):165–71.

59. Khan M, Ambady P, Kimbrough D, et al. Radiation-induced myelitis: initial and follow-up MRI and clinical features in patients at a single tertiary care institution during 20 years. AJNR Am J Neuroradiol 2018;39(8):1576–81.

60. Alfonso ER, De Gregorio MA, Mateo P, et al. Radiation myelopathy in over-irradiated patients: MR imaging findings. Eur Radiol 1997;7(3):400–4.

61. Okada S, Okeda R. Pathology of radiation myelopathy. Neuropathology 2001;21(4):247–65.

62. Flanagan EP, Keegan BM. Paraneoplastic myelopathy. Neurol Clin 2013;31(1):307–18.

63. Dalmau J, Graus F. Antibody-mediated encephalitis. N Engl J Med 2018;378(9):840–51.

64. Flanagan EP, McKeon A, Lennon VA, et al. Paraneoplastic isolated myelopathy: clinical course and neuroimaging clues. Neurology 2011;76(24):2089–95.

65. Klein NP, Ray P, Carpenter D, et al. Rates of autoimmune diseases in Kaiser Permanente for use in vaccine adverse event safety studies. Vaccine 2010;28(4):1062–8.

66. Schellinger KA, Propp JM, Villano JL, et al. Descriptive epidemiology of primary spinal cord tumors. J Neurooncol 2008;87(2):173–9.

67. Koeller KK, Rosenblum RS, Morrison AL. Neoplasms of the spinal cord and filum terminale: radiologic-pathologic correlation. Radiographics 2000;20(6):1721–49.

68. Miller DJ, McCutcheon IE. Hemangioblastomas and other uncommon intramedullary tumors. J Neurooncol 2000;47(3):253–70.

69. Celano E, Salehani A, Malcolm JG, et al. Spinal cord ependymoma: a review of the literature and case series of ten patients. J Neurooncol 2016;128(3):377–86.

70. Klekamp J. Spinal ependymomas. Part 1: intramedullary ependymomas. Neurosurg Focus 2015;39(2):E6.

71. Fine MJ, Kricheff II, Freed D, et al. Spinal cord ependymomas: MR imaging features. Radiology 1995;197(3):655–8.

72. Babu R, Karikari IO, Owens TR, et al. Spinal cord astrocytomas: a modern 20-year experience at a single institution. Spine (Phila Pa 1976) 2014;39(7):533–40.

73. Roonprapunt C, Houten JK. Spinal cord astrocytomas: presentation, management, and outcome. Neurosurg Clin N Am 2006;17(1):29–36.

Spinal Manifestations of Systemic Disease

Sean C. Dodson, MD[a], Nicholas A. Koontz, MD[b],*

KEYWORDS

- Systemic disease • Spine pathology • Neuroimaging • Infectious • Inflammatory • Metabolic
- Rheumatologic • Neoplastic

KEY POINTS

- Identifying the predominant pattern of disease (musculoskeletal system vs nervous system) helps generate an appropriate differential diagnosis.
- Radiologists must thoroughly review the electronic medical record and prior imaging (including nonspine imaging) to add specificity to the differential diagnosis.
- CT and MR imaging are often complementary in assessment of spinal manifestations of system disease.

INTRODUCTION

The spine is commonly involved in systemic disease and may include either musculoskeletal system or nervous system manifestations. An understanding of the common imaging findings of spinal involvement in systemic disease helps interpreting radiologists generate an appropriate, succinct differential diagnosis. As with other facets of neuroimaging, spine imaging cannot occur in a vacuum. The importance of the interpreting radiologist correlating with available clinical history to provide greater diagnostic specificity is stressed—this includes reviewing additional nonspine imaging studies found in a patient's medical record to synthesize an appropriate diagnosis.

NORMAL ANATOMY AND IMAGING TECHNIQUES

Spinal involvement in systemic disease is markedly varied but often disease-specific, which may include bones, synovial joints, intervertebral disks, paraspinal soft tissue, epidural space, meninges, or spinal cord. Thus, interpreting radiologists must be familiar with spinal anatomy. Identifying the space of origin of a spinal lesion (intradural extramedullary, prevertebral, osseous, and so forth.) may help generate a succinct, appropriate differential diagnosis. Additionally, it is critical to realize that CT and MR imaging provide complementary information useful for synthesizing an appropriate differential diagnosis.

IMAGING PROTOCOLS

A 1-size-fits-all approach to imaging protocols may not be optimal when approaching potential cases of spinal manifestations of systemic disease, although using a routine spine protocol may simplify workflow (Table 1). Given the necessity for total neuraxis imaging in many of these patients, acquisition of volumetric pulse sequences (thus allowing high-fidelity multiplanar reconstructions) versus acquiring equal field-of-view cervicothoracic and thoracolumbar sagittal sequences may reduce scanner time. This article advocates judicious use of intravenous gadolinium-based contrast medium, which may increase the sensitivity of MR imaging. This must be weighed against

The authors report no conflicts of interest, financial or otherwise, with regard to this article.
[a] Radiology Specialists of Florida, 2600 Westhall Lane, Maitland, FL 32751, USA; [b] Indiana University School of Medicine, 340 West 10th Street, Fairbanks Hall, Suite 6200, Indianapolis, IN 46202-3082, USA
* Corresponding author.
E-mail address: nakoontz@iupui.edu

Radiol Clin N Am 57 (2019) 281–306
https://doi.org/10.1016/j.rcl.2018.10.005

Table 1	
Suggested spine MR imaging protocol	
Sagittal	**Axial**
T1WI C−	T1WI C−
T2WI	T2WI
STIR	T1WI C+ FS
T1WI C+ FS	
DWI	

Abbreviations: C−, precontrast; C+, postcontrast; FS, fat saturation.

[a] Use of volumetric pulse sequences or equal field-of-view sagittal total spine protocol may reduce scanner time.

potential risks of nephrogenic systemic fibrosis and gadolinium deposition. Advanced sequences, such as diffusion-weighted imaging (DWI), can increase sensitivity for detecting marrow replacement and detection of cord derangement from sundry etiologies.

IMAGING FINDINGS/PATHOLOGY
Musculoskeletal System

Spinal neuroarthropathy
Background Spinal neuroarthropathy uncommonly occurs in patients with loss of sensation, proprioception, and abnormal range of motion, resulting in destruction of the joint capsule and ligaments.[1,2] Repeated stress produces microfractures, callus formation, joint dislocation, and bone destruction.

Presentation Patients present late in the disease process with spinal instability. A high index of suspicion is required to make a diagnosis early in the disease process, because pain is typically much less severe than expected. This condition is most commonly seen in traumatic spinal cord injury; in particular, patients who have undergone spinal fusion account for up to 70% of reported cases.[2–4] Other potential and systemic etiologies are detailed in **Box 1**.[1–3]

Imaging features Although of nervous system origin, the imaging hallmarks of spinal neuroarthropathy are best recognized with respect to musculoskeletal involvement. Involvement of the anterior and posterior columns can help distinguish spinal neuroarthropathy from other destructive spine conditions. Classically, neuroarthropathy is often described by the 6 Ds (**Box 2**). In the spine, this corresponds to disk space expansion, often with vacuum disk phenomenon; fragmentation of bone; increased bone density; and spondylolisthesis (**Fig. 1**). The lumbar spine is most commonly affected. Early in the

Box 1	
Etiologies of spinal neuroarthropathy	
Posttraumatic
Diabetes mellitus
Syringohydromyelia
Neurosyphilis
GBS
Transverse myelitis
Charcot-Marie-Tooth
Friedreich ataxia
Congenital insensitivity to pain

disease process, spinal neuroarthropathy can be difficult to distinguish from degenerative disk disease. Later in the disease process, an adjacent fluid collection mimicking an abscess may be seen, making diagnosis more challenging.

Crystalline arthropathy
Background Crystalline arthropathy constitutes a group of disorders with crystal deposition in and around joints ultimately leading to joint destruction. In the spine, the most commonly encountered condition is calcium pyrophosphate dihydrate (CPPD) crystal deposition disease. Less commonly, hydroxyapatite deposition disease or gout may be encountered. It is not uncommon for the same patient to have coexisting crystalline arthropathy, rheumatologic disease, and osteoarthritis, which can make diagnosis challenging.

Presentation The clinical presentation can be variable. In the acute setting, patients can present with fever, mild leukocytosis, focal pain, radiculopathy, or myelopathy. Middle-aged and elderly patients are more commonly affected. CPPD arthropathy becomes significantly more prevalent with age, with greater than 17% of the population affected by the age of 80.[5] CPPD arthropathy and hydroxyapatite deposition disease have no gender

Box 2	
6 Ds of spinal neuroarthropathy	
Increased *Density* of subchondral bone
Bone *Destruction*
Debris
Dislocation
Joint *Distention*
Disorganization

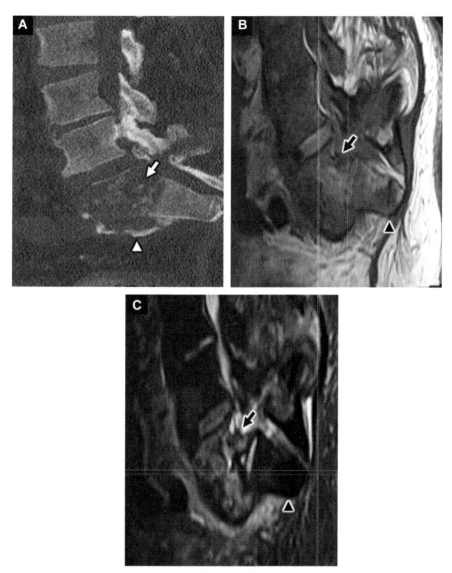

Fig. 1. Spinal neuroarthropathy in a diabetic patient. Sagittal non–contrast-enhanced CT (NECT) (*A*) shows destruction of the L5 and S1 vertebral bodies (*white arrow*) with subchondral sclerosis of the adjacent L4 vertebral body, calcific debris (*white arrowhead*), disorganization, and spondylolisthesis. Sagittal T1WI MR imaging (*B*) and sagittal STIR MR imaging (*C*) show vertebral destruction and debris (*black arrows*) as well as prior sacral resection due to decubitus ulcer and chronic infection (*black arrowheads*).

predilection, whereas gout affects men 3 times to 4 times more commonly than women.[6]

Imaging features The common imaging findings of crystalline arthropathies are summarized in **Box 3**. The hallmark of CPPD arthropathy is chondrocalcinosis with linear calcifications in cartilage, ligaments, tendons, bursae, and joint capsules, which are best seen on CT or radiography.[7] Small erosions may be seen along the dens and vertebral endplates and partially calcified retrodental pseudopannus may be encountered, often with

calcification within the cruciform, alar, and apical ligaments (**Fig. 2**). Nonsteroidal anti-inflammatory drugs (NSAIDs) are the mainstay of management, including treatment of acute flares of crowned dens syndrome, but cervical cord compression may require surgical intervention.[7,8]

Spinal hydroxyapatite deposition disease frequently results in the deposition of calcium hydroxyapatite crystals in the superior oblique fibers of the longus colli muscles.[9] Patients may develop acute calcific longus colli tendinitis, presenting with neck pain, fever, reduced range of motion,

---

Box 3
Key spine imaging findings of crystalline arthropathies

CPPD arthropathy
Chondrocalcinosis
Small erosions
Partially calcified retrodental pseudopannus

Hydroxyapatite deposition
Amorphous longus colli calcification near anterior C1
Retropharyngeal edema

Gout
Erosions with overhanging margins
Tophi

---

odynophagia, and/or dysphagia. Imaging shows amorphous calcification at the longus colli attachment near the anterior tubercle of C1, best seen on CT, as well as retropharyngeal and intramuscular edema and enhancement (**Fig. 3**).[9] This is often self-limited with symptoms managed by NSAIDs.

Spinal gout results from monosodium urate crystal deposition in disk spaces, facet joints, and the paravertebral soft tissues. Axial skeletal involvement is found more commonly in patients with peripheral tophi.[10] The lumbar spine is most commonly affected, followed by the thoracic spine and the sacroiliac (SI) joints. CT shows demarcated, punched-out, lytic lesions within the vertebral endplates, facet, and SI joints. Tophi present as soft tissue masses with or without faint calcifications (**Fig. 4**). On MR imaging, tophi are T1 hypointense and hypointense to isointense on T2-weighted imaging (T2WI) with heterogeneous enhancement.[11] The tophi often project into the extradural spinal canal or neural foramina producing spinal cord or nerve root compression.[11] Treatment typically involves a combination of NSAIDs, colchicine, allopurinol, and probenecid, although spinal cord or nerve root compression may require surgical intervention.

Hyperparathyroidism
Background There are 3 forms of hyperparathyroidism—primary, secondary, and tertiary. Primary is defined by excess parathyroid hormone (PTH) secretion in the absence of negative inhibition from calcium, usually indicative of an underlying adenoma or less likely glandular hyperplasia. Secondary hyperparathyroidism is the most common subtype and is often seen in the setting of chronic kidney disease and rarely vitamin D deficiency. A complex series of metabolic derangements leads to glandular hyperplasia, increased serum PTH, and resultant bone resorption.[12,13] Secondary hyperparathyroidism is the most common cause of renal osteodystrophy. Tertiary hyperparathyroidism results from long-standing secondary hyperparathyroidism in which PTH secretion goes unregulated even in the setting of treated secondary hyperparathyroidism. The resultant bone disease is referred to as osteitis fibrosa cystica.[14]

Presentation Patients typically present with diffuse bone pain, skeletal deformities, pathologic fractures, proximal muscle weakness, and hyperreflexia.[14]

Imaging findings Patients demonstrate diffuse osteopenia with excess osteoid accumulation along the endplates and a lucent band at the center of each vertebral body, resulting in a rugger jersey spine (**Fig. 5**).[12,15] There is an increased risk of pathologic fractures, and intravertebral disk herniations (Schmorl nodes) are common. Rarely, patients develop osteoclastomas (brown tumors), which are expansile, lytic lesions that are histologically identical to giant cell tumors (see **Fig. 5**).[12,16] On MR imaging, osteoclastomas are heterogeneous with solid enhancing and cystic components. Fluid-fluid levels may be present.

Hemodialysis spondyloarthropathy
Background Hemodialysis (HD) spondyloarthropathy is an uncommon destructive spondyloarthropathy related to either hydroxyapatite or amyloid deposition, although amyloid deposition is becoming less common with modern HD.[17] Patients are at increased risk of developing adynamic bone disease, a condition related to either resistance of PTH or oversuppression of PTH release, leading to bone fragility and insufficiency fractures.[18]

Presentation Patients are often asymptomatic although may present with pain and instability in the setting of a fracture.

Imaging findings HD spondyloarthropathy is usually a disk-centric pathology. Spinal imaging typically demonstrates multilevel vertebral endplate sclerosis with well-defined erosions with or without vertebral body collapse (**Fig. 6**). Amyloid deposits present as soft tissue masses centered on the disk or facet joint and are classically T1 hypointense and T2 hypointense to mildly hyperintense.[19] Signal abnormality within the endplates and adjacent disk space is less than expected in

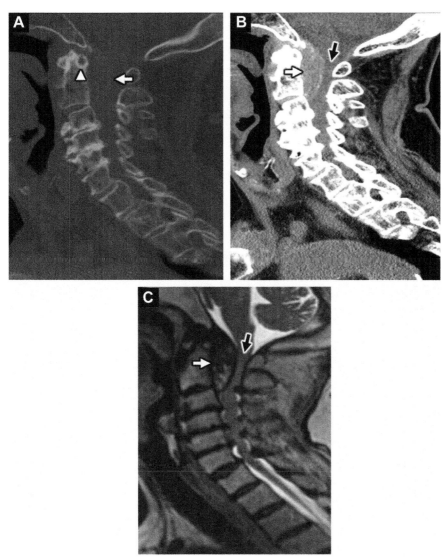

Fig. 2. CPPD. Sagittal bone algorithm NECT (*A*) shows characteristic large, partially calcified retrodental pseudo-pannus (*white arrow*) and subchondral cyst (*white arrowhead*). Sagittal soft tissue algorithm NECT (*B*) reveals cord compression (*black arrow*) due to the pseudopannus (*white arrow*). Sagittal T2WI MR imaging (*C*) shows the characteristic T2 dark pseudopannus (*white arrow*) yielding severe spinal canal stenosis with cord compression (*black arrow*).

the setting of an infectious process.[20] Unfortunately, these 2 entities can be difficult to distinguish based solely on imaging and require correlation with clinical findings, laboratory values, and occasional biopsy to exclude an infectious process.

Langerhans cell histiocytosis
Background Langerhans cell histiocytosis (LCH) is a multisystem disease of clonal proliferation and accumulation of dendritic cells.[21] Children and young adults are most frequently impacted, with 2:1 male predilection.[22] Skeletal

involvement is most common, but the skin, pituitary gland, liver, spleen, lungs, and hematopoietic system also may be affected.[21,22]

Presentation LCH spinal involvement may be asymptomatic or present with pain due to medullary involvement or pathologic fracture, restricted range of motion, myelopathy, or radiculopathy. Additional symptoms may include fever, leukocytosis, anemia, shortness of breath, hepatosplenomegaly, lymphadenopathy, or rash. Patients with pituitary dysfunction may present with diabetes insipidus.

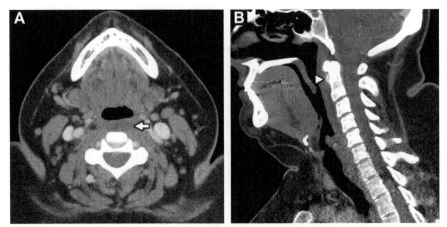

Fig. 3. Acute calcific longus colli tendinitis. Axial contrast-enhanced CT (*A*) shows bland retropharyngeal edema (*white arrow*). Sagittal contrast-enhanced CT (*B*) shows hallmark amorphous calcification (*white arrowhead*) at the longus colli attachment below the anterior tubercle of C1, confirming the diagnosis.

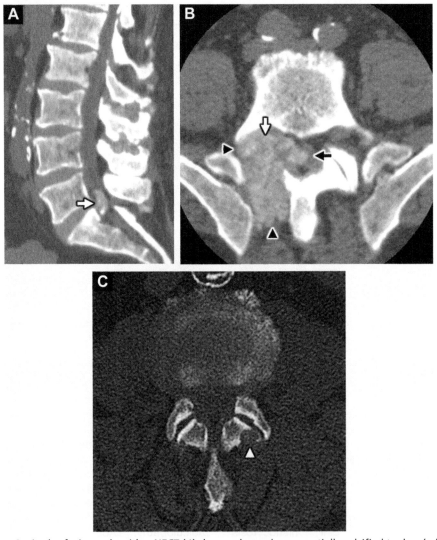

Fig. 4. Gout. Sagittal soft tissue algorithm NECT (*A*) shows a hyperdense, partially calcified tophus (*white arrow*) within the lumbar epidural space. Axial soft tissue algorithm NECT (*B*) in the same patient shows a hyperdense tophus (*white arrow*) centered in the region of the right facet joint, extending into the epidural space (*black arrow*), right neuroforamen, and extraspinal soft tissues (*black arrowheads*) via an eroded lamina. Axial bone algorithm NECT (*C*) in another patient with gout shows a periarticular erosion with classic overhanging margin (*white arrowhead*) at the left facet joint. (*Courtesy of* L. Shah, MD, Salt Lake City, UT.)

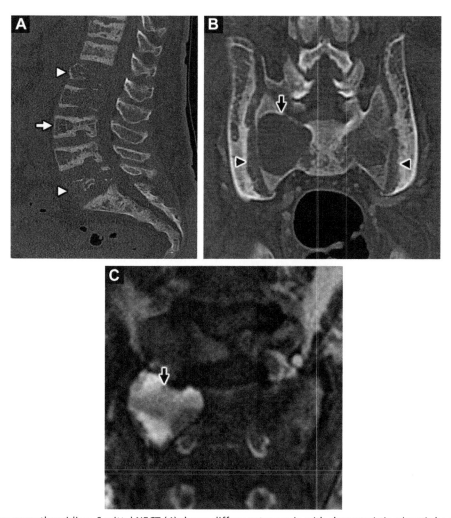

Fig. 5. Hyperparathyroidism. Sagittal NECT (*A*) shows diffuse osteopenia with characteristic sclerotic bands along the superior and inferior endplates with central lucency (*white arrow*), so-called rugger jersey spine. Note commonly associated pathologic fractures (*white arrowheads*) and intravertebral herniations. Coronal NECT (*B*) shows a large lytic lesion in the right sacral ala (*black arrow*) and bilateral SI joint erosions (*black arrowheads*). Coronal T2WI FS MR imaging (*C*) shows heterogeneously bright signal within the right sacral ala lesion (*black arrow*), a biopsy-proved osteoclastoma.

Imaging findings The most common spinal manifestation is vertebra plana with sparing of the posterior elements and associated enhancing soft tissue component (**Fig. 7**).[23] Additional findings including a lytic bone lesion with enhancing soft tissue, which may extend into the spinal canal or paravertebral soft tissues.[23,24] With appropriate therapy, the enhancing soft tissue component often resolves completely.[24]

Rheumatoid arthritis

Background Rheumatoid arthritis (RA) is an autoimmune, inflammatory arthropathy that classically affects young adult and middle-aged patients. As the prototypical seropositive spondyloarthropathy, most RA patients manifest elevated levels of autoantibodies directed at the fragment crystallizable portion of IgG, so-called rheumatoid factor. Women are 2 times to 4 times more commonly affected than men.[25] Spinal involvement is seen in approximately half of patients with RA.

Presentation Patients with spinal involvement often present with radiculopathy, myelopathy, and autonomic symptoms due to the propensity for cervical spine involvement. Neurologic symptoms portend a poor prognosis and are associated with increased mortality rates in RA patients.[26]

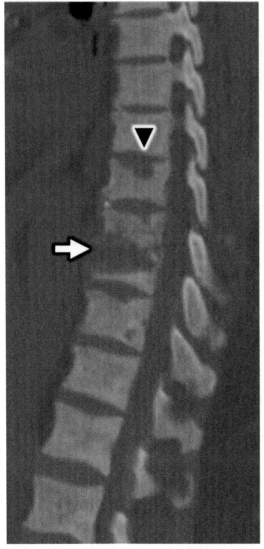

Fig. 6. HD spondyloarthropathy. Sagittal NECT shows diffuse sclerosis of the thoracic vertebrae. Note a disk-centric disease process with endplate erosions (*black arrowhead*) and associated vertebral collapse (*white arrow*) in a chronic HD patient. Symptomatology, laboratory assessment, and possible disc biopsy may be required to differentiate HD spondyloarthropathy from infectious discitis-osteomyelitis. (*Courtesy of* L. Shah, MD, Salt Lake City, UT.)

Imaging findings RA involvement of the cervical spine includes erosive changes at the dens, facets, and uncovertebral joints. Characteristic pannus formation surrounds the dens and may eventually destroy the adjacent ligamentous structures, leading to atlantoaxial instability and cranial settling with basilar invagination (**Fig. 8**).[25,27] The lack of calcifications within the pannus, disk spaces, and ligaments helps distinguish RA from CPPD arthropathy. The pannus may cause spinal

cord compression and compressive myelopathy. Due to the increased morbidity and mortality associated with atlantoaxial instability, imaging should include carefully supervised flexion and extension radiographs. If there is suggestion of vertical subluxation, MR imaging should be performed to evaluate for spinal cord compression.[27]

Juvenile idiopathic arthritis
Background Juvenile idiopathic arthritis (JIA), the most common arthritis and rheumatologic condition in children, is a heterogeneous group of inflammatory arthropathies. Multiple forms of JIA exist, including oligoarticular, polyarticular, systemic onset, psoriatic arthritis, and enthesitis-related JIA.[28]

Presentation The clinical presentation depends on the individual subtype. Patients with oligoarticular JIA typically present prior to 6 years of age with swelling, stiffness, and reduced range of motion in less than 5 joints.[28,29] Typically, patients have little to no pain at presentation and girls are more commonly affected than boys.

Children with polyarticular JIA present in the toddler to preschool age group, which is more common in girls than in boys. Arthritis may be asymmetric or symmetric, involving greater than 5 joints. Systemic symptoms are common and include fever, hepatosplenomegaly, lymphadenopathy, uveitis, serositis, and tenosynovitis

Systemic JIA differs in that patients typically present with at least 2 weeks of daily fever, rash, lymphadenopathy, hepatosplenomegaly, and/or serositis. Arthritis is only seen at the time of presentation in up to one-third of patients and develops over several months.

Juvenile psoriatic arthritis is defined as arthritis and psoriasis or arthritis plus 2 of the following: psoriasis in a first-degree relative, dactylitis, nail pitting, or onycholysis.

Enthesitis-related JIA is defined as arthritis or enthesitis plus 2 of the following: low back pain, personal of family history of HLA-B27 positivity, anterior uveitis, and onset in a boy over the age of 6. Boys are more commonly affected than girls.[29]

Imaging findings Historically, imaging of JIA relied heavily on radiography. Although this approach is valuable in excluding other potential etiologies for a child's symptoms, it does a poor job at identifying the early findings of JIA.[28–30] MR imaging is more sensitive at detecting synovitis, marrow edema, developing erosions, and enthesitis (**Fig. 9**).[29,30] With advanced disease, there is often bone production due to synovial hyperemia and pannus formation. Erosions can be seen at the

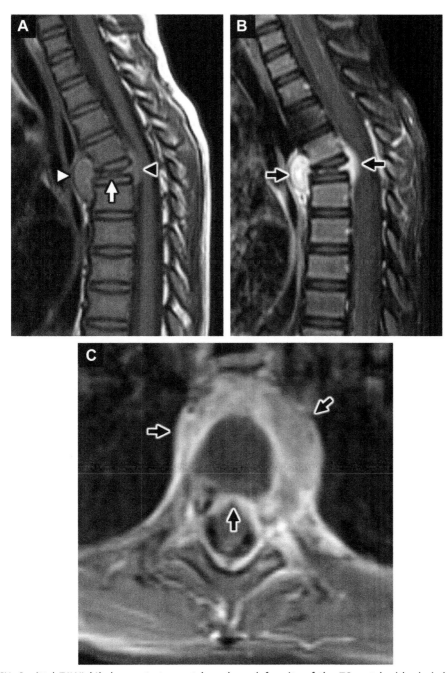

Fig. 7. LCH. Sagittal T1WI (*A*) demonstrates vertebra plana deformity of the T6 vertebral body (*white arrow*) sparing the posterior elements. Note a soft tissue component extending into the prevertebral soft tissues (*white arrowhead*) and ventral epidural space (*black arrowhead*). Sagittal (*B*) and axial (*C*) T1WI C+ MR imaging shows the soft tissue component to be avidly enhancing (*black arrows*).

odontoid process and joints throughout the spine, although these are less common than in adults with rheumatoid arthritis.[28–30] Cervical subluxation, cranial settling, basilar invagination, and ankylosis are common (see **Fig. 9**).[28–30] JIA patients are at risk of osteopenia and insufficiency fractures.

Seronegative spondyloarthropathy
Background Seronegative spondyloarthropathies constitute a heterogeneous group of disorders that are rheumatoid factor seronegative but often HLA-B27 seropositive. The 4 main conditions classified as seronegative spondyloarthropathies include ankylosing spondylitis (AS), reactive

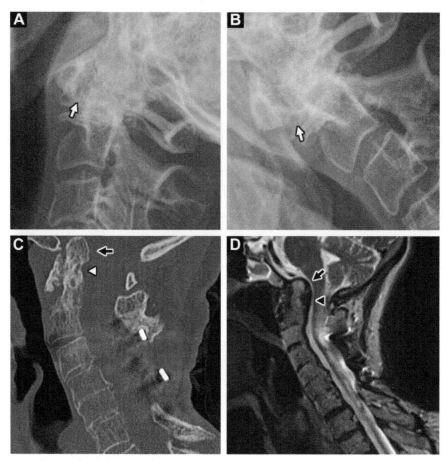

Fig. 8. RA. Lateral cervical radiographs of an RA patient in neutral (*A*) and flexion (*B*) positions reveal dynamic instability with abnormal widening of the atlantoaxial joint (*white arrows*). Sagittal NECT in a different RA patient (*C*) shows diffuse osteopenia with erosions of the dens (*white arrowhead*) and basilar invagination (*black arrow*). Sagittal T2WI MR imaging (*D*) shows a T2 dark retrodental pannus (*black arrowhead*) overlying the erosions and better delineates the basilar invagination (*black arrow*).

arthritis, psoriatic arthritis, and enteropathic spondyloarthropathy.

Presentation The clinical presentation is highly variable among the seronegative spondyloarthropathies. Men are more commonly affected than women, and patients typically present in early adulthood to midadulthood. Each condition is often accompanied by systemic symptoms, including fatigue, malaise, rash, gastrointestinal (GI) distress, uveitis, and dactylitis.

Patients with AS classically present with sacroiliitis that is worse when waking in the morning. As the ankylosis progresses, there is an increased risk of spine fractures and ligamentous or cord injuries with even mild trauma. Reactive spondyloarthropathy is typically preceded by a sexually transmitted disease (*Chlamydia*) or GI infection (*Campylobacter*, *Salmonella*, *Shigella*, or *Yersinia*). Patients present with a postinfectious triad of

arthritis, conjunctivitis, and urethritis. Spinal involvement occurs in up to 20% of patients. Patients with psoriatic arthritis and spinal involvement nearly always have characteristic skin plaques. Finally, enteropathic spondyloarthropathy is most commonly seen in patients with ulcerative colitis or Crohn disease.

Imaging findings Patients with AS typically present with bilaterally symmetric sacroiliitis, which begins with resorption of subchondral bone and erosions along the iliac side of the synovial portions of the SI joints. SI joints initially widen, then narrow and eventually fuse.[31,32] Focal inflammation of the vertebral body corners manifests as MR imaging signal abnormality (Romanus lesion), which progresses to erosions and vertebral body squaring (**Fig. 10**).[31] Patients often manifest aseptic discitis involving the adjacent vertebral endplates.[31,32] Later in the disease process,

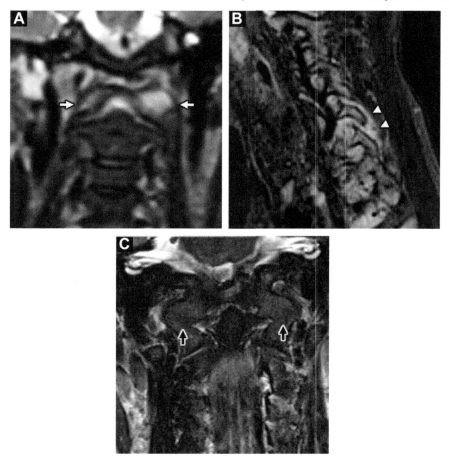

Fig. 9. JIA. Coronal T2WI FS MR imaging (*A*) shows edema within the lateral masses of C1 (*white arrows*) and adjacent joint spaces in the acute phase of disease. Sagittal STIR MR imaging (*B*) shows cervical facet and perifacet edema (*white arrowheads*). Coronal T2WI FS MR imaging (*C*) obtained 5 years later shows ankylosis of the occipital condyles and lateral masses of C1 (*black arrows*) in the chronic phase of disease.

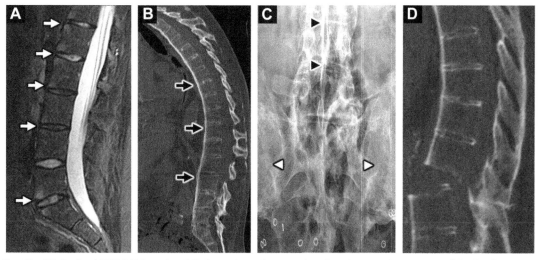

Fig. 10. AS. Sagittal STIR MR imaging (*A*) shows hyperintense signal at the anterior corners of the lumbar vertebral bodies (*white arrows*), so-called Romanus lesions in early disease. Sagittal NECT (*B*) in advanced AS shows a bamboo spine with multilevel vertebral body and facet ankyloses (*black arrows*). AP pelvis radiograph (*C*) in advanced AS shows bilateral SI joint ankylosis (*white arrowheads*), as well as ossification of the supraspinous ligaments (*black arrowheads*) producing a dagger sign. AS patients are at high risk for fracture-dislocation with even mild trauma, as seen on sagittal NECT (*D*).

patients develop thin vertical syndesmophytes and facet fusion, creating the classic bamboo spine appearance.[31,32] Additionally, patients develop ossification of the spinal ligaments, including the interspinous ligament, producing a dagger sign.[31]

Spinal involvement is only seen in up to 20% of patients with reactive arthritis[33,34] with common findings including juxta-articular osteopenia, erosions, periostitis, syndesmophytes, and ankylosis late in the disease process. Involvement of the SI joints is common (**Fig. 11**) and progresses from asymmetric to symmetric.[33]

Spinal imaging findings of psoriatic arthritis include asymmetric, often unilateral syndesmophyte formation, paravertebral ossifications, and ligamentous calcification (**Fig. 12**).[35] Facet joints are affected to a lesser extent and may not be involved. Sacroiliitis is bilateral and asymmetric.[35] Unlike AS and reactive arthritis, psoriatic arthritis involves both the synovial and syndesmotic portions of the SI joint.[35]

Patients with enteropathic spondyloarthropathy have imaging findings similar to those in patients with AS (**Fig. 13**). Clinical history and associated imaging findings of inflammatory bowel disease, as well as appendicular arthritis, help distinguish the 2 conditions.

Serous atrophy

Background Serous atrophy is an underdiagnosed condition characterized by atrophy of fatty marrow that is replaced by extracellular gelatinous material in patients with chronic illness and poor nutritional status.[36–38]

Presentation This condition has been reported in patients with severe malnutrition (including anorexia nervosa), malignancy, chronic systemic disease, chronic infection (such as HIV-AIDS),

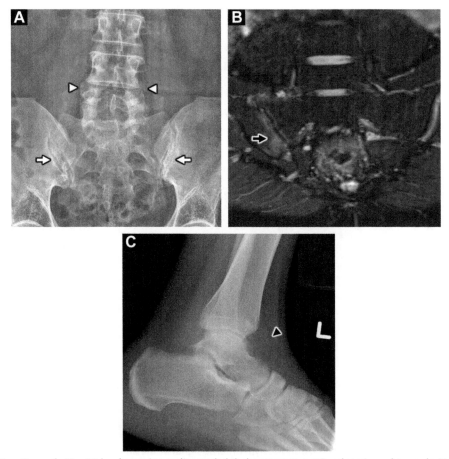

Fig. 11. Reactive arthritis. AP lumbar spine radiograph (*A*) shows asymmetric sclerosis and irregularity of the SI joints (*white arrows*) as well as parasyndesmophytes (*white arrowheads*). Coronal STIR MR imaging (*B*) in a different patient with reactive arthritis shows periarticular edema on the iliac side of the right SI joint (*black arrow*). Lateral ankle radiograph (*C*) in the same patient shows a nontraumatic ankle joint effusion (*black arrowhead*) due to synovitis.

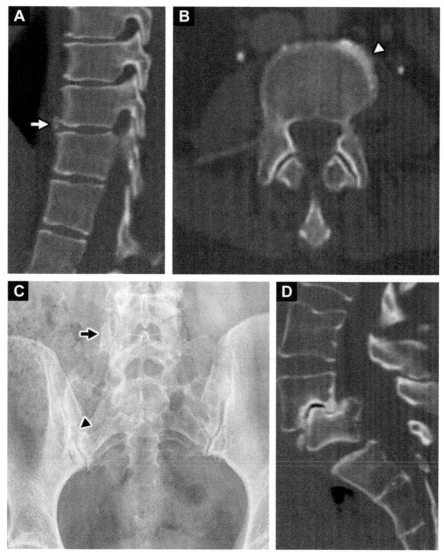

Fig. 12. Psoriatic arthritis. Sagittal NECT (*A*) shows a parasyndesmophyte (*white arrow*) with sparing of the facet joints. Axial CT (*B*) in the same patient shows fluffy paravertebral ossification (*white arrowhead*). AP pelvis radiograph (*C*) in a different patient with psoriatic arthritis shows asymmetric sclerosis and erosion of the right SI joint (*black arrowhead*) as well as bulky lower lumbar syndesmophytes (*black arrow*). Sagittal NECT (*D*) in a different psoriatic arthritis patient with chronic aseptic discitis shows a pencil-in-cup deformity at L4-L5 akin to the morphology of erosions classically seen the fingers of psoriatic arthritis patients.

and alcoholism. Patients present with severe weight loss and anemia.

Imaging findings MR imaging demonstrates heterogeneous marrow signal that is typically T1 hypointense and bright on fluid-sensitive sequences (**Fig. 14**).[36–38] Similar signal characteristics are often demonstrated in the adjacent soft tissues (see **Fig. 14**).[36–38] The depleted subcutaneous fat may also demonstrate short-tau inversion recovery (STIR) hyperintensity. Distinguishing serous atrophy from other marrow replacing processes is done by analyzing where the marrow changes begin. Unlike most marrow replacing processes, serous atrophy begins in the distal appendicular skeleton.[36–38] Conversion to gelatinous marrow predisposes these patients to insufficiency fractures, thus CT and MR imaging are often complementary modalities in this patient population.

Sickle cell disease
Background Sickle cell disease (SCD) is an autosomal recessive condition characterized by an

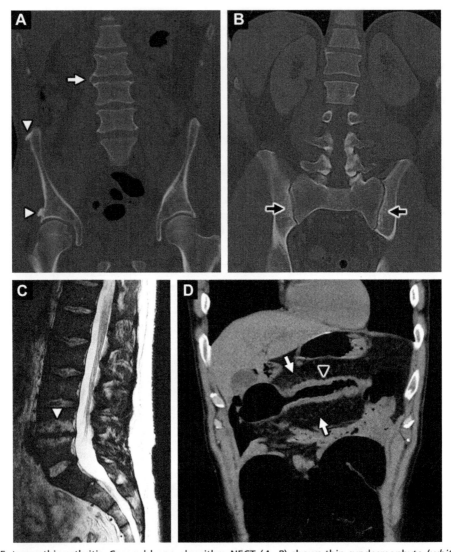

Fig. 13. Enteropathic arthritis. Coronal bone algorithm NECT (*A, B*) shows thin syndesmophyte (*white arrow*), multiple pelvic enthesophytes (*white arrowheads*), and symmetric sacroiliitis (*black arrows*), nonspecific findings that should raise suspicion for an inflammatory spondyloarthropathy. Sagittal T2WI MR imaging (*C*) shows end-plate and marrow edema from sterile spondylodiscitis, so-called Andersson lesion (*white arrowhead*). Coronal soft tissue algorithm contrast-enhanced CT (*D*) in same patient shows classic findings of Crohn disease with segmental bowel wall thickening (*black arrowhead*) and luminal narrowing of the transverse colon with comb sign (*white arrows*) of mesenteric hyperemia.

abnormality of the β-hemoglobin chain that deforms in low oxygen states. The abnormal structure of the hemoglobin leads to capillary obstruction, downstream ischemia, and infarctions.

Presentation SCD typically has an impact on patients of African, Hispanic, Middle Eastern, Asian, Indian, and Mediterranean descent. Patients present early in life, often earlier than 5 years of age, with sickle cell crisis—a condition characterized by severe acute pain secondary to bone

infarction.[39] Multisystem infarctions include cerebral, bone (with epiphyseal osteonecrosis resulting in growth disturbance), lung, liver, splenic, and renal. There is an increased risk of developing systemic infections. The abnormal configuration of the hemoglobin molecules leads to hemolysis and subsequent hemolytic anemia.[39]

Imaging findings Patients with SCD have decreased bone mineral density secondary to chronic anemia, which leads to erythroid hyperplasia and osteopenia and manifests as decreased

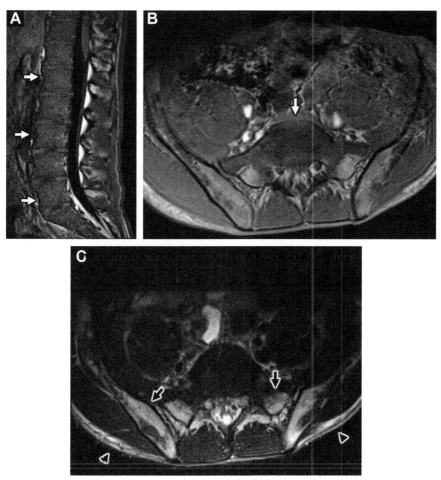

Fig. 14. Serous atrophy in an HIV patient. Sagittal (*A*) and axial (*B*) T1WI MR imaging shows heterogeneously decreased signal throughout the marrow spaces (*white arrows*). Axial STIR MR imaging (*C*) shows heterogeneous marrow signal, including bright signal within the pelvic bones and sacrum (*black arrows*). It is easy to confuse the true T2 bright signal abnormality within the subcutaneous fat (*black arrowheads*) for incomplete fat saturation.

trabecular bone on imaging.[40] Osteopenia increases the risk of vertebral compression fractures. Spine imaging often demonstrates central vertebral body collapse with peripheral sparing—commonly referred to as H-shaped vertebrae (Fig. 15). The central collapse is secondary to the underlying vascular supply of the vertebral endplates, because the long branches of the vertebral nutrient arteries are more susceptible to vascular occlusion than the short perforating branches of the periosteal vessels.[40] Rarely, compensatory vertical elongation of the adjacent vertebrae may be encountered, a finding first described as tower vertebra.[41] Marrow signal is decreased on both T1-weighted imaging (T1WI) and T2WI secondary to erythroid hyperplasia, chronic bone infarctions, and iron deposition in transfusion-dependent patients (see Fig. 15). Superimposed increased T2 signal is seen in the setting of acute infarction or

osteomyelitis (see Fig. 15). Contrast can be helpful to distinguish between the 2, because bone infarcts classically demonstrate a thin, serpentine rim of enhancement whereas osteomyelitis is more classically associated with diffuse marrow enhancement.

Nervous System

Acute transverse myelitis
Background Acute transverse myelitis (ATM) is an inflammatory myelitis that encompasses a heterogeneous group of disorders characterized by noncompressive myelopathy. The disorders are split into 2 broad categories—idiopathic and disease associated. Disease-associated ATM includes infectious or parainfectious etiologies, demyelinating disorders, systemic autoimmune, and paraneoplastic.[42,43]

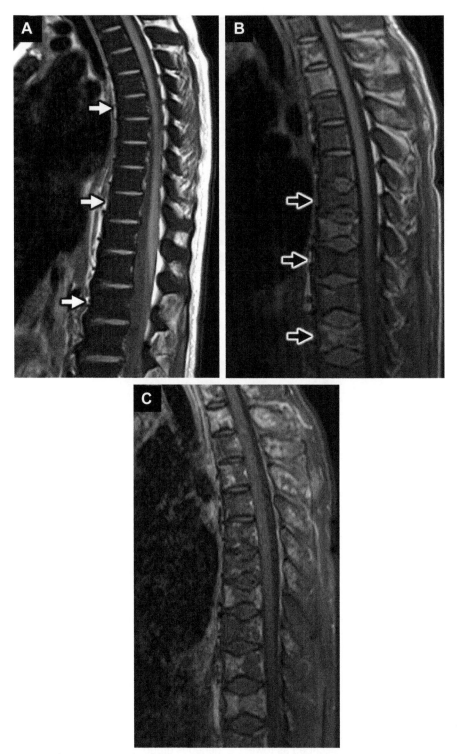

Fig. 15. SCD. Sagittal T1WI MR imaging (*A*) in a child with SCD shows diffusely hypointense marrow signal (*white arrows*), a nonspecific finding indicating anemia of chronic disease or iron deposition from transfusions. Sagittal T1WI MR imaging (*B*) in a different child shows heterogeneously dark signal throughout the marrow spaces and multiple tell-tale H-shaped vertebrae (*black arrows*). Sagittal T1WI C+ FS MR imaging (*C*) in the same child shows patchy areas of enhancement corresponding to evolving bone infarctions.

Presentation The clinical presentation is variable, typically including a combination of back pain, radiculopathy, sensory deficits, bowel and bladder dysfunction, or paralysis. Differentiation is ultimately achieved by symptomatology, laboratory analysis of blood and cerebrospinal fluid, and further imaging to assess for a more specific diagnosis.

In the setting of an underlying acute infectious process, patients are typically systemically ill, presenting with fever and meningismus. Parainfectious myelitis usually presents after a recent febrile illness or upper respiratory tract infection. Viral, bacterial, fungal, and parasitic infections can also produce ATM, but sometimes a specific pathogen is not identified.[44]

Demyelinating diseases, including multiple sclerosis (MS), neuromyelitis optica spectrum disorder (NMOSD), and acute disseminated encephalomyelitis (ADEM), may be difficult to distinguish from

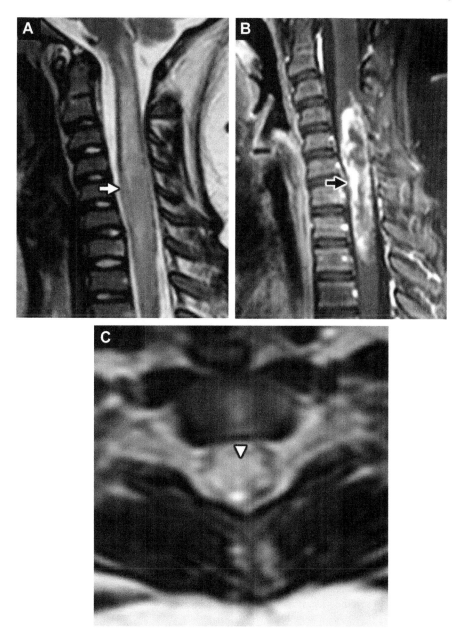

Fig. 16. Acute idiopathic transverse myelitis. Sagittal T2WI MR imaging (*A*) shows long-segment increased signal within the expanded cervical cord (*white arrow*). Sagittal T1WI C+ FS MR imaging (*B*) shows avid, leading edge enhancement at the periphery of the signal abnormality (*black arrow*). Axial T2WI MR imaging (*C*) shows diffuse cord involvement with greater than two-thirds of the cross-sectional area affected (*white arrowhead*).

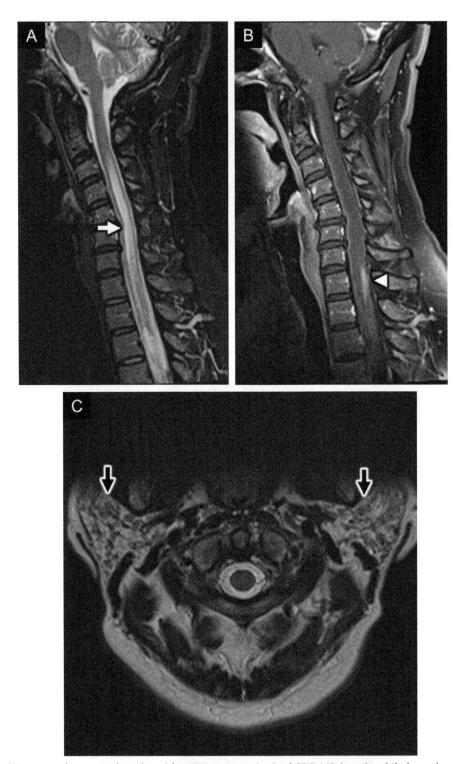

Fig. 17. Sjögren syndrome myelopathy with LETM pattern. Sagittal STIR MR imaging (A) shows long segment cord signal abnormality (*white arrow*) spanning the cervical and thoracic levels. Sagittal T1WI C+ FS MR imaging (B) shows patchy enhancement (*white arrowhead*) in the dorsal cord. The authors advise looking beyond the cord for diagnostic clues in these otherwise nonspecific LETM patients. In this case, axial T2WI MR imaging (C) showed a micronodular appearance of the parotid glands (*black arrows*) and solidified the primary differential diagnosis of Sjögren syndrome myelopathy, which was confirmed with serology.

other causes of transverse myelitis. MS and NMOSD are both often associated with optic neuritis, paresthesias, muscle weakness, hyperreflexia, gait disturbance, and bowel and bladder dysfunction. Differentiation is often best accomplished with clinical history, laboratory analysis, and MR imaging. ADEM may have a similar imaging appearance to MS but is often seen in younger patients after a recent viral illness or immunization.

ATM is an uncommon presentation of systemic autoimmune and paraneoplastic conditions. Typically, patients have systemic findings or laboratory results that help identify the specific etiology.[43]

Imaging findings Imaging findings of ATM are often nonspecific, including T2 hyperintense lesions that expand the cord and involve more than two-thirds its cross-sectional area (**Figs. 16 and 17**). MS and ADEM often present with short (fewer than 3) vertebral segment signal abnormality located peripherally in the cord and involving less than half the cross-sectional area of the cord. Enhancement is variable with all forms of transverse myelitis and may be seen in the acute/active setting. Three distinct patterns of cord involvement have been described in the setting of infectious and parainfectious myelitis: focal segmental, ascending, and disseminated myelitis.[44] Enhancement of the cauda equina may also be seen in the setting of infectious, para infectious, autoimmune-associated, and paraneoplastic myelitis. Evaluation of the entire neuraxis is recommended to evaluate for intracranial manifestations that may assist in narrowing the differential diagnosis.

Special consideration must be given to so-called longitudinally extensive transverse myelitis (LETM), in which cord signal abnormality or enhancement extends over a craniocaudal length greater than 3 vertebral segments. This is not a specific pathologic process (and should never be construed as such in a radiology report) but rather a useful imaging appearance that can confer some specificity to the differential diagnosis (**Box 4**).

Guillain-Barré syndrome

Background Guillain-Barré Syndrome (GBS) is a rare autoimmune, ascending, inflammatory demyelination usually preceded by an infection (respiratory or GI) or immunization.[45,46] Multiple GBS variants exist, likely related to the specific nerve fibers that are involved. The 3 most common subtypes are acute inflammatory demyelinating polyneuropathy (AIDP), Miller Fisher syndrome, and acute motor axonal neuropathy.[46]

Presentation Patients typically present with a rapidly progressive, ascending, symmetric paralysis of the extremities with associated hyporeflexia or areflexia. Weakness ranges from mild to severe with flaccid quadriplegia and respiratory failure in up to 30% of patients.[46] When there is cranial nerve involvement (Miller Fisher variant), patients classically present with ophthalmoplegia, ataxia, and areflexia. Although nonspecific, anti-GQ1b is present in the serum of greater than 85% of patients the Miller Fisher variant.[47]

Box 4
Longitudinally extensive transverse myelitis differential diagnosis

Rheumatologic
  Neuromyelitis optica/NMOSD
  Sjögren syndrome
  Systemic lupus erythematosus
  Antiphospholipid syndrome
Inflammatory/demyelinating
  Multiple sclerosis
  ADEM
  Sarcoid
  Behçet disease
  Postradiation
Metabolic
  Vitamin B_{12} deficiency
  Copper deficiency
Neoplastic/paraneoplastic
  Primary cord tumor
  Metastatic disease
  Paraneoplastic syndrome
Infectious/parainfectious
  Viral (HIV, HTLV-1, EBV, CMV, and VZV)
  Syphilis
  Tuberculosis
  Parasitic (*Toxocara* and *Ascaris*)
Vascular
  Infarction
  Dural arteriovenous fistula
  Vasculitis
Idiopathic

Abbreviations: CMV, cytomegalovirus; EBV, Epstein-Barr virus; HTLV-1, human T-lymphotrophic virus type 1; VZV, varicella zoster virus.

Children and young adults are most commonly affected, and older patients have a worse prognosis. Symptoms peak at 4 weeks, but prognosis is highly variable, with 65% of patients having minor residual symptoms at 1 year. Major residual deficits are seen in up to 15% of patients with 1 study demonstrating mortality rates up to 8%.[48]

Imaging findings Contrast-enhanced MR imaging shows smooth enhancement of the cauda equina with preferential involvement of the ventral nerve roots, which are often mildly thickened (**Fig. 18**).[45–47] Brain imaging may demonstrate enhancement of the cranial nerves, most commonly affecting the trigeminal nerves.[47]

Chronic inflammatory demyelinating polyneuropathy

Background Chronic inflammatory demyelinating polyneuropathy (CIDP) is an autoimmune demyelinating polyneuropathy that is considered the chronic counterpart to GBS. There is a temporal continuum between AIDP and CIDP, with the former reaching its nadir within 3 weeks to 4 weeks and the latter continuing to progress for greater than 8 weeks. The immunologic cause(s) of most forms of CIDP remain unclear, because specific provoking antigens have not previously been identified. Antibodies to different isoforms of neurofascin or to contactin, however, have been detected in small numbers of patients with CIDP.[49,50]

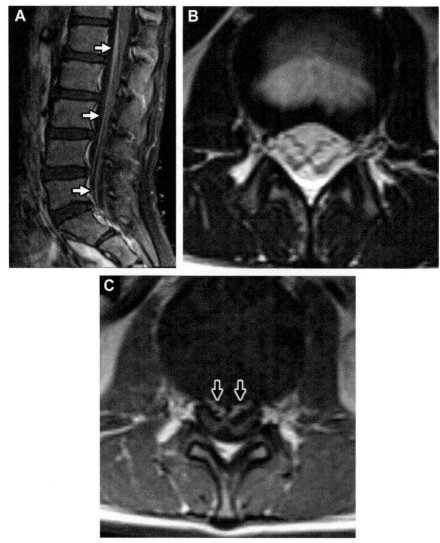

Fig. 18. AIDP. Sagittal T1WI C+ FS MR imaging (*A*) shows abnormal smooth enhancement of the cauda equina (*white arrows*). Axial T2WI MR imaging (*B*) shows mild thickening of the cauda equina nerve roots. On axial T1WI C+ MR imaging (*C*) note the disproportionate hyperenhancement of the ventral nerve roots (*black arrows*), commonly seen in AIDP.

Presentation CIDP is clinically heterogeneous with grossly symmetric, sensory, and motor neuropathy evolving as a monophasic, relapsing, or progressive disorder. It is classically associated with symmetric progressive limb weakness (more commonly involving proximal muscle groups), sensory disturbances, and hyporeflexia or areflexia with a relapsing

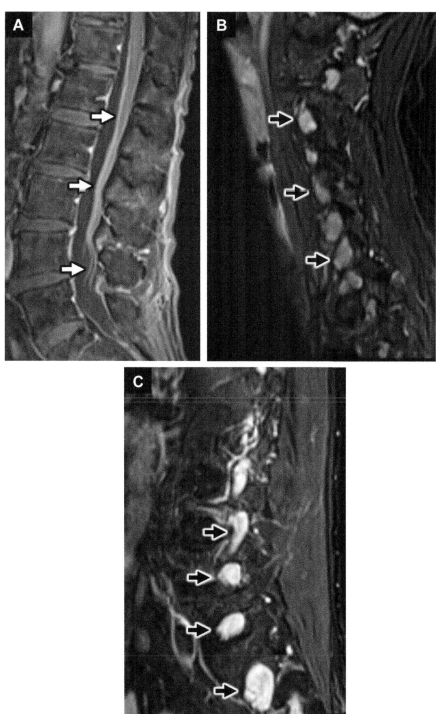

Fig. 19. CIDP. Sagittal T1W C+ FS MR imaging (A) shows homogeneously enhancing, thickened cauda equina nerve roots (*white arrows*) in a patient with progressive limb weakness and hyporeflexia. The appearance of the cauda equina mimics AIDP, but progressive symptoms beyond 8 weeks in this case indicated CIDP. Sagittal STIR MR imaging of the cervical (B) and lumbar spine (C) demonstrates markedly enlarged, hyperintense extradural nerve roots (*black arrows*) in a patient with CIDP.

or progressive course.[51] CIDP is most common in adults between the 40 years and 60 years of age, with a slight male predominance.[51]

Imaging findings Spinal imaging demonstrates significantly enlarged, enhancing nerve roots (lumbar > cervical > thoracic), peripheral nerves, and plexuses (brachial and lumbar), which are best seen on MR imaging (**Fig. 19**). The extradural component of the nerve roots is more commonly impacted than the intradural component.[52] Cranial nerves also may be affected.

Box 5
Key spine imaging findings of metastatic disease

Osseous metastases

CT

- Lytic or sclerotic lesions, usually multiple
- Pathologic fracture

MR imaging

- Marrow replacement, usually multifocal, T1 dark/STIR bright, and enhancing
- Localized bright marrow DWI signal (normally dark in adults due to fat saturation nulling marrow signal on echoplanar-based DWI)

Epidural metastases

CT

- Soft tissue replacement of epidural fat

MR imaging

- Soft tissue replacement of epidural fat with enhancing mass
- Extension of tumor into neural foramina and paravertebral space
- Spinal cord compression
- Localized bright DWI signal in epidural fat (normally DWI dark from fat saturation)

Spinal cord metastases

CT

- Insensitive

MR imaging

- Enhancing intramedullary nodule
- Marked edema disproportionate to size of metastasis
- Reduced diffusivity (high cellularity tumor)
- Rare hemorrhage or cystic change[59,60]
- Rim and flame signs[59,60]

Leptomeningeal metastases

CT

- Insensitive

MR imaging

- Localized or multifocal enhancement
- Sugarcoating of cord surface
- Enhancing cauda equina nerve roots
- Soft tissue mass in distal thecal sac
- Corresponding bright DWI signal (high cellularity tumor)

Metastatic disease

Background Spinal metastatic disease is commonly encountered and may include osseous, epidural, spinal cord, or leptomeningeal disease. As cancer treatment evolves, life expectancy prolongs and the prevalence of spinal metastases increases, although this is malignancy-specific and likely underreported.[53,54] Metastatic

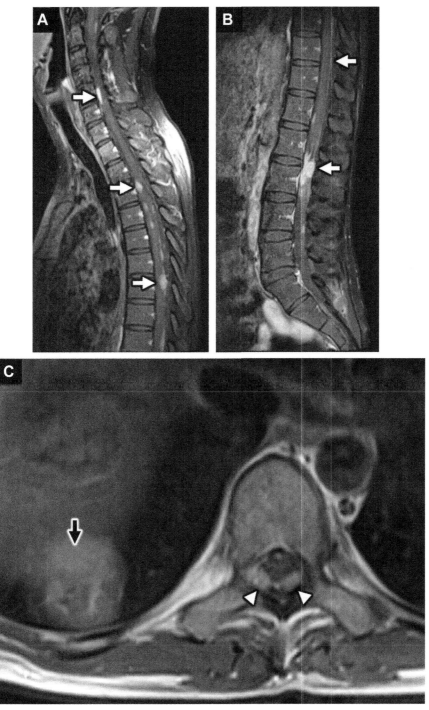

Fig. 20. Leptomeningeal metastases in melanoma patient. Sagittal T1WI C+ FS MR imaging of the cervicothoracic (*A*) and thoracolumbar spine (*B*) demonstrates nodular leptomeningeal enhancement (*white arrows*). Axial T1WI C+ MR imaging (*C*) shows leptomeningeal enhancement (*white arrowheads*) along the dorsal thecal sac. It is critical to review the extraspinal soft tissues on all spinal imaging, which in this case revealed a suspicious mass within the right lower lobe (*black arrow*), subsequently biopsy-confirmed as metastatic melanoma.

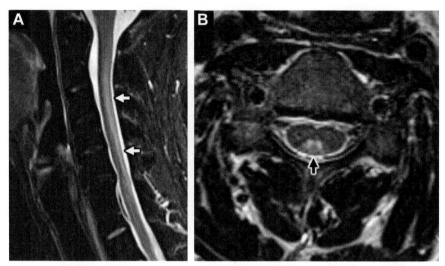

Fig. 21. Subacute combined degeneration. Sagittal STIR MR imaging (*A*) shows long segment hyperintense signal within the dorsal aspect of the cord (*white arrows*). Axial T2WI MR imaging (*B*) shows signal abnormality in the dorsal columns (*black arrow*), often referred to as the inverted V sign.

disease may occur from hematogenous spread, direct extension, cerebrospinal fluid seeding in the setting of a primary central nervous system malignancy, or through lymphatic channels.

Presentation The clinical presentation is variable and depends on the site of involvement. Patients may present with weakness, sensory disturbances, pain, radiculopathy, and bowel or bladder dysfunction. Intracranial involvement may present as altered mental status, headache, cranial nerve dysfunction, and seizures.

Imaging findings CT and MR imaging are complementary modalities in assessment of spinal metastatic disease (**Box 5**). CT may identify lytic or sclerotic lesions as well as offer superior assessment of underlying osseous integrity in the setting of pathologic fractures. Contrast-enhanced MR imaging is the best imaging modality to evaluate for metastatic marrow replacement, cord metastases, leptomeningeal metastatic disease (**Fig. 20**), and cord compression. Lumbar puncture confers specificity to the diagnosis in the setting of suspected leptomeningeal metastases.

Subacute combined degeneration
Background Subacute combined degeneration is a treatable and often reversible myelopathy characterized by selective degeneration of the dorsal and lateral spinal cord columns in the setting of vitamin B$_{12}$ deficiency. It is most commonly seen in the setting of malnutrition although can be encountered in patients with pernicious anemia, prior gastric bypass or gastrectomy, bacterial overgrowth in intestinal blind loops, inflammatory

bowel disease, celiac disease, and recreational nitrous oxide abuse.[55] The underlying mechanism relates to inactivation of methylcobalamin, limiting methionine synthesis.[56]

Presentation Patients typically present with symmetric paresthesia in the hands and feet. The disease course is insidious early on with rapid decline and severe disability over the next few months. Symptoms include altered sensation, gait ataxia, and distal leg weakness. Physical examination may demonstrate loss of vibratory and position sense, weakness, spasticity, hyperreflexia, and extensor plantar responses.[55] Early diagnosis is critical, because outcomes are related to the duration of symptomatology.

Imaging findings MR imaging demonstrates mild cord expansion with abnormal, increased T2 signal in the dorsal columns, which has been referred to as the inverted V sign in the cervical cord (**Fig. 21**).[56–58] In the thoracic cord, the abnormal bilateral paired nodular T2 hyperintensity has been described as looking like a dumbbell or binoculars.[58] Rarely there may be faint contrast enhancement.[55]

SUMMARY

Numerous systemic diseases may manifest with spinal involvement, which makes approaching these cases a challenge for the interpreting radiologist. By compartmentalizing the imaging findings into musculoskeletal versus nervous system processes, digging into the electronic medical record, and carefully examining extraspinal imaging findings (including those found in nonspine imaging examinations), a succinct, appropriate differential diagnosis usually can be synthesized, if a single correct diagnosis is not arrived at, in these challenging cases.

REFERENCES

1. Lacout A, Lebreton C, Mompoint D, et al. CT and MRI of spinal neuroarthropathy. AJR Am J Roentgenol 2009;193:W505–14.
2. Ledbetter LN, Salzman KL, Sanders RK, et al. Spinal neuroarthropathy: pathophysiology, clinical and imaging features, and differential diagnosis. RadioGraphics 2016;36:783–99.
3. Barrey C, Massourides H, Cotton F, et al. Charcot spine: two new case reports and a systematic review of 109 clinical cases from the literature. Ann Phys Rehabil Med 2010;53(3):200–20.
4. Lee D, Dahdaleh NS. Charcot spinal arthropathy. J Craniovertebr Junction Spine 2018;9(1):9–19.
5. Richette P, Bardin T, Doherty M. An update on the epidemiology of calcium pyrophosphate dihydrate crystal deposition disease. Rheumatology 2009;48: 711–5.
6. Doherty M. New insights into the epidemiology of gout. Rheumatology 2009;48(2):ii2–8.
7. Chang EY, Lim WY, Wolfson T, et al. Frequency of atlantoaxial calcium pyrophosphate dihydrate deposition at CT. Radiology 2013;269(2):519–24.
8. Inokuchi R, Ohshima K, Yamamoto M, et al. Crowned dens syndrome. Spine J 2015;15(6): 1499–500.
9. Shawky A, Elnady B, El-Morshidy E, et al. Longus colli tendinitis - a review of literature and case series. SICOT J 2017;3:48.
10. de Mello FM, Helito PV, Bordalo-Rodrigues M, et al. Axial gout is frequently associated with the presence of current tophi, although not with spinal symptoms. Spine (Phila Pa 1976) 2014;39:E1531–6.
11. Elgafy H, Liu X, Herron J. Spinal gout: a review with case illustration. World J Orthop 2018;7(11): 766–75.
12. Chang CY, Rosenthal DI, Mitchell DM, et al. Imaging findings of metabolic bone disease. Radiographics 2016;36:1871–87.
13. Slatopolsky E, Brown A, Dusso A. Pathogenesis of secondary hyperparathyroidism. Kidney Int 1999; 56(73):S14–9.
14. Bandeira F, Cusano N, Silva B, et al. Bone disease in primary hyperparathyroidism. Arq Bras Endocrinol Metabol 2014;58(5):553–61.
15. Wittenberg A. The Rugger Jersey spine sign. Radiology 2004;230:491–2.
16. Arsalanizadeh B, Westacott R. Osteoclastomas ('brown tumors') and spinal cord compression: a review. Clin Kidney J 2013;6:220–3.
17. Kaneko S, Yamagata K. Hemodialysis-related amyloidosis: is it still relevant? Semin Dial 2018; 1–7. https://doi.org/10.1111/sdi.12720.
18. Sista SK, Arum SM. Management of adynamic bone disease in chronic kidney disease: a brief review. J Clin Transl Endocrinol 2016;5:32–5.
19. Kiss E, Keusch G, Zanetti M, et al. Dialysis-related amyloidosis revisited. AJR Am J Roentgenol 2005; 185(6):1460–7.
20. Theodorou DJ, Theodorouc SJ, Resnick D. Imaging in dialysis spondyloarthropathy. Semin Dial 2002; 15(4):290–6.
21. Haupt R, Minkov M, Astigarraga I, et al. Langerhans cell histiocytosis (LCH): guidelines for diagnosis, clinical work-up, and treatment for patients til the age of 18 years. Pediatr Blood Cancer 2013;60: 175–84.
22. Liu YH, Fan XH, Fang K. Langerhans' cell histiocytosis with multisystem involvement in an adult. Clin Exp Dermatol 2007;32(6):765–8.
23. Khung S, Budzik JF, Amzallag-Bellenger E, et al. Skeletal involvement in Langerhans cell histiocytosis. Insights Imaging 2013;4:569–79.
24. Peng XS, Pan T, Chen LY, et al. Langerhans' cell histiocytosis of the spine in children with soft tissue extension and chemotherapy. Int Orthop 2009;33:731–6.
25. Joaquim AF, Ghizoni E, Tedeschi H, et al. Radiological evaluation of cervical spine involvement in rheumatoid arthritis. Neurosurg Focus 2015;38(4):E4–11.
26. Nguyen HV, Ludwig SC, Silber J, et al. Rheumatoid arthritis of the cervical spine. Spine J 2004;4(3): 329–34.
27. Jurik AG. Imaging the spine in arthritis – a pictorial review. Insights Imaging 2011;2:177–91.
28. Sheybani EF, Khanna G, White AJ, et al. Imaging of juvenile idiopathic arthritis: a multimodality approach. Radiographics 2013;33:1253–73.
29. Sudol-Szopinska I, Matuszewska G, Gietka P, et al. Imaging of juvenile idiopathic arthritis. Part 1: clinical classifications and radiographs. J Ultrason 2016; 16(66):225–36.
30. Sudol-Szopinska I, Matuszewska G, Gietka P, et al. Imaging of juvenile idiopathic arthritis. Part 2: clinical classifications and radiographs. J Ultrason 2016; 16(66):225–36.
31. Jang JH, Ward MM, Rucker AN, et al. Ankylosing spondylitis: patterns of radiographic involvement. Radiology 2011;258:192–8.
32. Cawley MI, Chalmers TM, Ball J. Destructive lesions of vertebral bodies in ankylosing spondylitis. Ann Rheum Dis 1971;30(5):539–40.
33. Klecker RJ, Weissman BN. Imaging features of psoriatic arthritis and Reiter's syndrome. Semin Musculoskelet Radiol 2003;7(2):115–26.
34. Jacobson JA, Girish G, Jiang Y, et al. Radiographic evaluation of arthritis: inflammatory conditions. Radiology 2008;248(2):378–89.

35. Rogelio A, Pugh DG, Slocum CH, et al. Psoriatic arthritis: a Roentgenologic study. Radiology 1960; 75(5):691–702.

36. Boutin RD, White LM, Laor T, et al. MRI findings of serous atrophy of bone marrow and associated complications. Eur Radiol 2015;25:2771–8.

37. Shergill KK, Shergill GS, Pillai HJ. Gelatinous transformation of bone marrow: rare or underdiagnosed? Autops Case Rep 2017;7(4):8–17.

38. Sung CW, Hsieh K, Lin YH, et al. Serous degeneration of bone marrow mimics spinal tumor. Eur Spine J 2017;26(1):S80–4.

39. Lonergan GJ, Cline DB, Abbondanzo SL. From the archives of the AFIP: sickle cell anemia. Radiographics 2001;21:971–94.

40. Vaishya R, Agarwal AK, Edomwonyi EO, et al. Musculoskeletal manifestations of sickle cell disease: a review. Cureus 2015;7(10):e358.

41. Marlow TJ, Brunson CY, Jackson S, et al. "Tower vertebra": a new observation in sickle cell disease. Skeletal Radiol 1998;27(4):195–8.

42. Barnes G, Kaplin A, Kerr D, et al. Proposed diagnostic criteria and nosology of acute transverse myelitis. Neurology 2002;59:499–505.

43. Jacob A, Weinshenker BG. An approach to the diagnosis of acute transverse myelitis. Semin Liver Dis 2008;28(1):105–20.

44. Pradhan S, Gupta RK, Ghosh D. Parinfectious myelitis: three distinct clinic-imagiological patterns with prognostic implications. Acta Neurol Scand 1997;95:241–7.

45. Alkan O, Yildirim T, Tokmak N, et al. Spinal MRI findings of Guillain-Barré syndrome. J Radiol Case Rep 2009;3(3):25–8.

46. Dimachkie MM, Barohn RJ. Guillain-Barré syndrome and variants. Neurol Clin 2013;31(2):491–510.

47. Snyder LA, Rismondo V, Miller NR. The fisher variant of Guillain-Barré syndrome (Fischer syndrome). J Neuroophthalmol 2009;29:312–24.

48. Rees JH, Thompson RD, Smeeton NC, et al. Epidemiological study of Guillain-Barré syndrome in south east England. J Neurol Neurosurg Psychiatry 1998; 64(1):74–7.

49. Querol L, Nogales-Gadea G, Rojas-Garcia R, et al. Antibodies to contactin-1 in chronic inflammatory demyelinating polyneuropathy. Ann Neurol 2013; 73(3):370–80.

50. Ng JK, Malotka J, Kawakami N, et al. Neurofascin as a target for autoantibodies in peripheral neuropathies. Neurology 2012;79(23):2241–8.

51. Gorson KC. An update on the management of chronic inflammatory demyelinating polyneuropathy. Ther Adv Neurol Disord 2012;5(6):359–73.

52. Fletcher GP, Roberts CC. AJR teaching file: progressive polyradiculopathy. AJR Am J Roentgenol 2006; 186:S230–2.

53. Nayar G, Ejikeme T, Chongsathidkiet P, et al. Leptomeningeal disease: current diagnostic and therapeutic strategies. Oncotarget 2017;8(42):73312–28.

54. Pavlidis N. The diagnostic and therapeutic management of leptomeningeal carcinomatosis. Ann Oncol 2004;15(4):iv285–91.

55. Ravina B, Loevner LA, Bank W. MR findings in subacute combined degeneration of the spinal cord: a case of reversible cervical myelopathy. AJR Am J Roentgenol 2000;174:863–5.

56. Yuan JL, Wang SK, Jiang T, et al. Nitrous oxide induced subacute combined degeneration with longitudinally extensive myelopathy with inverted V-sign on spine MRI: a case report and literature review. BMC Neurol 2017;17:222–5.

57. Narra R, Mandapalli A, Jukuri N, et al. "Inverted V sign" in sub-acute combined degeneration of cord. J Clin Diagn Res 2015;9(5):TJ01.

58. Sun HY, Lee JW, Park KS, et al. Spine MR imaging features of subacute combined degeneration patients. Eur Spine J 2014;23(5):1052–8.

59. Rykken JB, Dien FE, Hunt CH, et al. Intramedullary spinal cord metastases: MRI and relevant clinical features from a 13-year institutional case series. AJNR Am J Neuroradiol 2013;34(10):2043–9.

60. Rykken JB, Diehn FE, Hunt CH, et al. Rim and flame signs: postgadolinium MRI findings specific for non-CNS intramedullary spinal cord metastases. AJNR AM J Neuroradiol 2013;34(4):908–15.

Imaging of Vascular Disorders of the Spine

Miriam E. Peckham, MD*, Troy A. Hutchins, MD

KEYWORDS

- Spine • MR imaging • Angiography • Spinal vascular malformation • Spinal cord infarction
- Spinal aneurysm • Hemangioblastoma • Vertebral hemangioma

KEY POINTS

- Spinal vascular malformations can be divided into shunting and nonshunting lesions, with shunting lesions classified by their type of arterial connection.
- Spinal artery aneurysms present as fusiform lesions and likely represent dissecting pseudoaneurysms, unlike the brain where most aneurysms form at branch points.
- MR imaging changes can be delayed in spinal cord infarction. The presence of a bone infarct can be a helpful feature in determining whether T2 changes in the cord are due to ischemia.
- Large hemangioblastomas should present with flow voids, and if they are not present, another diagnosis should be considered.
- Aggressive hemangiomas can be distinguished by their characteristic trabeculation pattern on radiographic imaging.

INTRODUCTION

Spinal vascular disorders are much less common than vascular entities affecting the brain; however, they can result in significant morbidity. The radiologist plays an important role in the diagnosis of these conditions, some of which can mimic nonvascular entities both clinically and radiographically. Conventional MR imaging is the workhorse for initial diagnosis, followed by angiographic imaging. We review imaging characteristics of these disorders, which we have divided into 3 categories: vascular malformations, vascular emergencies, and vascular masses.

SPINAL VASCULAR ANATOMY

The segmental arteries, arising in pairs from the aorta in the thoracic (intercostal and subcostal) and lumbar (lumbar segmental) spine, supply the spinal column, paraspinal muscles, dura, and spinal cord.[1,2] The thoracic spine above T3 is often supplied by a common arterial trunk (supreme intercostal), usually arising from the aorta, costocervical trunk, or, rarely, the vertebral artery.[1,2] Cervical supply is variable with feeders from vertebral, deep cervical (from the costocervical trunk), ascending cervical (from the thyrocervical trunk), and sometimes ascending pharyngeal and occipital arteries.[1,2] Below L4, lumbosacral arterial supply comes from internal iliac artery branches and the median sacral artery (origin at the aortoiliac bifurcation).[1,2]

At each level, the segmental arteries give rise to the spinal arteries, which divide into ventral, middle, and dorsal branches within the intervertebral foramen.[3] Ventral and dorsal branches (anterior and posterior spinal canal arteries) provide vertebral, ligamentous, and partial dural supply.[1,2,4] The middle branch feeds the

Disclosures: The authors have no conflicts of interest or financial disclosures.
Neuroradiology Division, Department of Radiology and Imaging Sciences, University of Utah Health Sciences Center, 30 North, 1900 East, #1A071, Salt Lake City, UT 84132-2140, USA
* Corresponding author.
E-mail address: Miriam.Peckham@hsc.utah.edu

Radiol Clin N Am 57 (2019) 307–318
https://doi.org/10.1016/j.rcl.2018.09.005
0033-8389/19/© 2018 Elsevier Inc. All rights reserved.

dura and nerve root at each level before bifurcating to become anterior and posterior radicular, radiculopial, or radiculomedullary arteries (**Fig. 1**).[1–4]

The anterior two-thirds of the spinal cord is supplied by the anterior spinal artery (ASA), which originates from the intracranial vertebral arteries and is reinforced along its length by an average of 6 anterior radiculomedullary arteries, the largest of which is known as the artery of Adamkiewicz (AKA).[1,5] AKA most often arises between T8 and L2 (75%) on the left side (80%).[1,5] The paired posterior spinal arteries (PSAs) form a discontinuous anastomotic network that feeds the posterior one-third of the spinal cord, arising from ipsilateral intracranial vertebral or posterior inferior cerebellar arteries, and are reinforced along their lengths by 10 to 20 posterior radiculomedullary arteries.[1,2,6] Although there is a rich peripheral anastomotic network along the cord pial surface (vasa corona), there are no deep communications between the ASA and PSA.[1,6] This accounts for the involvement of the central gray matter with peripheral sparing in cases of spinal cord infarction.[6,7]

Spinal cord venous drainage is variable but tends to follow arterial anatomy with many more anastomoses. Drainage is from radiculomedullary veins to the internal vertebral (epidural) venous plexus. This drains to the external venous plexus, and eventually to the caval system predominantly through the innominate veins in the cervical levels, the azygous/hemiazygous systems in the thoracic levels, and the ascending lumbar vein in the lumbar levels.[3,8] The spinal veins are valveless, explaining why spinal cord congestion and edema are seen diffusely in cases of spinal dural arteriovenous fistula, regardless of fistula location.[3,8,9]

VASCULAR DISORDERS
Spinal Vascular Malformations

Multiple classification systems exist for these lesions based on vascular supply, surgical findings, and genetic inheritance.[10–12] If classifying by vascular connections, lesions can be divided as shunting (arteriovenous malformation [AVM] and dural arteriovenous fistula [dAVF]) or nonshunting (cavernous malformation [CM]).[13–15] The shunting lesions can be categorized by arterial supply: dAVFs arise from radiculomeningeal branches, similar to meningeal supply of these lesions in the brain, and AVMs arise through radiculomedullary or radiculopial arteries, similar to neural tissue supply of these lesions in the brain.[12,13,16,17] This classification scheme, delineated by Krings,[13] is followed for simplicity.

Dural arteriovenous fistula
The dAVFs comprise most shunting spinal vascular malformations (~70%) and are supplied by radiculomeningeal arteries, similar to their counterpart in the brain.[16,17] Unlike AVMs, these lesions are acquired and seen most commonly in middle-aged men. The shunt is located along the dura mater where the radiculomeningeal artery, which feeds the nerve root and dura, creates a shunt with a radicular vein. This leads to venous congestion and hypertension and eventually edematous changes within the cord.[18–20] The clinical presentation is that of a stepwise decline in function, with bilateral leg weakness found in the most cases.[21]

MR imaging frequently demonstrates prominent perimedullary flow voids with multilevel expansion and T2 hyperintensity of the cord (**Fig. 2**A). The thoracolumbar region is the most frequently

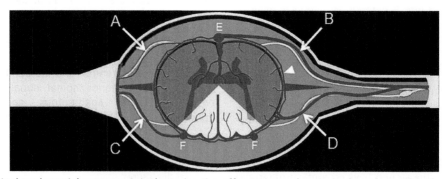

Fig. 1. Spinal cord arterial anatomy. Spinal arteries give off anterior and posterior branches within the foramina, which become radicular (A) (feed nerve root and dura), anterior radiculomedullary (B) (reinforce ASA), posterior radiculomedullary (C) (reinforce PSAs), or radiculopial (D) (feed cord pial surface). ASA (E) supplies the anterior two-thirds of the spinal cord (*brown shaded area*) and PSAs (F) supply the posterior one-third. Vasa corona (*white arrowhead*) provides a rich superficial anastomotic network. There are no deep communications between the ASA and PSA tributaries.

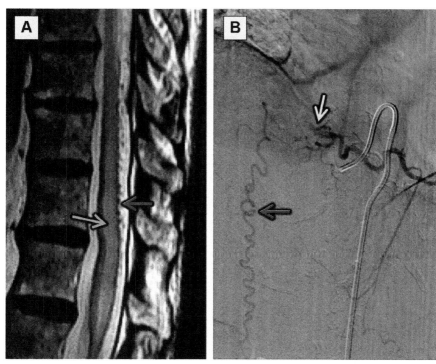

Fig. 2. Dural arteriovenous fistula. T2-weighted sagittal image of the thoracic spine (*A*) shows prominent perimedullary flow voids (*red arrow*) and extensive cord edema (*blue arrow*). DSA (*B*) demonstrates a fistulous connection between a radiculomeningeal artery and radicular vein (*yellow arrow*), with reflux into dilated posterior spinal veins (*red arrow*).

affected site.[22] T2 hypointensity along the periphery of the cord has been observed, which may represent susceptibility changes related to venous deoxygenation.[23] Variable enhancement can be seen with breakdown of the blood-cord barrier.[16]

Digital subtraction angiography (DSA) remains the standard for localization of the fistula site and is used for preoperative or embolization planning (**Fig. 2**B).[19,24] MR angiography (MRA) has been found to have variable accuracy for localizing the fistula site, found to be successful in only 43% of cases in one large case series.[21] MRA can be helpful to guide DSA to levels of suspicious vascularity.[25]

Arteriovenous malformation

Similar to cerebral lesions, AVMs are fed by the vascular supply to neural tissue.[16] AVMs can be categorized by their arteriovenous connection, with a network of vessels considered glomerular and the presence of a shunt considered fistulous. Glomerular lesions are the most common AVMs and present predominantly in an intramedullary location, with feeders derived from both anterior and posterior circulations and drainage to large veins.[15,16] Fistulous AVMs are intradural and perimedullary in location rather than intramedullary.[13,15] These are divided into 3 types based on

size of the feeding vessel, shunt volume, and pattern of drainage. Type 1 has nondilated feeders and draining veins, type 2 has mildly dilated feeders and 1 to 2 prominent draining veins, and type 3 has large tortuous arterial feeders and draining veins with a large shunt volume.[13,16]

AVMs are predominantly found in the thoracolumbar spine with symptoms usually due to venous congestion and hemorrhage. On MR imaging, the lesion subtype cannot be differentiated. AVMs usually present as grouped intramedullary or perimedullary vessels with prominent draining veins, which are frequently accompanied by T2 signal changes from venous congestion as well as hemorrhage (**Fig. 3**A). These changes eventually can lead to ischemia.[16,17] AVMs also can have associated aneurysms, with rupture resulting in subarachnoid hemorrhage.[26] Conventional angiography is essential for diagnosis of these lesions, allowing localization of the nidus and delineation of the feeding arteries and draining veins (**Fig. 3**B).[17,27] MRA has been used for preoperative planning with varying results.[28]

Cavernous malformations

Spinal cord CMs are uncommon, seen in only 5% of all cases in the central nervous system.[29] These

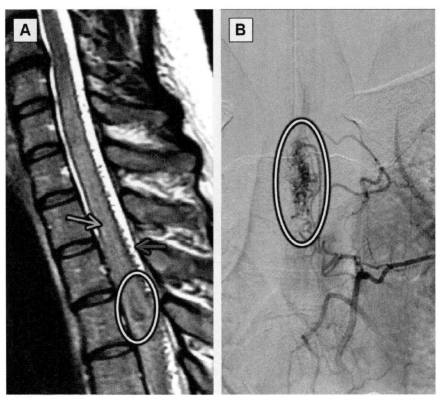

Fig. 3. Glomerular arteriovenous malformation. T2-weighted sagittal image of the thoracic spine (*A*) demonstrates prominent perimedullary flow voids (*red arrow*) and cord edema (*blue arrow*), similar to what is seen in a dAVF; however, a differentiating feature is the "tangle" of intramedullary flow voids (*yellow circle*). DSA (*B*) is confirmatory of a glomerular arteriovenous malformation (*yellow circle*).

slow-flow, predominantly intramedullary, vascular lesions have low pressure and can be occult, taking years to present clinically with hemorrhage, causing either gradual or more immediate neurologic deficits.[30,31] The thoracic cord is the most common location for CMs, with the cervical cord the second most common.[32] Very rarely, these lesions can present in an extradural location with involvement of the neural foramina.[33,34]

Similar to their MR imaging presentation in the brain, spinal cord CMs present as lobulated lesions containing perilesional hemosiderin deposition that is hypointense on T1-weighted and T2-weighted sequences, and heterogeneous internal T1 and T2 signal with an overall appearance likened to "popcorn" (**Fig. 4**A, B).[35,36] Susceptibility (T2*/gradient recalled echo/susceptibility weighted imaging) sequences are sensitive to CMs because of their extensive hemosiderin deposition. CMs can rarely demonstrate internal calcifications, less commonly than cerebral CMs. Perilesional edema is present only in cases of recent hemorrhage and is otherwise absent. CMs do not avidly enhance and are occult on angiographic imaging.[17,32,37,38]

CMs that arise in an extradural location do not share the same imaging characteristics as intramedullary lesions. Reported cases have demonstrated avidly enhancing epidural lesions that are T1 hypo-isointense and T2 hyperintense. As they often involve the neural foramen, nerve sheath tumor and meningioma are often in the leading preoperative diagnoses in multiple cases. The classic finding of perilesional hemosiderin deposition has only rarely been seen in these lesions.[33] Epidural lesions also have been found to cause widening of the neural foramina as well as erosion of adjacent bones (**Fig. 4**C, D).[39]

Spinal Vascular Emergencies

Spinal cord ischemia

Spinal cord infarction is much less common than cerebral infarction and has a larger spectrum of causes.[16,17] It has often been reported as a complication of aortic surgery, although association with other procedures such as coronary artery bypass graft surgery, thoracic spine surgery, angiography, embolization, and even epidural injection and selective nerve blocks has been reported.[40–42]

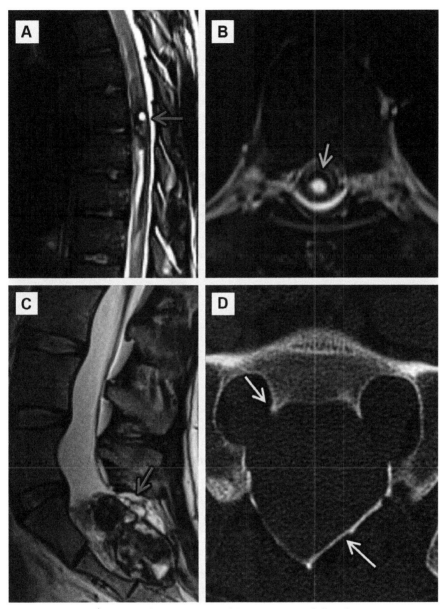

Fig. 4. Two examples of spinal CM. The first patient (*A, B*) has an intramedullary heterogeneous "popcorn"-like lesion (*red arrow*) seen on T2-weighted sagittal (*A*) and axial (*B*) sequences. Peripheral hemosiderin deposition is noted (*blue arrow*). A second patient (*C, D*) demonstrates an extradural lesion, which is large and heterogeneous on T2-weighted sagittal imaging (*red arrow, C*) and causes osseous erosion and remodeling of the canal and neural foramina as seen on CT (*yellow arrows, D*). This rare form of extradural CM was confirmed after surgical excision.

Spinal cord infarction also has been seen in the nonoperative setting with drug use, aortic aneurysm rupture, and spinal vascular malformation making up a few of the multiple reported causes.[43–45]

MR imaging is the modality of choice for spinal cord ischemia, although in up to 50% of cases it can be negative within the first 24 hours.[46]

Because the ASA territory is most often affected, early T2 signal changes are predominantly present in the anterior and central aspects of the cord with peripheral sparing, creating an "anterior pencil" sign on sagittal T2-weighted sequences in most cases, often accompanied by cord swelling.[47,48] On axial images, involvement of the gray matter regions in the anterior cord can have the appearance of "owl's eyes" (**Fig. 5**A).[40,49] Because of variation in surface anastomotic connections of the ASA, the amount and laterality of central cord involvement can vary.[16]

The thoracic cord is the most commonly affected region, with less frequent involvement of the cervical cord.[50] Diffusion-weighted imaging is an important part of evaluation, which can demonstrate restriction in the area of infarction approximately 8 hours after symptom onset, with pseudo-normalization occurring after 1 week (**Fig. 5**B).[51,52] Enhancement is frequently seen in more subacute insults, typically after 5 days, and can persist for up to 3 weeks after symptom onset.[46] In confounding cases, the presence of concomitant bone infarctions can be helpful in establishing the ischemia diagnosis (**Fig. 5**C, D).[53]

Spinal aneurysm

Fewer than 1% of spontaneous subarachnoid hemorrhages (SAHs) originate from the spine, with most cases arising from AVMs, dAVFs, and hemorrhage from spinal tumors.[54,55] Spinal SAH also can be caused by rupture of an isolated spinal

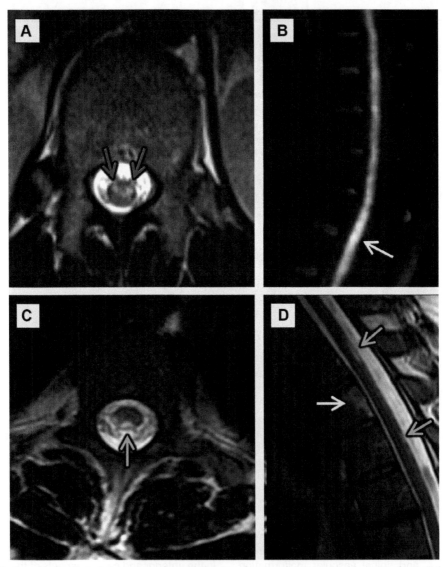

Fig. 5. Spinal cord infarction. Anterior spinal cord infarction frequently presents with an "owl-eyes" sign on axial T2-weighted imaging (*red arrows, A*) due to involvement of the anterior and central gray matter. Diffusion-weighted imaging (*B*) demonstrates corresponding diffusion restriction (*yellow arrow*). Posterior spinal cord infarction demonstrates T2 signal change involving the posterior aspect of the cord (*blue arrow, C*). Sagittal T2-weighted image (*D*) of the same patient demonstrates linear dorsal cord involvement (*blue arrows*), as well as a bone infarct (*yellow arrow*).

artery aneurysm (SAA); these rare lesions have been found to lack an internal elastic lamina, suggesting they are in fact pseudoaneurysms secondary to intimal dissection.[56,57] These aneurysms appear to arise secondary to hyperdynamic flow, as has been seen in cases of coarctation of the aorta and AVMs.[26,58]

On computed tomography (CT), MR imaging, and conventional angiography, SAAs present as sites of focal fusiform dilatation within an intradural spinal vessel (radiculomedullary or radiculopial) and demonstrate focal enhancement (**Fig. 6**). This is unlike their intracranial counterparts, which most often arise at vessel branch points.[56,57] SAAs tend to be small in size, which is also in distinction to the variable sizes of intracranial aneurysms.[55] In cases of subarachnoid hemorrhage with negative cranial angiography, ruptured SAAs should be considered and further imaging workup should be performed.[59,60]

Spinal Vascular Masses

Hemangioblastoma
Accounting for up to 5% of spinal cord tumors, hemangioblastoma is an intramedullary, richly vascular, lesion associated with Von-Hippel Lindau Syndrome (VHL).[61–64] One large case series demonstrated that two-thirds of spinal cord hemangioblastomas were sporadic, with another large series demonstrating increased prevalence in VHL than in a nonsyndromic population.[61,65] Most cases present with a single lesion, with the exception of patients with VHL, who can present with multiple lesions. The thoracic cord is the most common site of presentation followed by the cervical cord.[62,66] Approximately two-thirds of hemangioblastomas are subpial in location, involving the superficial aspect of the posterior spinal cord that is frequently seen intraoperatively[62,67]; 25% are entirely intramedullary. An extramedullary presentation is extremely rare in these lesions, which have been reported to involve the cauda equine and filum terminale.[68–71]

Hemangioblastomas are well-demarcated and avidly enhance. Smaller lesions can demonstrate more homogeneous signal characteristics with diffuse enhancement and T2 hyperintensity and T1 hypointensity. Larger lesions can demonstrate more heterogeneous enhancement (**Fig. 7**).[62,67] Contrast administration is essential for evaluation, as small lesions can be T1 isointense with respect to the spinal cord and, therefore, difficult to appreciate.[67] Prominent flow voids are seen associated with larger lesions (greater than 15 mm in size) and appear to reflect prominent feeding arteries and draining veins (see **Fig. 7**B). If no associated flow voids are present in a lesion larger than 2.5 cm, then other diagnostic possibilities should be explored.[62] Syrinx or cyst formation is also a frequent by-product of this lesion, seen in just more than half of cases.[67] This has been hypothesized to be related to transudation from tumor vessels or related to secretion of tumor cells, rather than to mass effect from these frequently small lesions.[62]

Angiographically, intense contrast staining is noted at the site of the tumor, with prominent

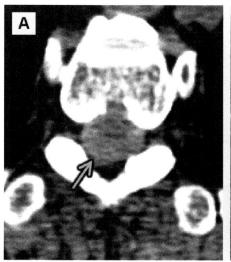
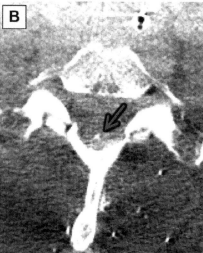

Fig. 6. SAA. A patient with sudden onset of back pain is found to have extensive subarachnoid hemorrhage within the spinal canal on CT (*blue arrow, A*). Rotational angiography acquired during DSA (*B*) confirms an aneurysm along the dorsal aspect of the spinal cord (*red arrow*).

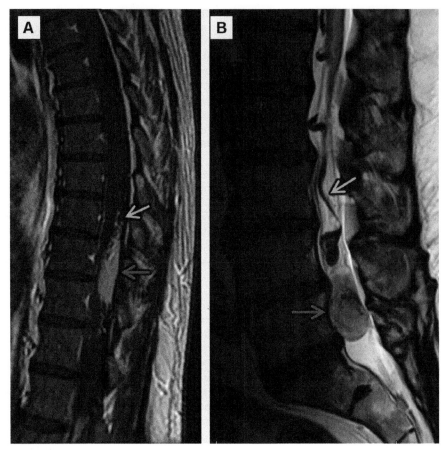

Fig. 7. Hemangioblastoma. An enhancing lesion along the dorsal aspect of the spinal cord avidly enhances on postcontrast T1-weighted imaging (*A, red arrow*). The associated prominent vessels (*blue arrow*) support hemangioblastoma as a leading imaging diagnosis, which was confirmed postoperatively. A second patient presents with a lesion along the cauda equina nerve fibers on T2-weighted imaging (*B, red arrow*) with surrounding large and tortuous flow voids (*blue arrow*). Hemangioblastoma was confirmed postoperatively.

arterial feeders and draining veins a frequent finding in larger lesions.[62] Additionally, 3-dimensional CT angiography (CTA) has been found to be helpful for preoperative planning and can accurately delineate feeding arteries.[72]

Vertebral hemangioma

Vertebral hemangioma (VH) is the most common vertebral lesion (prevalence of up to 26%), and is multiple in up to one-third of cases.[73,74] These benign vascular neoplasms are composed of normally formed blood vessels with the absence of arteriovenous shunts.[75,76] A small percentage of patients may experience painful symptoms related to neural compression from lesion expansion, fracture, hematoma, and cortical erosion.[77–80] Expansile VHs have been termed "aggressive," and have several features including involvement of the whole vertebral body, irregular honeycomb pattern, and extension to the posterior elements.[77,81,82]

Characteristic imaging is of a fat-containing, T1-hyperintense lesion with well-circumscribed margins, which is also hyperintense on T2-weighted sequences due to slow flow within vascular channels and interstitial edema.[83] These lesions may not completely saturate on STIR (short tau inversion recovery), as the overall signal on T1, T2, and STIR images depends on the percentage of fatty, stromal, and vascular elements within the lesion.[75] VHs with a more vascular component tend to show more avid enhancement, whereas fat-predominant lesions tend to enhance less.[75] Most of VHs have been found to have a coarse trabeculated "corduroy cloth" appearance in the sagittal and coronal planes and a "honeycomb" or "polka-dot" appearance in the axial plane related to vascular channels intermixed with vertically oriented thickened trabeculae to provide support.[75,76]

Atypical, "aggressive" VHs can demonstrate a more confounding imaging appearance: more T2 hyperintensity, less T1 hyperintense signal, avid enhancement, and hypervascularity on spinal angiographic imaging.[79] These lesions can be expansile and contain a prominent soft tissue component, making their appearance concerning for an aggressive mass. For these lesions, CT or radiographs can be helpful in demonstrating the underlying trabeculated "corduroy" osseous pattern (**Fig. 8**).

VHs with low fat content can also be differentiated from primary malignancy or metastatic disease by MR imaging perfusion. One study used T1 dynamic contrast-enhanced perfusion

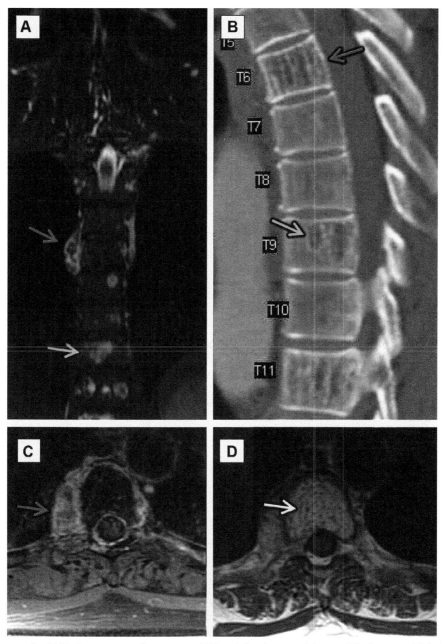

Fig. 8. "Aggressive" VH. Postcontrast fat-saturated T1-weighted coronal image (*A*) shows multiple irregularly enhancing osseous lesions, which have a well-circumscribed appearance (*blue arrow*). One lesion demonstrates extraosseous extension (*red arrow, A*). On CT (*B*), coarse trabeculation in a linear pattern corresponds with these lesions (*red* and *blue arrows*). Axial postcontrast T1-weighted imaging (*C*) confirms extraosseous extension (*red arrow*). On axial T1-weighted imaging (*D*), the osseous trabeculation makes a "polka-dot" pattern (*yellow arrow*). These imaging findings are consistent with an expansile VH with a soft tissue component.

time-intensity curves, with 88% of atypical VHs demonstrating minimal delayed enhancement as compared with the sharp rise and washout seen with metastatic lesions.[84]

SUMMARY

The radiologist plays an important role in the diagnosis of spinal vascular disorders. Although these entities are rare, they frequently present with distinguishing imaging features that can guide diagnosis and treatment.

REFERENCES

1. Santillan A, Nacarino V, Greenberg E, et al. Vascular anatomy of the spinal cord. J Neurointerv Surg 2012; 4(1):67–74.
2. Melissano G, Civilini E, Bertoglio L, et al. Angio-CT imaging of the spinal cord vascularisation: a pictorial essay. Eur J Vasc Endovasc Surg 2010;39(4): 436–40.
3. Miyasaka K, Asano T, Ushikoshi S, et al. Vascular anatomy of the spinal cord and classification of spinal arteriovenous malformations. Interv Neuroradiol 2000;6(Suppl 1):195–8.
4. Shimizu S, Tanaka R, Kan S, et al. Origins of the segmental arteries in the aorta: an anatomic study for selective catheterization with spinal arteriography. AJNR Am J Neuroradiol 2005;26(4): 922–8.
5. Yoshioka K, Niinuma H, Ehara S, et al. MR angiography and CT angiography of the artery of Adamkiewicz: state of the art. Radiographics 2006;26(Suppl 1):S63–73.
6. Vargas MI, Gariani J, Sztajzel R, et al. Spinal cord ischemia: practical imaging tips, pearls, and pitfalls. AJNR Am J Neuroradiol 2015;36(5):825–30.
7. Mascalchi M, Cosottini M, Ferrito G, et al. Posterior spinal artery infarct. AJNR Am J Neuroradiol 1998; 19(2):361–3.
8. Griessenauer CJ, Raborn J, Foreman P, et al. Venous drainage of the spine and spinal cord: a comprehensive review of its history, embryology, anatomy, physiology, and pathology. Clin Anat 2015;28(1):75–87.
9. Krings T, Geibprasert S. Spinal dural arteriovenous fistulas. AJNR Am J Neuroradiol 2009;30(4):639–48.
10. Kim LJ, Spetzler RF. Classification and surgical management of spinal arteriovenous lesions: arteriovenous fistulae and arteriovenous malformations. Neurosurgery 2006;59(5 Suppl 3):S195–201 [discussion: S3–13].
11. Rodesch G, Hurth M, Alvarez H, et al. Classification of spinal cord arteriovenous shunts: proposal for a reappraisal—the Bicetre experience with 155 consecutive patients treated between 1981 and 1999. Neurosurgery 2002;51(2):374–9 [discussion: 379–80].
12. Rosenblum B, Oldfield EH, Doppman JL, et al. Spinal arteriovenous malformations: a comparison of dural arteriovenous fistulas and intradural AVM's in 81 patients. J Neurosurg 1987;67(6):795–802.
13. Krings T. Vascular malformations of the spine and spinal cord*: anatomy, classification, treatment. Clin Neuroradiol 2010;20(1):5–24.
14. Abecassis IJ, Osbun JW, Kim L. Classification and pathophysiology of spinal vascular malformations. Handb Clin Neurol 2017;143:135–43.
15. Bao YH, Ling F. Classification and therapeutic modalities of spinal vascular malformations in 80 patients. Neurosurgery 1997;40(1):75–81.
16. Krings T, Lasjaunias PL, Hans FJ, et al. Imaging in spinal vascular disease. Neuroimaging Clin N Am 2007;17(1):57–72.
17. Rubin MN, Rabinstein AA. Vascular diseases of the spinal cord. Neurol Clin 2013;31(1):153–81.
18. Hurst RW, Kenyon LC, Lavi E, et al. Spinal dural arteriovenous fistula: the pathology of venous hypertensive myelopathy. Neurology 1995;45(7):1309–13.
19. Brown PA, Zomorodi AR, Gonzalez LF. Endovascular management of spinal dural arteriovenous fistulas. Handb Clin Neurol 2017;143:199–213.
20. Hacein-Bey L, Konstas AA, Pile-Spellman J. Natural history, current concepts, classification, factors impacting endovascular therapy, and pathophysiology of cerebral and spinal dural arteriovenous fistulas. Clin Neurol Neurosurg 2014;121:64–75.
21. Muralidharan R, Saladino A, Lanzino G, et al. The clinical and radiological presentation of spinal dural arteriovenous fistula. Spine 2011;36(25): E1641–7.
22. Koenig E, Thron A, Schrader V, et al. Spinal arteriovenous malformations and fistulae: clinical, neuroradiological and neurophysiological findings. J Neurol 1989;236(5):260–6.
23. Hurst RW, Grossman RI. Peripheral spinal cord hypointensity on T2-weighted MR images: a reliable imaging sign of venous hypertensive myelopathy. AJNR Am J Neuroradiol 2000;21(4):781–6.
24. Kiyosue H, Matsumaru Y, Niimi Y, et al. Angiographic and clinical characteristics of thoracolumbar spinal epidural and dural arteriovenous fistulas. Stroke 2017;48(12):3215–22.
25. Mull M, Nijenhuis RJ, Backes WH, et al. Value and limitations of contrast-enhanced MR angiography in spinal arteriovenous malformations and dural arteriovenous fistulas. AJNR Am J Neuroradiol 2007;28(7):1249–58.
26. Nakagawa I, Park HS, Hironaka Y, et al. Cervical spinal epidural arteriovenous fistula with coexisting spinal anterior spinal artery aneurysm presenting as subarachnoid hemorrhage—case report. J Stroke Cerebrovasc Dis 2014;23(10):e461–5.

27. Steinmetz MP, Chow MM, Krishnaney AA, et al. Outcome after the treatment of spinal dural arteriovenous fistulae: a contemporary single-institution series and meta-analysis. Neurosurgery 2004;55(1): 77–87 [discussion: 87–8].

28. Morris JM, Kaufmann TJ, Campeau NG, et al. Volumetric myelographic magnetic resonance imaging to localize difficult-to-find spinal dural arteriovenous fistulas. J Neurosurg Spine 2011;14(3):398–404.

29. Azad TD, Veeravagu A, Li A, et al. Long-term effectiveness of gross-total resection for symptomatic spinal cord cavernous malformations. Neurosurgery 2018. https://doi.org/10.1093/neuros/nyx610.

30. Otten M, McCormick P. Natural history of spinal cavernous malformations. Handb Clin Neurol 2017; 143:233–9.

31. Clark AJ, Wang DD, Lawton MT. Spinal cavernous malformations. Handb Clin Neurol 2017;143:303–8.

32. Zevgaridis D, Medele RJ, Hamburger C, et al. Cavernous haemangiomas of the spinal cord. A review of 117 cases. Acta Neurochir (Wien) 1999; 141(3):237–45.

33. Killeen T, Czaplinski A, Cesnulis E. Extradural spinal cavernous malformation: a rare but important mimic. Br J Neurosurg 2014;28(3):340–6.

34. Mataliotakis G, Perera S, Nagaraju S, et al. Intradural extramedullary cavernoma of a lumbar nerve root mimicking neurofibroma. A report of a rare case and the differential diagnosis. Spine J 2014;14(12): e1–7.

35. Hegde AN, Mohan S, Lim CC. CNS cavernous haemangioma: "popcorn" in the brain and spinal cord. Clin Radiol 2012;67(4):380–8.

36. Hegde A, Mohan S, Tan KK, et al. Spinal cavernous malformations: magnetic resonance imaging and associated findings. Singapore Med J 2012;53(9): 582–6.

37. Do-Dai DD, Brooks MK, Goldkamp A, et al. Magnetic resonance imaging of intramedullary spinal cord lesions: a pictorial review. Curr Probl Diagn Radiol 2010;39(4):160–85.

38. Fontaine S, Melanson D, Cosgrove R, et al. Cavernous hemangiomas of the spinal cord: MR imaging. Radiology 1988;166(3):839–41.

39. Feng J, Xu YK, Li L, et al. MRI diagnosis and preoperative evaluation for pure epidural cavernous hemangiomas. Neuroradiology 2009;51(11):741–7.

40. Zalewski NL, Rabinstein AA, Krecke KN, et al. Spinal cord infarction: clinical and imaging insights from the periprocedural setting. J Neurol Sci 2018;388: 162–7.

41. Picone AL, Green RM, Ricotta JR, et al. Spinal cord ischemia following operations on the abdominal aorta. J Vasc Surg 1986;3(1):94–103.

42. Ross RT. Spinal cord infarction in disease and surgery of the aorta. Can J Neurol Sci 1985;12(4): 289–95.

43. Yogendranathan N, Herath H, Jayamali WD, et al. A case of anterior spinal cord syndrome in a patient with unruptured thoracic aortic aneurysm with a mural thrombus. BMC Cardiovasc Disord 2018; 18(1):48.

44. Huntley GD, Ruff MW, Hicks SB, et al. Ascending spinal cord infarction secondary to recurrent spinal cord cavernous malformation hemorrhage. J Stroke Cerebrovasc Dis 2017;26(4):e72–3.

45. Farrell CM, Cucu DF. Cocaine-related acute spinal cord infarction. R I Med J (2013) 2018;101(1):28–9.

46. Mull M, Thron A. Spinal infarcts. In: von Kummer R, Back T, editors. Magnetic resonance imaging in ischemic stroke. Berlin: Springer Berlin Heidelberg; 2006. p. 251–67.

47. Weidauer S, Nichtweiss M, Lanfermann H, et al. Spinal cord infarction: MR imaging and clinical features in 16 cases. Neuroradiology 2002;44(10):851–7.

48. Weidauer S, Nichtweiss M, Hattingen E, et al. Spinal cord ischemia: aetiology, clinical syndromes and imaging features. Neuroradiology 2015;57(3): 241–57.

49. Harada K, Chiko Y, Toyokawa T. Anterior spinal cord syndrome—"owl's eye sign". J Gen Fam Med 2018; 19(2):63–4.

50. Robertson CE, Brown RD Jr, Wijdicks EF, et al. Recovery after spinal cord infarcts: long-term outcome in 115 patients. Neurology 2012;78(2):114–21.

51. Kuker W, Weller M, Klose U, et al. Diffusion-weighted MRI of spinal cord infarction—high resolution imaging and time course of diffusion abnormality. J Neurol 2004;251(7):818–24.

52. Gass A, Back T, Behrens S, et al. MRI of spinal cord infarction. Neurology 2000;54(11):2195.

53. Pawar NH, Loke E, Aw DC. Spinal cord infarction mimicking acute transverse myelitis. Cureus 2017; 9(12):e1911.

54. van Gijn J, Kerr RS, Rinkel GJ. Subarachnoid haemorrhage. Lancet 2007;369(9558):306–18.

55. Sung TH, Leung WK, Lai BM, et al. Isolated spinal artery aneurysm: a rare culprit of subarachnoid haemorrhage. Hong Kong Med J 2015;21(2):179–82.

56. Geibprasert S, Krings T, Apitzsch J, et al. Subarachnoid hemorrhage following posterior spinal artery aneurysm. A case report and review of the literature. Interv Neuroradiol 2010;16(2):183–90.

57. Johnson J, Patel S, Saraf-Lavi E, et al. Posterior spinal artery aneurysm rupture after 'Ecstasy' abuse. BMJ Case Rep 2014;2014 [pii:bcr2014011248].

58. Aoun SG, El Ahmadieh TY, Soltanolkotabi M, et al. Ruptured spinal artery aneurysm associated with coarctation of the aorta. World Neurosurg 2014; 81(2):441.e17-22.

59. Madhugiri VS, Ambekar S, Roopesh Kumar VR, et al. Spinal aneurysms: clinicoradiological features and management paradigms. J Neurosurg Spine 2013;19(1):34–48.

60. Gonzalez LF, Zabramski JM, Tabrizi P, et al. Spontaneous spinal subarachnoid hemorrhage secondary to spinal aneurysms: diagnosis and treatment paradigm. Neurosurgery 2005;57(6):1127–31 [discussion: 1127-31].

61. Browne TR, Adams RD, Roberson GH. Hemangioblastoma of the spinal cord. Review and report of five cases. Arch Neurol 1976;33(6):435–41.

62. Chu BC, Terae S, Hida K, et al. MR findings in spinal hemangioblastoma: correlation with symptoms and with angiographic and surgical findings. AJNR Am J Neuroradiol 2001;22(1):206–17.

63. Butman JA, Linehan WM, Lonser RR. Neurologic manifestations of von Hippel-Lindau disease. Grand Rounds at the Clinical Center of the National Institutes of Health. JAMA 2008;300(11):1334–42.

64. Vortmeyer AO, Gnarra JR, Emmert-Buck MR, et al. von Hippel-Lindau gene deletion detected in the stromal cell component of a cerebellar hemangioblastoma associated with von Hippel-Lindau disease. Hum Pathol 1997;28(5):540–3.

65. Conway JE, Chou D, Clatterbuck RE, et al. Hemangioblastomas of the central nervous system in von Hippel-Lindau syndrome and sporadic disease. Neurosurgery 2001;48(1):55–62 [discussion: 62–3].

66. Vo DT, Cravens GF, Germann RE. Isolated hemangioblastoma of the cervical spinal cord: a case report and literature review. Int J Surg Case Rep 2016;26:7–11.

67. Baker KB, Moran CJ, Wippold FJ 2nd, et al. MR imaging of spinal hemangioblastoma. AJR Am J Roentgenol 2000;174(2):377–82.

68. Blaty D, Malos M, Palmrose T, et al. Sporadic intradural extramedullary hemangioblastoma of the cauda equina: case report and literature review. World Neurosurg 2018;109:436–41.

69. Kunihiro N, Takami T, Yamagata T, et al. Spinal hemangioblastoma of cauda equina origin not associated with von Hippel-Lindau syndrome—case report. Neurol Med Chir (Tokyo) 2011;51(10):732–5.

70. da Costa LB Jr, de Andrade A, Braga BP, et al. Cauda equina hemangioblastoma: case report. Arq Neuropsiquiatr 2003;61(2b):456–8.

71. Tucer B, Ekici MA, Kazanci B, et al. Hemangioblastoma of the filum terminale associated with von Hippel-Lindau disease: a case report. Turk Neurosurg 2013;23(5):672–5.

72. Deng X, Wang K, Wu L, et al. Intraspinal hemangioblastomas: analysis of 92 cases in a single institution: clinical article. J Neurosurg Spine 2014;21(2):260–9.

73. Slon V, Stein D, Cohen H, et al. Vertebral hemangiomas: their demographical characteristics, location along the spine and position within the vertebral body. Eur Spine J 2015;24(10):2189–95.

74. Karlin CA, Brower AC. Multiple primary hemangiomas of bone. AJR Am J Roentgenol 1977;129(1):162–4.

75. McEvoy SH, Farrell M, Brett F, et al. Haemangioma, an uncommon cause of an extradural or intradural extramedullary mass: case series with radiological pathological correlation. Insights Imaging 2016;7(1):87–98.

76. Pastushyn AI, Slin'ko EI, Mirzoyeva GM. Vertebral hemangiomas: diagnosis, management, natural history and clinicopathological correlates in 86 patients. Surg Neurol 1998;50(6):535–47.

77. Vasudeva VS, Chi JH, Groff MW. Surgical treatment of aggressive vertebral hemangiomas. Neurosurg Focus 2016;41(2):E7.

78. Fox MW, Onofrio BM. The natural history and management of symptomatic and asymptomatic vertebral hemangiomas. J Neurosurg 1993;78(1):36–45.

79. Friedman DP. Symptomatic vertebral hemangiomas: MR findings. AJR Am J Roentgenol 1996;167(2):359–64.

80. Eisenstein S, Spiro F, Browde S, et al. The treatment of a symptomatic vertebral hemangioma by radiotherapy. A case report. Spine 1986;11(6):640–2.

81. Gaudino S, Martucci M, Colantonio R, et al. A systematic approach to vertebral hemangioma. Skeletal Radiol 2015;44(1):25–36.

82. Laredo JD, Reizine D, Bard M, et al. Vertebral hemangiomas: radiologic evaluation. Radiology 1986;161(1):183–9.

83. Winfield JM, Poillucci G, Blackledge MD, et al. Apparent diffusion coefficient of vertebral haemangiomas allows differentiation from malignant focal deposits in whole-body diffusion-weighted MRI. Eur Radiol 2018;28(4):1687–91.

84. Morales KA, Arevalo-Perez J, Peck KK, et al. Differentiating atypical hemangiomas and metastatic vertebral lesions: the role of T1-weighted dynamic contrast-enhanced MRI. AJNR Am J Neuroradiol 2018;39(5):968–73.

MR Imaging for Assessing Injury Severity and Prognosis in Acute Traumatic Spinal Cord Injury

Jason F. Talbott, MD, PhD[a,b,*], John Russell Huie, PhD[b,c], Adam R. Ferguson, PhD[b,c], Jacqueline C. Bresnahan, PhD[b,d], Michael S. Beattie, PhD[b,d], Sanjay S. Dhall, MD[e,f]

KEYWORDS

- MRI • Spinal cord • Contusion • Central cord injury • Diffusion • Tensor • SCIWORA • Hemorrhage

KEY POINTS

- T2-weighted (T2W) imaging is the most important sequence for detection of acute traumatic spinal cord pathology in clinical practice.
- Intramedullary hemorrhage on T2W imaging is universally associated with some component of irreversible injury and arguably the most robust MR imaging predictor of injury severity.
- The MR imaging appearance of the injured spinal cord in the early stages of injury is highly dynamic and the time delay from injury to imaging must be considered in image interpretation.
- Diffusion imaging offers promise as specific tool for interrogating spinal cord integrity, although well-designed, prospective clinical studies validating its application remain limited.
- There is a continued need for well-designed prospective longitudinal studies to definitively validate the prognostic significance of conventional and advanced MR imaging biomarkers in acute traumatic spinal cord injury.

INTRODUCTION

Written knowledge of spinal cord injury (SCI) dates to antiquity, with descriptions of paraplegic injuries of the spine recorded in the Edwin Smith surgical papyrus of Ancient Egypt circa 2500 BC.[1] The grave prognosis for severe SCI was known to the ancient Egyptian author(s) of these scrolls who described SCI as "an ailment not to be treated."[1] Although little progress in understanding or treatment of this devastating injury was made over subsequent millennia, the past 4 decades have witnessed an explosion in knowledge of injury pathophysiology and management.[2–4] With its

Support: DOD grant SC150198.
[a] Department of Radiology and Biomedical Imaging, Zuckerberg San Francisco General Hospital, 1001 Potrero Avenue, Room 1X57C, San Francisco, CA 94110, USA; [b] Department of Neurological Surgery, University of California, San Francisco, 400 Parnassus Avenue, San Francisco, CA 94122, USA; [c] Brain and Spinal Injury Center, Zuckerberg San Francisco General Hospital, 1001 Potrero Avenue, Building 1, Room 101, San Francisco, CA 94110, USA; [d] Brain and Spinal Injury Center, Zuckerberg San Francisco General Hospital, 1001 Potrero Avenue, Building 1, Room 101, San Francisco, CA 94114, USA; [e] Department of Neurological Surgery, University of California, San Francisco, 505 Parnassus Avenue, Room M779, San Francisco, CA 94143, USA; [f] Brain and Spinal Injury Center, Zuckerberg San Francisco General Hospital, 1001 Potrero Avenue, San Francisco, CA 94110, USA
* Corresponding author. Department of Radiology and Biomedical Imaging, Zuckerberg San Francisco General Hospital, 1001 Potrero Avenue, Room 1X57C, San Francisco, CA 94110.
E-mail address: Jason.talbott@ucsf.edu

exquisite soft tissue contrast, the advent of MR imaging for clinical spine trauma evaluation beginning in the late 1980s has coincided with these advances and played a significant role in enhancing clinical diagnosis and triage of SCI patients. This article reviews the epidemiology and pathophysiologic mechanisms of traumatic SCI. The primary focus is on the role of MR imaging with conventional techniques for evaluating SCI patients during the acute phase of injury, with emphasis on specific imaging features and injury classification systems that may aid in diagnosing injury severity and predicting clinical outcome (**Figs. 1** and **2**). More recent advances in diffusion imaging for spinal cord evaluation in trauma also are reviewed.

SPINAL CORD INJURY EPIDEMIOLOGY AND PATHOPHSYIOLOGY

In the United States, the annual incidence of SCI has been estimated at approximately 54 cases per 1 million people, resulting in approximately 17,700 new injuries per year.[5] SCI prevalence is approximately 288,000 persons with SCI in the United States (range 247,000–358,000).[5] The past several decades have witnessed a shift in SCI demographics, with increasingly older patients suffering injury. The average age of injury is currently 43 years, compared with 29 years during the 1970s.[5] Boys and men remain disproportionately affected, accounting for 78% of new cases. Most common mechanisms of injury include vehicular crashes (38%), falls (31%), and acts of violence, including gunshot wounds (14%).[5]

The financial burden related to these injuries is tremendous given the young age of the affected population and high cost of associated health care and living expenses. For example, direct health care and living expense costs for a 25 year old with high tetraplegia is on average $4.9 million, excluding indirect costs, such as losses in wages and productivity.[5] Although the overall financial burden is staggering, the physical, emotional, and psychological burden of functional

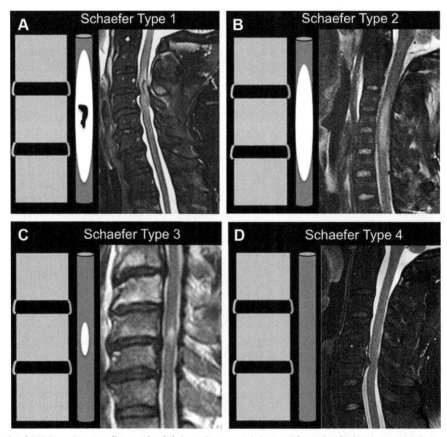

Fig. 1. Sagittal MR imaging grading scale. (*A*) Sample type 1 injury with sagittal T2W image and cartoon depiction showing central T2 hypointensity consistent with hemorrhage, surrounding by hyperintense edema. (*B*) Sample type 2 injury with T2-hyperintense edema spanning greater than 1 vertebral body in the sagittal plane. (*C*) Sample type 3 injury with T2-hyperintense edema spanning less than 1 vertebral body in sagittal plane. (*D*) Sample type 4 injury were no abnormal T2 signal abnormality is present.

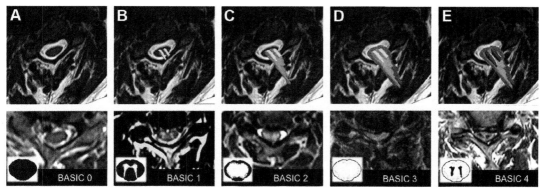

Fig. 2. Axial T2W BASIC scoring system for acute SCI. (*A*) BASIC grade 0 injury with no appreciable T2 signal abnormality (upper and lower panels). (*B*) BASIC grade 1 injury with 3-D volumetric approximation of injury projected in yellow on axial T2 image in the upper panel. Sample axial T2 image from injury epicenter in lower panel with cartoon depiction of BASIC-1 pattern the left lower corner inset. Pathologic T2 hyperintensity is approximately confined to central gray matter. (*C*) BASIC grade 2 injury with 3 D volumetric approximation of injury (*upper panel in yellow mesh*) and sample axial T2 image from injury epicenter in lower panel with cartoon depiction in left lower inset. Pathologic T2 hyperintensity involves central gray matter and adjacent white matter with peripheral cord sparing. (*D*) BASIC grade 3 injury with 3-D volumetric approximation of injury (*upper panel in gray mesh*) and lower panel with sample axial T2 image from injury epicenter and cartoon depiction in left lower inset. T2 hyperintensity involves the entire transverse extent of the cord. (*E*) BASIC grade 4 injury with 3-D volumetric approximation of injury (*upper panel in both gray mesh and solid black*). Lower panel shows sample axial T2W image at injury epicenter with T2 hyperintensity involving entire cord with central hypointensity consistent with intramedullary hemorrhage. Cartoon depiction in left lower inset.

disability for patients and their families is immeasurable.

SCI pathophysiology can be divided into primary and secondary injury mechanisms.[6,7] With primary injury, deformation and mechanical disruption of the spinal cord related to transient or fixed deformities of the spinal column result in direct and mostly irreversible injury to axons, glia, blood vessels, and neuronal cell bodies in the form of contusion, laceration, or transection injury. Immediate neurologic deficits relate to the severity of primary spinal injury with disruption of axonal transmission, hemorrhage, and massive shifts in membrane potentials disrupting normal spinal cord function.[6]

Secondary injury mechanisms are complex, multifactorial, and occur immediately after primary insult but may progress for years after primary injury.[8–10] In the acute phase, endothelial damage leads to increased vascular permeability with resulting vasogenic edema and initiation of a complex inflammatory cascade involving infiltrating leukocytes and activation of native microglia.[7,11,12] Release of inflammatory cytokines, such as tumor necrosis factor α, interleukin (IL)-1, and IL-6 perpetuate this maladaptive and largely destructive inflammatory cycle.[13,14] Compromised spinal cord perfusion from direct vascular injury and decreased perfusion pressures, precipitated by cord edema and compression, leads to secondary ischemic injury.[12,15] Concurrently, cellular ionic homeostasis is compromised with failure of cell membrane ionic gradients and loss of regulated extracellular glutamate, sodium, and other ionic concentrations triggering altered gene regulation, glutamate excitotoxicity, free radical production, and apoptosis.[6] In later stages of injury, astrocytic proliferation contributes to formation of a glial scar, which may impair axonal regeneration.[16] Oligodendrocyte apoptosis with resultant axonal demyelination occurs throughout the secondary injury process.[17,18]

CLINICAL ASSESSMENT

Thorough clinical evaluation remains the mainstay of initial assessment for diagnosis and management of acute SCI. A variety of neurologic and functional assessment instruments have been developed to classify injury severity and prognosticate future outcome. The American Spinal Injury Association (ASIA) has published International Standards for Neurological Classification of Spinal Cord Injury, including a neurologic examination updated in 2011 for classification of SCI based on sensory and motor examination findings.[19] This examination is the most studied and validated examination for clinical evaluation of acute SCI patients. The examination evaluates sensory function (light touch and pinprick) for the C2 through S4-5 dermatomes. Motor scores ranging from 0 to 5 for each of 10 paired upper and lower extremity key muscle groups are also obtained, with a maximum motor score of 100. A neurologic level of injury (NLI) is established based on the sensory and motor levels. Furthermore, the completeness of injury can then be classified by the ASIA Impairment Scale (AIS), a 5-point ordinal metric ranging from grade A (complete spinal cord injury) to grade E (normal examination). ASIA motor and sensory scores as well as AIS grade have been validated as useful clinical predictors of functional recovery at 1 year and are frequently reported in the literature. Numerous functional scales have also been described for assessing functional skills in chronic SCI patients. These include the Spinal Cord Independence Measure Version III, Spinal cord Injury Functional Ambulation Inventory, and Walking Index for Spinal Cord Injury.

MR IMAGING FOR ACUTE SPINAL CORD INJURY

Although initial clinical assessment remains a central component of injury determination and prognostication, notable limitations can complicate early clinical evaluation. For example, comorbid conditions, such as traumatic brain injury, long-bone fractures, severe pain, intubation, and sedative medications, among others, all potentially interfere with specific clinical assessment of spinal cord function. During this acute phase of injury, MR imaging offers great promise as a specific and objective assessment of the injured spinal cord. Guidelines published by the American College of Radiology in 2007 recommend MR imaging for patients with suspected spine trauma who present with new myelopathy.[20] MR imaging is also recommended for patients who are unevaluable for more than 48 hours from admission and for patients who may have vascular injury or spinal instability for which sensitive imaging evaluation of the spine is desired.[20,21] The benefits of MR imaging must be considered against possible complications related to clearing, transferring and monitoring a potentially neurologically and medically unstable patient in the magnetic resonance environment.[21]

The optimal magnetic resonance protocol for an acute SCI patient varies, depending on a patient's clinical condition. For example, it may be necessary to delay or abbreviate a magnetic resonance examination in some patients if they are neurologically unstable and/or require emergent surgical decompression. With these considerations in mind, the magnetic resonance examination should be structured so that it can optimally detect emergent spinal cord pathology, including cord compression, extra-axial hemorrhage, and unstable spinal column injuries. To accomplish this, a standard MR imaging protocol comprises sagittal fast spin-echo (FSE) T1-weighted (T1W) imaging, axial and sagittal FSE T2W, sagittal short tau inversion recovery (or other T2W fat-suppressed sequence), and axial T2*W sequences.[21] Increasingly, axial or sagittal diffusion-weighted imaging (DWI) sequences are being incorporated into routine clinical spine trauma protocols.

T2W FSE imaging is the workhorse for spinal cord evaluation because it is highly sensitive to intramedullary pathology, despite its nonspecificity with respect to underlying pathophysiologic mechanisms of injury.[22] Both axial and sagittal depictions of T2 cord signal abnormality provide complementary information with respect to injury characterization (see **Figs. 1** and **2**; **Fig. 3**).[23] T2W imaging is sensitive to the paramagnetic effects of iron from blood products in the form of deoxyhemoglobin and hemosiderin, with well-validated prognostic implications of hemorrhage detection.[22,24,25] Phase dispersion results in accelerated T2 shortening with resultant hypointense signal in areas of intramedullary hemorrhage[26,27] (**Fig. 4**).

T2*W and more recently developed susceptibility-weighted imaging sequences have increased sensitivity for intramedullary blood

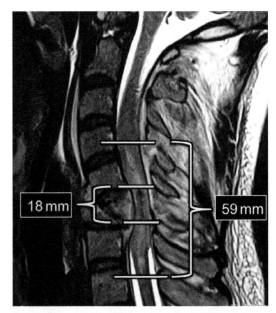

Fig. 3. Example measurements of upper and lower bounds of edema and hemorrhage in SCI. Horizontal white lines approximate the upper and lower margins of T2-hyperintense edema spanning 59 mm whereas the horizontal yellow lines approximate the upper and lower margins of cord hemorrhage, spanning 18 mm.

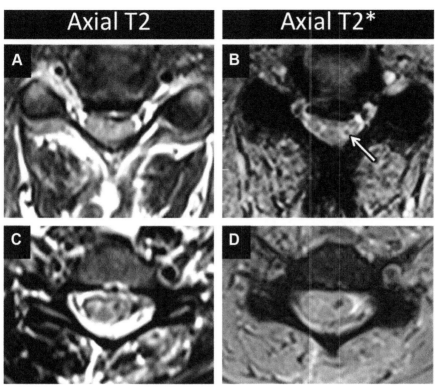

Fig. 4. T2W and T2*W imaging for hemorrhage detection. (A) Axial T2W image at epicenter of acute SCI shows subtle centromedullary T2 hyperintensity without evidence for hypointense hemorrhage. Axial T2*W image from the same patient at the same axial level (B) reveals a punctate hypointense focus of hemorrhage in the left lateral cord (white arrow [B]), not apparent on the T2W image. (C) Axial T2W and (D) axial T2*W images from a different patient both demonstrate hypointense hemorrhage within the left frontal horn of the spinal cord, although hemorrhage is more conspicuous in the T2*W image (D).

products (see Fig. 4); however, the associated prognostic implications of hemorrhage detection on these sequences are less well described.[28] Axial T2*W sequences also enhance intrinsic gray-white matter contrast with relative gray-matter hyperintensity in the normal spinal cord.[29] The intrinsic normal gray matter hyperintensity with the axial T2*W sequence may mask mild central cord pathologic edema, limiting its application for detecting traumatic central cord edema.

Increasing effort has recently focused on standardized collection and reporting of data for SCI with the first set of SCI-specific common data elements published in 2015.[30] A subgroup of experts in spinal cord imaging have defined guidelines for traumatic SCI imaging, including standardized MR imaging protocols for 1.5 T and 3 T.[31]

CONVENTIONAL MR IMAGING FOR SPINAL CORD INJURY EVALUATION AND PROGNOSTICATION

Numerous studies published within the first decade of MR imaging introduction to clinical practice evaluated the clinical association between injury severity and detection of spinal cord signal abnormalities on MR imaging.[24,32–40] Among these, the 4-level sagittal scoring scheme initially proposed by Schaefer and colleagues[33] has persisted as a primary framework for MR imaging classification for acute SCI to this day. In a study of 78 acute SCI patients, Schaefer and colleagues[33] describe 4 distinct injury patterns and their correlation with initial injury severity (see Fig. 1). The investigators observed complete motor and sensory dysfunction in 13/14 patients (93%) with central intramedullary cord hemorrhage, designated as type 1 injury (see Figs. 1 and 3; Fig. 5). Far more variable clinical disabilities were observed in patients with nonhemorrhagic type 2 injury, reflected on MR imaging by T2-hyperintense contusion extending longitudinally greater than 1 vertebral body length (see Fig. 1; Figs. 6 and 7). These patients had more severe deficits than those with type 3 injury, whose T2-hyperintense contusion was confined to a single metamer (Fig. 8). Not surprisingly, patients without evidence of cord injury on MR imaging

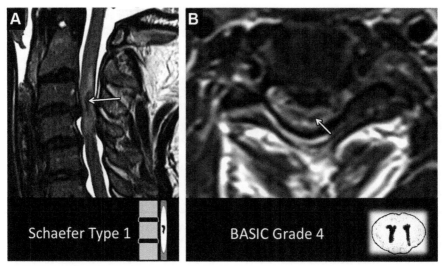

Fig. 5. Hemorrhagic contusion injury. A72-year-old woman status post–motor vehicle accident with initial motor and sensory complete SCI. (*A*) Sagittal and (*B*) axial T2W images show centromedullary T2 hypointensity (*white arrows* [*A* and *B*]) with surrounding hyperintense edema consistent with Schaefer type 1 and BASIC grade 4 injury. Lower panels show cartoon depiction of injury pattern. This patient had no functional recovery at 1-year follow-up.

(type 4 injury) did well clinically, with a large majority displaying no or only mild transient motor and sensory deficits.

Injury prognostication has long been the holy grail of applications for MR imaging in acute SCI. To date, however, data supporting MR imaging

for prognostication are mixed and no randomized clinical trial has been conducted to evaluate MR imaging for clinical management or prognostication.[41–44] Schaefer and colleagues[33] found that injury classification on MR imaging, as described in their earlier work, was highly prognostic with

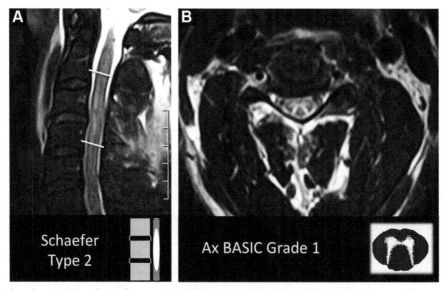

Fig. 6. Axial and sagittal grading of acute SCI. (*A*) Sagittal T2W MR imaging in this 37-year-old man presenting with quadriplegia after bodysurfing accident shows longitudinally extensive spinal cord edema spanning more than 2 vertebral segments, consistent with Schaefer type 2 injury (upper and lower limits of edema delineated by parallel white lines). (*B*) Axial T2W image, however, shows T2 hyperintense signal is largely confined to central gray matter, consistent with BASIC grade 1 injury, portending a good prognosis for this patient who recovered to ASIA D by time of discharge from rehabilitation facility. Lower panels show cartoon depiction of injury pattern.

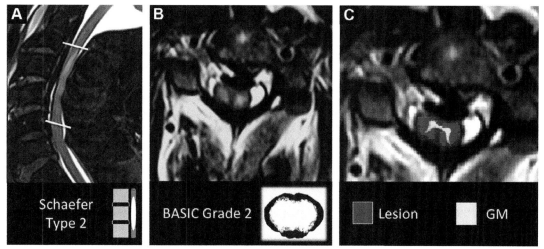

Fig. 7. Moderate acute SCI. (*A*) Sagittal T2W MR imaging in this 50-year-old woman presenting with quadriplegia after a helmeted scooter accident shows longitudinally extensive spinal cord edema spanning more than 2 vertebral segments, consistent with Schaefer type 2 injury (*white lines* [A]) approximate longitudinal extend of contusion. (*B*) Axial T2W image at the epicenter reveals T2 hyperintense signal involving central gray matter and surrounding white matter with sparing of peripheral cord, consistent with BASIC grade 2 injury. Lower panels show cartoon depiction of injury pattern. (*C*) Same image as in (*B*) with hyperintense edema outlined in 'red' and probabilistic gray matter overlay from spinal cord toolbox atlas in yellow.

respect to motor score recovery, with 9% median motor recovery for type 1 pattern, 41% for type 2 pattern, and 72% for type 3 pattern. Baseline neurologic status was not controlled for, however, in their analysis.[45]

In a meta-analysis, Bozzo and colleagues[22] reviewed the literature between 1988 and 2009

relevant to MR imaging for short-term and long-term SCI prognostication. The investigators identified 4 studies comprising a total of 205 patients for which MR imaging findings were correlated with improvement in neurologic examination.[22,32,46–48] Together, these studies suggest MR imaging is most accurate at predicting outcomes when

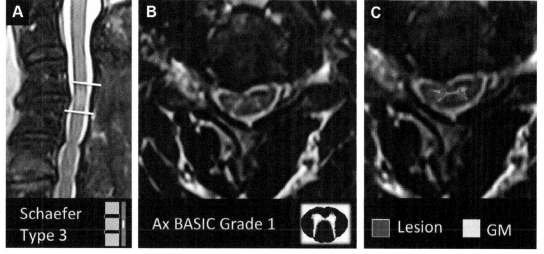

Fig. 8. Mild acute SCI. (*A*) Sagittal T2W MR imaging obtained for a 62-year-old man presenting with bilateral upper extremity paresthesias and hand weakness after a fall shows short segment spinal cord edema spanning less than a single vertebral segment, consistent with Schaefer type 3 injury (upper and lower limits of edema delineated by parallel white lines). (*B*) Axial T2W image at the epicenter reveals T2 hyperintense signal isolated to central gray matter, consistent with BASIC grade 1 injury. Lower panels show cartoon depiction of injury pattern. (*C*) Same image as in (*B*) with hyperintense edema outlined in red and probabilistic gray matter from spinal cord toolbox atlas in yellow.

patients have evidence for very mild (normal cord signal) or very severe (intramedullary hemorrhage) injury. In contrast, tremendous outcome variability was observed with intermediate degrees of injury. Among the 49 patients who demonstrated nonhemorrhagic cord edema spanning greater than 1 vertebral body segment in length (Schaefer type 2 injury), there was a near equal probability that the neurologic outcome would be ASIA A (26%), ASIA B (22%), ASIA C (24%), or ASIA D (24%).[22] Thus, for approximately one-third of acute SCI patients in this analysis, initial MR imaging did no better than blind guessing for predicting ASIA grade.

In a recent evidence-based guidelines statement, published under the auspices of AOSpine North America, AOSpine International, and the American Association of Neurological Surgeons, and the Congress of Neurological Surgeons, MR imaging was recommended in the acute stages of SCI, although the quality of evidence and level of recommendation for injury prognostication were rated as very low and weak, respectively.[41,42] Recommendations for MR imaging prognostication were based on review of acute MR imaging and clinical outcome data from 7 studies, which corrected for baseline clinical data in their analysis.[25,41,42,49–54] This includes work from Shepard and Bracken,[52] where evaluation of 191 patients enrolled in the National Acute Spinal Cord Injury Study III between 1991 and 1995 found that MR imaging did not add to prognostic yield of the initial clinical evaluation. In this study, however, magnetic resonance was an elective component of the study protocol and MR imaging results were collected from multiple centers as a post hoc analysis with heterogeneous MR imaging interpretation methods. Furthermore, some of the results from that study warrant close scrutiny. For example, significant motor deficits (average motor score of 33 out of 70) were reported for patients without spinal cord edema, results conflicting with numerous prior and subsequent studies.[22,23,33,35] In a relatively large cohort study of 104 SCI patients with follow-up motor scores obtained up to 1 year after injury, Flanders and colleagues[25] used stepwise multiple regression analysis to show that MR imaging features of cord hemorrhage and edema length (see **Fig. 3**) enhanced predictive modeling of motor recovery by 16% to 33%, compared with initial clinical assessment alone. In a separate study, including 42 patients with acute central cord syndrome, length of T2 signal abnormality was significantly correlated with manual dexterity and dysesthetic pain but not with ASIA motor score.[54] In a large study of 376 SCI patients, intramedullary signal characteristics on MR imaging within 3 days of injury categorized as (1) normal, (2) edema, or (3) hemorrhage, did not independently predict functional independence motor scores at 1 year.[50] MR imaging signal was incorporated into a multidimensional prediction model that outperformed initial AIS grade alone for predicting 1 year functional independence motor scores.[50] Boldin and colleagues[53] found that hemorrhage of less than 4 mm in length was associated with a good prognosis, whereas longer segments of intramedullary hemorrhage were associated with complete injury. A more recent study comparing concentrations of inflammatory and structural proteins obtained from cerebrospinal fluid (CSF) specimens within the first 24 hours of injury with preoperative MR imaging measures of cord injury found that CSF and MR imaging biomarkers performed similarly for predicting initial injury severity. CSF biomarkers outperformed standard MR imaging features for predicting neurologic improvement during the first 6 months after injury.[55]

Until recently, the T2 MR imaging appearance of injury in the axial plane was thought to lack prognostic value.[22] Animal and human pathology studies, however, have demonstrated that the transverse extent of SCI in the axial plane reflects relative white matter sparing and serves as a major determinant of functional outcome.[15,56–58] Axial MR evaluation allows definition of anatomically relevant spinal involvement in a graded manner. Clinical outcomes were recently correlated with transverse extent of MR imaging T2 signal abnormality in the axial plane at the injury epicenter with a 5-point classification scheme called the Brain and Spinal Injury Center (BASIC) score[59] (see **Fig. 2**). Absence of any cord signal abnormality (BASIC grade 0) portended an excellent prognosis with all patients demonstrating little or no clinical deficit at time of hospital discharge. With BASIC grade 1 injury, T2 hyperintensity is approximately confined to the central spinal cord gray matter. The relatively good clinical outcomes at discharge for these patients (87% are discharged with either ASIA grade D or E) suggest mild central vasogenic edema or petechial microhemorrhage without significant coagulative necrosis, similar to Schaefer type 3 injury. When T2 hyperintense signal extends beyond the approximate confines of gray matter, patients have a worse prognosis. Distinguishing those patients, who have some spared peripheral white matter signal (BASIC 2), from those with diffuse transverse T2 hyperintensity (BASIC 3), allows for more granular distinction among patients who would otherwise all be classified as multilevel hyperintensity according to the Schaefer sagittal T2 classification.[33] BASIC score 2 patients fared better than those with BASIC 3 score, with 88% of BASIC 2 patients achieving ASIA grade C or D and no ASIA grade A at follow-up, as opposed to 63% of BASIC grade 3 patients discharged as ASIA grade A or B. Thus, discretization of nonhemorrhagic edema patterns based on varying extent of white matter injury as evidenced on axial T2W imaging with the BASIC 1, 2, and 3 scores seems to enhance prognosis of patients where sagittal grading performs more poorly. Consistent with prior studies, the presence of macroscopic intramedullary hemorrhage as seen In BASIC 4 grade injury predicted a poor prognosis with all patients having ASIA grade A at time of discharge. Preliminary validation of the BASIC score for injury prognosis compared with other systems of MR imaging–based injury classification has been recently published.[23,60,61]

In summarizing the current literature, Fehlings and colleagues[41] conclude that intramedullary hemorrhage is the most robust prognostic magnetic resonance biomarker with moderate evidence associating intramedullary hematoma length with scores of neurologic and functional recovery. The investigators conclude, however, that there is insufficient evidence to support other individual MR imaging features, including cord edema, swelling, and lesion length, for predicting neurologic outcomes. With similar conclusions, Kurpad and colleagues[42] attempted to grade the prognostic validity of numerous conventional MR imaging features while acknowledging severe limitations based on variable study design and data reporting in the current literature. This analysis focused on prognostic validity of individual MR parameters rather than more comprehensive classification systems, which incorporate multiple parameters. Given the pathologic heterogeneity of the SCI syndrome, identification of a single predictive imaging variable for all patients seems unlikely. Multidimensional analysis approaches incorporating combined clinical and multiparametric imaging data are likely needed to improve prognosis.[50] In addition to shortcomings of the current literature, limitations of conventional MR imaging for injury prognostication in part relate to inherit limitations of the technique, which does not reliably distinguish between transient reversible pathology, such as vasogenic edema and irreversible cytotoxic injury observed with more severe contusion.[42] Nevertheless, there remains a need for further high-quality prospective longitudinal observation studies with sufficient sample sizes that

incorporate high-quality MR imaging with standardized imaging delays after injury, consistent methodologies for reporting MR imaging injury features, and standardized clinical data collection to definitively validate the prognostic significance of conventional MR imaging biomarkers in acute traumatic SCI.[41,42]

CRANIOCAUDAL LEVEL OF INJURY

In addition to the pattern of T2 signal abnormality, the craniocaudal level of injury observed on MR imaging has been correlated with injury severity, prognosis, need for ventilatory support, and clinical NLI. Flanders and colleagues[62] introduced a method for more precisely localizing the craniocaudal level of injury wherein each vertebral body and its adjacent inferior disc are subdivided into 3 segments. Using this system, the investigators found a dramatic effect of injury level and hemorrhage on functional measures of disability. Specifically, high cervical hemorrhagic injuries predicted complete reliance on caregivers and equipment for performance of activities of daily living.[62] In one of few studies to correlate MR imaging craniocaudal injury extent with clinical NLI, Zohrabian and colleagues[63] looked at the utility of upper and lower bounds of edema, upper and lower bounds of hemorrhage, and injury epicenter on MR imaging for predicting clinical NLI (see Fig. 3). Importantly, the upper and lower bounds of cord hemorrhage were found most predictive of clinical NLI, highlighting the value of MR imaging for objectively assessing injury level when early clinical examination may be precluded. The upper and lower bounds of T2 hyperintense cord edema were, however, imprecisely related to clinical NLI. Consideration of variations between vertebral and spinal cord segmental levels must also be accounted for when translating MR imaging observations to clinical levels of injury.[64] Given recent evidence that NLI and initial injury severity act jointly as primary determinants of motor function recovery,[65] precise determination of NLI with MR imaging will facilitate more personalized approach to diagnosis, treatment, prognosis, and clinical trial planning.

DYNAMIC MR IMAGING PATHOLOGY

The timing of MR imaging after injury can have a dramatic impact on findings, particularly in the early stages of injury when secondary processes are most dynamic. Although many studies have focused on MR imaging findings obtained at a single point in time during the acute phase of injury, select longitudinal studies have emphasized the dynamic range of MR imaging pathology over time.[45,47,66–71] In 48 SCI patients, Leypold and colleagues[69] evaluated rate of T2 signal evolution during the first 5 days after injury, using multiple regression analysis to show that time to MR imaging directly correlated with length of edema. The investigators calculated a rate of edema growth equal to 1 vertebral body segment length for every 1.2 days between injury and MR imaging.[69] Aarabi and colleagues[70] evaluated 42 patients with motor complete SCI who underwent consecutive magnetic resonance scans with initial MR imaging on average 6.2 hours after injury and follow-up MR imaging 54 hours after injury. The investigators report an average rate of craniocaudal lesion expansion of 0.9 mm ± 0.8 mm per hour, results greater than lesion expansion rate reported by Leypold and colleagues.[69] This difference likely relates to the fact that Aarabi and colleagues[70] evaluated only severely injured patients, and initial injury severity has been shown to positively correlate with rate of lesion expansion.[67,69] In the most standardized longitudinal MR imaging study published to date, Rutges and colleagues[71] prospectively examined MR imaging performed at 6 serial time-points within the first 3 weeks of injury in 19 cervical SCI patients. The first 48 hours to 72 hours postinjury were the most dynamic with respect to lesion expansion, indicating that this time interval reflects the most dramatic manifestation of secondary injury mechanisms and may be well-suited target period for neuroprotective interventions.[71] In light of the variable data supporting T2 hyperintense edema length as a biomarker of injury severity and outcome, these data highlight the importance of considering time from injury when interpreting MR imaging findings for both diagnostic and prognostic purposes. In determining the optimal time to image after injury, timing of MR imaging must be considered and controlled for as a critical covariate when imaging is used for injury stratification and/or to monitor injury as part of SCI clinical trials.

SPINAL CORD COMPRESSION

The prognostic significance of extrinsic spinal cord compression and spinal canal narrowing in SCI has been an active area of investigation over the past 2 decades.[49,50,54,72–75] Using reliable and standardized methods for determining midsagittal maximal spinal canal compromise (MCC) and maximal spinal cord compression (MSCC) (**Fig. 9**), Miyanji and colleagues[49] collected imaging and clinical data in 100

patients prospectively at admission and follow-up. Imaging data included quantitative measures MCC, MSCC, and longitudinal length of intramedullary cord signal abnormality in addition to 6 qualitative dichotomous variables, including presence or absence of intramedullary hemorrhage, cord swelling, cord edema, soft tissue injury, disc herniation, and preinjury stenosis. Using stepwise multivariable regression analysis, the investigators found that MSCC, intramedullary hemorrhage, and cord swelling were significant predictors of follow-up ASIA motor scores. After adjusting for initial ASIA score, however, only the qualitative variables of cord hemorrhage and cord swelling were significantly correlated with outcome. Using a similar multivariate approach, Haefeli and colleagues[23] recently assessed several MR imaging features of injury, including axial grade (BASIC score), Schaefer sagittal grade, length of injury, MCC, and MSCC.[23] These analyses showed that MR imaging measures of intrinsic cord signal abnormality were predictive of outcome whereas measures of extrinsic cord compression, including MCC and MSCC, were not. In contrast, Aarabi and colleagues[54] found a significant association between canal diameter, MCC, and functional motor scores in a cohort of 42 patients with acute traumatic central cord syndrome (ATCCS). Similar positive correlations between degree of spinal cord compression and likelihood of complete injury in thoracolumbar SCI were recently reported.[75] The heterogeneous nature of study cohorts with respect to ATCCS pathology and injury severity may explain some of the variability across these studies given the potential impact of preexisting stenosis and injury severity on the prognostic significance of these measures in acute SCI.

SPINAL CORD INJURY WITHOUT RADIOLOGIC ABNORMALITY AND CENTRAL CORD SYNDROME

SCI without radiologic abnormality (SCIWORA) is a term first coined by Pang and Wilberger in 1982,[76] predating the clinical application of MR imaging for acute SCI. The original description of this entity specifically referred to pediatric patients presenting with traumatic myelopathy but without evidence for traumatic spine injury on radiographs[76]; however, there is an evolving lexicography for this entity with the advent of CT and MR imaging and broadened application to adult populations.[77] In a large systematic literature review encompassing more than 1100 adult patients with SCIWORA, Boese and Lechler[78] define an

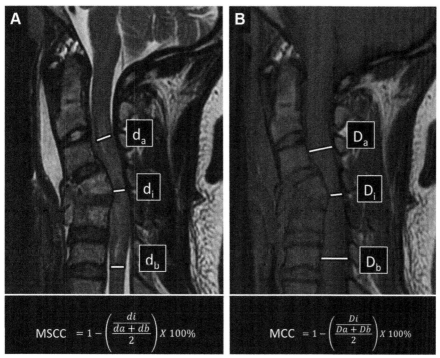

Fig. 9. Midsagittal evaluation of MCC and MSCC. (*A*) Midsagittal T2W image with sample measures for d_a, d_b, and d_i for calculation of spinal cord compression (MSCC equation at *bottom inset*). (*B*) Midsagittal T1W image with sample measures for D_a, D_b, and D_i for calculation of spinal canal compromise (MCC equation at *bottom inset*).

imaging classification system that dichotomizes patients based on the absence (type I) or presence (type II) of traumatic spine abnormality on MR imaging. Type II injuries predominate, comprising 93% of cases and are further subdivided based on MR imaging into those with isolated extraneural injury (type IIa), isolated intraneural injury (type IIb), and combined intraneural and extraneural injury (type IIc).[78] As expected, patients with MR imaging features of intrinsic spinal cord pathology (IIb and IIc) had worse outcomes. Given that traumatic spinal cord MR imaging findings in adult SCIWORA patients overlap with those described previously for the general SCI population,[79–82] the designation of SCIWORA in adults is arguably an antiquated and arbitrary designation that may simply encompass injuries with lower kinetic impact not sufficient to incur spinal column injury evident on radiographs.

ATCCS is another subtype designation for SCI patients. ATCCS diagnosis is reliant on unique clinical rather than imaging findings. ATCCS refers to an SCI syndrome wherein there is differential predominance of upper extremity weakness with relative lower extremity sparing and variable sensory and autonomic deficits.[83,84] Due to its unique clinical features including increased potential for spontaneous recovery independent of treatment, specific ATCCS management guidelines have been proposed.[85] In the mildest injuries, symptoms may be isolated to peripheral upper extremity burning sensation with a normal objective neurologic examination. Although early histopathologic studies implicated frontal horn motor neuron necrosis and selective medial corticospinal tract (CST) involvement as the etiology for upper extremity predominant weakness, more recent studies correlating MR imaging, and histopathologic, and clinical findings have challenged this hypothesis.[86–88] Combined MR imaging and histopathology studies were the first to demonstrate dorsolateral column predominant white matter injury diffusely involving the CSTs and lack of MR imaging or histopathologic evidence for intramedullary hemorrhage in postmortem specimens from ATCCS patients.[87,88] Furthermore, anatomic studies of the spinal cord dispute historical notions of somatopic organization of the lateral CST in the spinal cord of primates.[89,90] Despite decades of research, a unifying imaging diagnosis for central cord syndrome remains elusive as magnetic resonance features, including intramedullary edema and hemorrhage, spinal canal stenosis, and spinal fractures are observed in both ATCCS and non-ATCCS SCI patients.[41,54] With the advent of atlas-based MR imaging analysis techniques, the relative involvement of lateral CST in ATCCS could be potentially interrogated as a more specific imaging feature of ATCCS.[91]

DIFFUSION IMAGING AND SPINAL CORD INJURY

DWI is the best studied advanced quantitative MR imaging technique for application in human SCI. Other advanced functional, molecular, and microstructural imaging techniques for evaluating the traumatically injured spinal cord, including myelin water mapping, functional MR imaging, magnetic resonance spectroscopy, and magnetization transfer imaging, hold great promise but have yet to be sufficiently evaluated for assessing injury severity or prognosis in acute traumatic SCI patients and are not reviewed further.[92]

DWI uses magnetic gradients to probe the molecular motions of water molecules in tissue.[93] The diffusion pulse sequence is designed such that brownian motion of water contributes directly to attenuation of signal on a DWI image compared with a baseline T2W image, referred to as B0 or B naught.[93] From diffusion data, an approximation of the diffusion coefficient of water in tissues, the apparent diffusion coefficient (ADC), can be derived.[93] At the most basic level of clinical imaging, diffusion gradients applied along 3 orthogonal axes and a B0 image are sufficient to derive an average DW image and ADC map. In a case report of a single acute SCI patient, Sagiuchi and colleagues[94] were the first to use this basic 3-dir DWI technique to demonstrate a reduction in ADC values at the injury epicenter on initial MR imaging performed within 2 hours of acute high cervical SCI. In a larger study of 14 acute SCI patients, Tsuchiya and colleagues[95] identified hyperintense DWI signal with subjectively reduced ADC signal intensity in 9 patients when interrogating diffusion in a single direction (z axis). Although a trend toward significance was observed, this study did not show a statistically significant reduction in ADC values at the lesion epicenter compared with normal-appearing spinal cord.[95] Correlation of quantitative ADC values along the z axis with very coarse short-term outcome measures did not reveal statistically significant prognostic associations in this small, retrospective study.[95] More recently, Zhang and Huan[96] measured ADC values in 20 patients with acute SCI. In 10 cases of spinal cord edema without hemorrhage, ADC values at the injury epicenter were

significantly reduced compared with normal cord.[96] In a small retrospective cohort of 7 patients, Pouw and colleagues[97] showed that DWI and T2W imaging had similar sensitivity for detecting cord injury when performed within the first 24 hours of injury. Collectively, the results from these DWI studies suggests acute SCI is usually associated with an initial DWI hyperintensity and reduction in spinal cord ADC values (Fig. 10) compared with normal spinal cord. There is insufficient evidence to support DWI-derived ADC correlations with injury severity or outcome.[92] Although the precise molecular mechanisms of reduced ADC values in acute SCI are not completely understood,[98] the progression of injuries with low ADC values to cystic myelomalacia on follow-up MR imaging suggests some component of cytotoxic edema and irreversible tissue injury.[99]

Diffusion tensor imaging (DTI) was developed to more accurately reflect water diffusion in tissues with anisotropic geometry, such as white matter, where water motion is differentially hindered in 1 or more directions.[100,101] With DTI, a minimum of 6 noncollinear diffusion encoding gradients are applied and the rotationally invariant directionality of gaussian water motion can be modeled as an ellipse.[100,101] Quantitative scalar metrics, which reflect diffusion properties averaged over a voxel of tissue at the smallest scale, can be derived and serve as potential biomarkers of tissue disruption.[100] The most commonly used DTI parameters include (1) fractional anisotropy (FA), a unitless scalar metric ranging from 0 to 1 quantifying the fraction of the tensor that can be assigned to anisotropic water diffusion within a voxel (Fig. 11), and (2) mean diffusivity (MD), the magnitude of diffusivity averaged over all sampled directions. Unlike ADC values calculated from 3-dir DWI, MD is a more accurate measure of average diffusivity in all directions, particularly in anisotropic tissues like white matter, because it is rotationally invariant,[102] meaning the orientation of anisotropic tissue within the scanner does not alter the MD values. Other DTI parameters include axial diffusivity (AD), sometimes also referred to as longitudinal diffusivity or $\lambda_{\parallel}$. AD is a measurement of diffusivity along the long axis or primary eigenvector of the diffusion tensor ellipse. Radial diffusivity (RD), sometimes also referred to as transverse diffusivity or the symbol $\lambda_{\perp}$, is the averaged diffusivity along the 2 minor axes of the tensor ellipse. White matter anisotropy is largely attributed to barriers of water motion related to axon membranes and myelin sheaths.[103] AD then reflects the relatively unimpeded motion of extracellular water traveling parallel to white matter

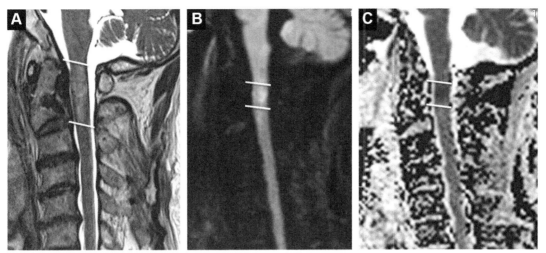

Fig. 10. DWI of acute SCI. (A) Sagittal T2W image of the cervical spinal cord in an 87-year-old woman with quadriplegia after fall reveals expansile cord edema with predominantly hyperintense T2 signal abnormality at C1-C2 without compression (upper and lower limits of edema delineated by parallel white lines). Sagittal DWI (B) and ADC map (C) reveals a corresponding more focal region of reduced diffusion conspicuously identified as hyperintensity on the DWI and hypointensity on the ADC image, delineated by horizontal white lines in (B) and (C).

bundles, whereas RD reflects the more hindered motion of water perpendicular to axons.[101] In preclinical models, AD and RD have been shown to correlate with microstructural white matter pathologies, including axonal injury and demyelination, respectively,[57,104,105] although their specificity for these injury subtypes has been challenged.[106] Nevertheless, the relatively regular and parallel orientation of white matter bundles in the spinal cord, along with the known functional significance of ascending and descending spinal cord white matter tracts, make SCI a potentially ideal

pathology for DTI-based interrogation of white matter integrity.[107,108]

In one of the earliest published studies to use DTI in acute SCI, Shanmuganathan and colleagues[109] found significantly lower MD, FA, and AD values at the injury site compared with values of the whole cervical spinal cord obtained from controls. In a follow-up study with 25 SCI patients, Cheran and colleagues[110] again demonstrated signficant reductions in FA and AD values between SCI and controls. Furthermore, in patients with nonhemorrhagic contusion, MD, FA, AD, and RD

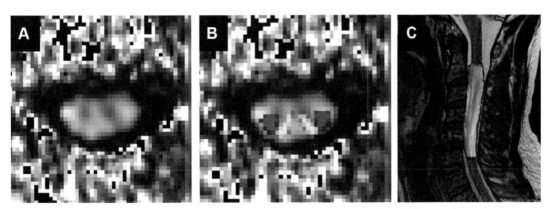

Fig. 11. DTI of the normal spinal cord. (A) Axial FA map of the cervical spinal cord shows relative hyperintense signal corresponding to the more anisotropic ascending and descending white matter tracts with relative hypointensity corresponding to the more isotropic central gray matter. (B) Atlas-based registration of normalized white matter tracts enables tract-based extraction of DTI metrics (lateral CSTs overlaid in red and cuneate fasciculus in yellow). (C) FA data also enable diffusion tensor fiber tracking with normal white matter tracts from the C2 to C6 levels projected over an anatomic sagittal T2W image.

Table 1
Summary of diffusion MR imaging for acute traumatic spinal cord injury in humans

Authors, Year	Study Design, Subjects	Diffusion Acquisition	Diffusion Metrics	Key Results
Sagiuchi et al,[94] 2002	• Case report • 1 pt imaged within 2 h of injury	• 1.5 T, sag 3-dir DWI, b =500, 700	• NA	• First report of DWI in clinical acute SCI • Hyperintense signal on DWI and hypointense ADC signal at injury epicenter • Quantitative ADC values not reported
Facon et al,[107] 2005	• Retrospective case series • 15 patients with compressive SCI, 2/15 acute • 11 HCs	• 1.5 T, sag 6-dir DTI, b = 500 • Manual ROI at epicenter	• FA, MD	• FA but not MD values significantly decreased at compression site compared with controls. • FA with high sensitivity and specificity for spinal cord abnormality compared with T2 and MD
Tsuchiya et al,[95] 2006	• Retrospective • 14 patients imaged 2 h to 3 d postinjury	• 1.5 T, sag 1-dir DWI (z axis), b = 400 • Manual ROI at epicenter	• ADC (z axis) calculated in 13 patients	• ADC values not significantly different between epicenter and normal-appearing cord
Shanmuganathan et al,[109] 2008	• Retrospective • 20 pts imaged 2 h to 15 d postinjury • 8 HCs	• 1.5 T, axial 6-dir DTI, b = 1000 • Manual whole card and epicenter ROIs	• MD, FA, RA, VR, E1 (AD), E2, E3	• Significant differences in MD and FA values at different cervical cord levels in HCs • Patient whole-cord ADC (but not FA) significantly different from HCs • Significantly lower MD, FA, RA, VR, E1, E2, and E3 values at injury site compared with HCs
Endo et al,[99] 2011	• Retrospective • 16 patients imaged within 24 h postinjury	• 1.5 T, axial 3-dir DWI, b = 1000	• ADC	• Low ADC values at epicenter associated with cavity formation on follow-up MR imaging

Study	Design/Population	Technique	Metrics	Findings
Cheran et al,[110] 2011	• Retrospective • 32 pts, 25 included, 13/25 with hemorrhage	• 1.5 T, axial 6-dir DTI, b = 1000	• MD, FA, RD, AD	• significant reductions in FA and AD values between SCI and controls. • When no hemorrhage, FA, AD, and RD measures at the injury site all correlated with initial ASIA motor score
Pouw et al,[97] 2012	• Prospective, 7 pts within 24 h of injury	• 1.5 T, sag 3-dir DWI, b = 1000	• ADC	• Qualitative T2 and DWI have comparable injury detection rate
Zhang et al,[96] 2014	• Retrospective • 20 pts within 72 h of injury	• 1.5 T, sag 3-dir DWI, b = 400 or 500	• ADC	• ADC significantly decreased at injury site in edema-type lesions, distinguishing cytotoxic and vasogenic edema • DWI assists in hemorrhage detection
Vedantam et al,[108] 2015	• Retrospective • 12 pts between 0 and 12 d of injury	• 1.5 T, axial 15-dir DTI at C1-C2, b = 600	• FA	• Significant associations between high cervical whole cord and CST FA values and upper limb motor scores and ASIA grade
Shen et al,[112] 2007	• Case series • 5 SCIWORA pts imaged within 48 h of injury	• 1.5 T, sag 1-dir DWI, b = 400	• NA	• DWI sensitive to cord contusion based on qualitative evaluation
D'Souza et al,[113] 2017	• Prospective cohort • 20 pts within 7 d of injury • 30 HCs	• 3T, axial 20-dir DTI, b = 700	• FA, MD	• FA significantly decreased and MD elevated at injury epicenter compared with HCs • FA significantly correlated with initial clinical severity
Shanmuganathan et al,[111] 2017	• Prospective cohort • 30 pts imaged within 5 d of injury • 15 HCs	• 1.5 T, axial 20-dir DTI, b = 700	• MD, AD, RD, FA	• AD best predictor of neurologic and functional outcomes at 1 y

Abbreviations: b, b-value (s/mm²); dir, direction; E, eigenvalue; HC, healthy control; NA, not applicable; pt, patient; RA, relative anisotropy; ROI, region of interest; sag, sagittal; VR, volume ratio.

measures at the injury site all correlated with initial injury severity as assessed with ASIA motor scores.[110] In light of the previously described limitations of T2W imaging for assessing injury severity in nonhemorrhagic SCI, these results are a potentially significant advance in SCI MR biomarker identification. In the first and only published prospective study to date to evaluate the prognostic validity of DTI in acute SCI, Shanmuganathan and colleagues[111] prospectively correlated normalized DTI metrics from acute MR imaging with AIS grade, motor scores, and Spinal Cord Independence Measure III at 1 year after injury. DTI

metrics were normalized to control values taken at a corresponding level of the spinal cord to account for potential craniocaudal variations and presented as Z-score values. Stepwise regression analysis revealed AD as the most robust DTI parameter for predicting neurologic and functional outcomes. Comparison with more conventional MR classifications schemes, such as the lesion length, sagittal grade, and BASIC score, was not performed; thus, superiority over conventional methods was not established. A summary of diffusion studies published for acute human SCI is provided in **Table 1**.

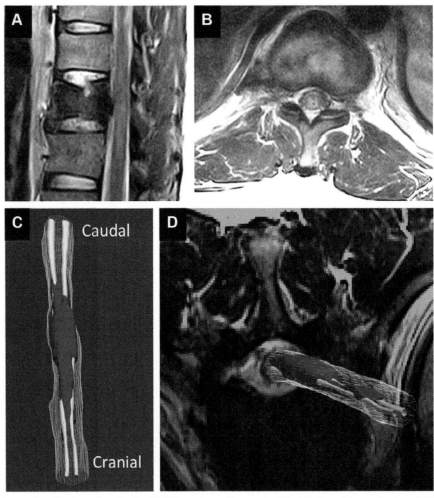

Fig. 12. Volumetric atlas-based analysis of MR imaging after acute SCI. (*A*) Coned-in sagittal and (*B*) axial T2W images of the spinal cord in a patient with acute lower thoracic SCI after fall. Conventional 2-D evaluation of injury somewhat limits appreciation of the volumetric distribution and anatomic involvement of injury. (*C*) After segmentation of the T2-hyperintense injury (*red*) and registration of imaging data to a spinal cord atlas using the spinal cord toolbox, the 3-D extent of lesion is more clearly defined and can be correlated with probabilistic atlases of the spinal cord for anatomic localization of injury. In this case, the bilateral ventral horns are projected in white solid mesh and their involvement with injury is clearly demonstrated. White mesh depicts volume rendering of the spinal cord. (*D*) Projection of 3-D models in (*C*) on axial T2W image near the injury epicenter.

SUMMARY

MR imaging is the established gold standard imaging modality for evaluating the traumatically injured spinal cord. Despite great advances in understanding the correlation between findings on MR imaging and acute injury severity and prognosis, few MR imaging biomarkers for injury prognostication are well validated in the current literature. Although the lack of well-validated MR biomarkers is partially based on variable study design and data reporting in the current literature, there are also inherit limitations with conventional MR imaging technique. For example, transient and reversible pathology, such as vasogenic edema and irreversible cytotoxic injury, are not always reliably distinguished with conventional T2W MR imaging.[4?] Intramedullary hemorrhage evidenced on T2W Imaging is universally associated with some component of irreversible injury and arguably the most robust predictor of injury severity. Diffusion imaging offers promise as a more specific tool for interrogating spinal cord integrity, although well-designed, prospective clinical studies remain limited.[112,113] There is a need for future high-quality prospective longitudinal observation studies with sufficient sample sizes that incorporate high-quality MR imaging data. Future studies should account for timing of imaging after injury and use consistent methodologies for reporting MR imaging injury features along with standardized clinical data collection to definitively validate the prognostic significance of conventional and advanced MR imaging biomarkers in acute traumatic SCI. Utilization of atlas-based analysis techniques will help reduce bias and enhance quantitative data extraction (**Fig. 12**). Advanced functional, molecular, and microstructural imaging techniques hold promise for overcoming limitations of conventional techniques but require validation in clinical practice. Correlation with standardized, high-quality neurologic and functional long-term outcome data are also essential.

REFERENCES

1. van Middendorp JJ, Sanchez GM, Burridge AL. The Edwin Smith papyrus: a clinical reappraisal of the oldest known document on spinal injuries. Eur Spine J 2010;19(11):1815–23.
2. Siddiqui AM, Khazaei M, Fehlings MG. Translating mechanisms of neuroprotection, regeneration, and repair to treatment of spinal cord injury. Prog Brain Res 2015;218:15–54.
3. Yue JK, Upadhyayula PS, Chan AK, et al. A review and update on the current and emerging clinical trials for the acute management of cervical spine and spinal cord injuries - Part III. J Neurosurg Sci 2016;60(4):529–42.
4. Yue JK, Winkler EA, Rick JW, et al. Update on critical care for acute spinal cord injury in the setting of polytrauma. Neurosurg Focus 2017;43(5):E19.
5. Birmingham UoAa, editor. National Spinal Cord Injury Statistical Center, Facts and Figures at a Glance. 2017. Available at: https://www.nscisc.uab.edu/Public/Facts%20and%20Figures%20-%202018.pdf. Accessed September 1, 2018.
6. Ahuja CS, Wilson JR, Nori S, et al. Traumatic spinal cord injury. Nat Rev Dis Primers 2017;3:17018.
7. Ahuja CS, Nori S, Tetreault L, et al. Traumatic spinal cord injury-repair and regeneration. Neurosurgery 2017;80(3S):S9–22.
8. Amar AP, Levy ML. Pathogenesis and pharmacological strategies for mitigating secondary damage in acute spinal cord injury. Neurosurgery 1999;44(5):1027–39 [discussion: 1039–40].
9. Karsy M, Hawryluk G. Pharmacologic management of acute spinal cord injury. Neurosurg Clin N Am 2017;28(1):49–62.
10. Baptiste DC, Fehlings MG. Pharmacological approaches to repair the injured spinal cord. J Neurotrauma 2006;23(3–4):318–34.
11. Gensel JC, Zhang B. Macrophage activation and its role in repair and pathology after spinal cord injury. Brain Res 2015;1619:1–11.
12. Tator CH, Fehlings MG. Review of the secondary injury theory of acute spinal cord trauma with emphasis on vascular mechanisms. J Neurosurg 1991;75(1):15–26.
13. Beattie MS, Ferguson AR, Bresnahan JC. AMPA-receptor trafficking and injury-induced cell death. Eur J Neurosci 2010;32(2):290–7.
14. Jones TB, McDaniel EE, Popovich PG. Inflammatory-mediated injury and repair in the traumatically injured spinal cord. Curr Pharm Des 2005;11(10):1223–36.
15. Tator CH. Update on the pathophysiology and pathology of acute spinal cord injury. Brain Pathol 1995;5(4):407–13.
16. Yuan YM, He C. The glial scar in spinal cord injury and repair. Neurosci Bull 2013;29(4):421–35.
17. Beattie MS, Hermann GE, Rogers RC, et al. Cell death in models of spinal cord injury. Prog Brain Res 2002;137:37–47.
18. Beattie MS, Li Q, Bresnahan JC. Cell death and plasticity after experimental spinal cord injury. Prog Brain Res 2000;128:9–21.
19. Kirshblum SC, Burns SP, Biering-Sorensen F, et al. International standards for neurological classification of spinal cord injury (revised 2011). J Spinal Cord Med 2011;34(6):535–46.
20. Daffner RH, Hackney DB. ACR appropriateness criteria on suspected spine trauma. J Am Coll Radiol 2007;4(11):762–75.

21. Shah LM, Ross JS. Imaging of spine trauma. Neurosurgery 2016;79(5):626–42.

22. Bozzo A, Marcoux J, Radhakrishna M, et al. The role of magnetic resonance imaging in the management of acute spinal cord injury. J Neurotrauma 2011; 28(8):1401–11.

23. Haefeli J, Mabray MC, Whetstone WD, et al. Multivariate analysis of MRI biomarkers for predicting neurologic impairment in cervical spinal cord injury. AJNR Am J Neuroradiol 2017;38(3):648–55.

24. Kulkarni MV, McArdle CB, Kopanicky D, et al. Acute spinal cord injury: MR imaging at 1.5 T. Radiology 1987;164(3):837–43.

25. Flanders AE, Spettell CM, Tartaglino LM, et al. Forecasting motor recovery after cervical spinal cord injury: value of MR imaging. Radiology 1996; 201(3):649–55.

26. Gomori JM, Grossman RI. Mechanisms responsible for the MR appearance and evolution of intracranial hemorrhage. Radiographics 1988;8(3):427–40.

27. Hackney DB, Asato R, Joseph PM, et al. Hemorrhage and edema in acute spinal cord compression: demonstration by MR imaging. Radiology 1986;161(2):387–90.

28. Wang M, Dai Y, Han Y, et al. Susceptibility weighted imaging in detecting hemorrhage in acute cervical spinal cord injury. Magn Reson Imaging 2011; 29(3):365–73.

29. Martin AR, De Leener B, Cohen-Adad J, et al. A novel MRI biomarker of spinal cord white matter injury: T2*-weighted white matter to gray matter signal intensity ratio. AJNR Am J Neuroradiol 2017;38(6):1266–73.

30. Biering-Sorensen F, Alai S, Anderson K, et al. Common data elements for spinal cord injury clinical research: a National Institute For Neurological Disorders And Stroke Project. Spinal Cord 2015;53(4): 265–77.

31. Available at: https://http://www.commondataelements. ninds.nih.gov/SCI.aspx - tab=Data_Standards. Accessed June, 1, 2018.

32. Bondurant FJ, Cotler HB, Kulkarni MV, et al. Acute spinal cord injury. A study using physical examination and magnetic resonance imaging. Spine 1990; 15(3):161–8.

33. Schaefer DM, Flanders A, Northrup BE, et al. Magnetic resonance imaging of acute cervical spine trauma. Correlation with severity of neurologic injury. Spine 1989;14(10):1090–5.

34. Marciello MA, Flanders AE, Herbison GJ, et al. Magnetic resonance imaging related to neurologic outcome in cervical spinal cord injury. Arch Phys Med Rehabil 1993;74(9):940–6.

35. Flanders AE, Schaefer DM, Doan HT, et al. Acute cervical spine trauma: correlation of MR imaging findings with degree of neurologic deficit. Radiology 1990;177(1):25–33.

36. Mirvis SE, Geisler FH, Jelinek JJ, et al. Acute cervical spine trauma: evaluation with 1.5-T MR imaging. Radiology 1988;166(3):807–16.

37. Kalfas I, Wilberger J, Goldberg A, et al. Magnetic resonance imaging in acute spinal cord trauma. Neurosurgery 1988;23(3):295–9.

38. Tarr RW, Drolshagen LF, Kerner TC, et al. MR imaging of recent spinal trauma. J Comput Assist Tomogr 1987;11(3):412–7.

39. Ohshio I, Hatayama A, Kaneda K, et al. Correlation between histopathologic features and magnetic resonance images of spinal cord lesions. Spine 1993;18(9):1140–9.

40. Goldberg AL, Rothfus WE, Deeb ZL, et al. The impact of magnetic resonance on the diagnostic evaluation of acute cervicothoracic spinal trauma. Skeletal Radiol 1988;17(2):89–95.

41. Fehlings MG, Tetreault LA, Wilson JR, et al. A clinical practice guideline for the management of patients with acute spinal cord injury and central cord syndrome: recommendations on the timing (</=24 hours versus >24 hours) of decompressive surgery. Global Spine J 2017;7(3 Suppl): 195S–202S.

42. Kurpad S, Martin AR, Tetreault LA, et al. Impact of baseline magnetic resonance imaging on neurologic, functional, and safety outcomes in patients with acute traumatic spinal cord injury. Global Spine J 2017;7(3 Suppl):151S–74S.

43. Parashari UC, Khanduri S, Bhadury S, et al. Diagnostic and prognostic role of MRI in spinal trauma, its comparison and correlation with clinical profile and neurological outcome, according to ASIA impairment scale. J Craniovertebr Junction Spine 2011;2(1):17–26.

44. Gupta R, Mittal P, Sandhu P, et al. Correlation of qualitative and quantitative MRI parameters with neurological status: a prospective study on patients with spinal trauma. J Clin Diagn Res 2014; 8(11):RC13–7.

45. Schaefer DM, Flanders AE, Osterholm JL, et al. Prognostic significance of magnetic resonance imaging in the acute phase of cervical spine injury. J Neurosurg 1992;76(2):218–23.

46. Andreoli C, Colaiacomo MC, Rojas Beccaglia M, et al. MRI in the acute phase of spinal cord traumatic lesions: relationship between MRI findings and neurological outcome. Radiol Med 2005; 110(5–6):636–45.

47. Shimada K, Tokioka T. Sequential MR studies of cervical cord injury: correlation with neurological damage and clinical outcome. Spinal Cord 1999; 37(6):410–5.

48. Ramon S, Dominguez R, Ramirez L, et al. Clinical and magnetic resonance imaging correlation in acute spinal cord injury. Spinal Cord 1997;35(10): 664–73.

49. Miyanji F, Furlan JC, Aarabi B, et al. Acute cervical traumatic spinal cord injury: MR imaging findings correlated with neurologic outcome–prospective study with 100 consecutive patients. Radiology 2007;243(3):820–7.

50. Wilson JR, Arnold PM, Singh A, et al. Clinical prediction model for acute inpatient complications after traumatic cervical spinal cord injury: a subanalysis from the Surgical Timing in Acute Spinal Cord Injury Study. J Neurosurg Spine 2012;17(1 Suppl):46–51.

51. Selden NR, Quint DJ, Patel N, et al. Emergency magnetic resonance imaging of cervical spinal cord injuries: clinical correlation and prognosis. Neurosurgery 1999;44(4):785–92 [discussion: 792–3].

52. Shepard MJ, Bracken MB. Magnetic resonance imaging and neurological recovery in acute spinal cord injury: observations from the National Acute Spinal Cord Injury Study 3. Spinal Cord 1999; 37(12):833–7.

53. Boldin C, Raith J, Fankhauser F, et al. Predicting neurologic recovery in cervical spinal cord injury with postoperative MR imaging. Spine 2006;31(5): 554–9.

54. Aarabi B, Alexander M, Mirvis SE, et al. Predictors of outcome in acute traumatic central cord syndrome due to spinal stenosis. J Neurosurg Spine 2011;14(1):122–30.

55. Dalkilic T, Fallah N, Noonan VK, et al. Predicting injury severity and neurological recovery after acute cervical spinal cord injury: a comparison of cerebrospinal fluid and magnetic resonance imaging biomarkers. J Neurotrauma 2018;35(3):435–45.

56. Bresnahan JC, Beattie MS, Todd FD 3rd, et al. A behavioral and anatomical analysis of spinal cord injury produced by a feedback-controlled impaction device. Exp Neurol 1987;95(3):548–70.

57. Budde MD, Kim JH, Liang HF, et al. Axonal injury detected by in vivo diffusion tensor imaging correlates with neurological disability in a mouse model of multiple sclerosis. NMR Biomed 2008;21(6): 589–97.

58. Loy DN, Kim JH, Xie M, et al. Diffusion tensor imaging predicts hyperacute spinal cord injury severity. J Neurotrauma 2007;24(6):979–90.

59. Talbott JF, Whetstone WD, Readdy WJ, et al. The Brain and Spinal Injury Center score: a novel, simple, and reproducible method for assessing the severity of acute cervical spinal cord injury with axial T2-weighted MRI findings. J Neurosurg Spine 2015;23(4):495–504.

60. Mabray MC, Talbott JF, Whetstone WD, et al. Multidimensional analysis of magnetic resonance imaging predicts early impairment in thoracic and thoracolumbar spinal cord injury. J Neurotrauma 2016;33(10):954–62.

61. Farhadi HF, Kukreja S, Minnema A, et al. Impact of admission imaging findings on neurological outcomes in acute cervical traumatic spinal cord injury. J Neurotrauma 2018;35(12):1398–406.

62. Flanders AE, Spettell CM, Friedman DP, et al. The relationship between the functional abilities of patients with cervical spinal cord injury and the severity of damage revealed by MR imaging. AJNR Am J Neuroradiol 1999;20(5):926–34.

63. Zohrabian VM, Parker L, Harrop JS, et al. Can anatomic level of injury on MRI predict neurological level in acute cervical spinal cord injury? Br J Neurosurg 2016;30(2):204–10.

64. Cadotte DW, Cadotte A, Cohen-Adad J, et al. Characterizing the location of spinal and vertebral levels in the human cervical spinal cord. AJNR Am J Neuroradiol 2015;36(4):803–10.

65. Dvorak MF, Noonan VK, Fallah N, et al. The influence of time from injury to surgery on motor recovery and length of hospital stay in acute traumatic spinal cord injury: an observational Canadian cohort study. J Neurotrauma 2015;32(9):645–54.

66. Silberstein M, Hennessy O. Implications of focal spinal cord lesions following trauma: evaluation with magnetic resonance imaging. Paraplegia 1993;31(3):160–7.

67. Le E, Aarabi B, Hersh DS, et al. Predictors of intramedullary lesion expansion rate on MR images of patients with subaxial spinal cord injury. J Neurosurg Spine 2015;22(6):611–21.

68. Taneichi H, Abumi K, Kaneda K, et al. Monitoring the evolution of intramedullary lesions in cervical spinal cord injury. Qualitative and quantitative analysis with sequential MR imaging. Paraplegia 1994; 32(1):9–18.

69. Leypold BG, Flanders AE, Burns AS. The early evolution of spinal cord lesions on MR imaging following traumatic spinal cord injury. AJNR Am J Neuroradiol 2008;29(5):1012–6.

70. Aarabi B, Simard JM, Kufera JA, et al. Intramedullary lesion expansion on magnetic resonance imaging in patients with motor complete cervical spinal cord injury. J Neurosurg Spine 2012;17(3):243–50.

71. Rutges J, Kwon BK, Heran M, et al. A prospective serial MRI study following acute traumatic cervical spinal cord injury. Eur Spine J 2017;26(9):2324–32.

72. Fehlings MG, Furlan JC, Massicotte EM, et al. Interobserver and intraobserver reliability of maximum canal compromise and spinal cord compression for evaluation of acute traumatic cervical spinal cord injury. Spine 2006;31(15):1719–25.

73. Ruegg TB, Wicki AG, Aebli N, et al. The diagnostic value of magnetic resonance imaging measurements for assessing cervical spinal canal stenosis. J Neurosurg Spine 2015;22(3):230–6.

74. Fehlings MG, Rao SC, Tator CH, et al. The optimal radiologic method for assessing spinal canal

compromise and cord compression in patients with cervical spinal cord injury. Part II: results of a multi-center study. Spine 1999;24(6):605–13.

75. Skeers P, Battistuzzo CR, Clark JM, et al. Acute thoracolumbar spinal cord injury: relationship of cord compression to neurological outcome. J Bone Joint Surg Am 2018;100(4):305–15.

76. Pang D, Wilberger JE Jr. Spinal cord injury without radiographic abnormalities in children. J Neurosurg 1982;57(1):114–29.

77. Dreizin D, Kim W, Kim JS, et al. Will the real SCI-WORA please stand up? exploring clinicoradiologic mismatch in closed spinal cord injuries. AJR Am J Roentgenol 2015;205(4):853–60.

78. Boese CK, Lechler P. Spinal cord injury without radiologic abnormalities in adults: a systematic review. J Trauma Acute Care Surg 2013;75(2):320–30.

79. Machino M, Yukawa Y, Ito K, et al. Can magnetic resonance imaging reflect the prognosis in patients of cervical spinal cord injury without radiographic abnormality? Spine 2011;36(24):E1568–72.

80. Mohanty SP, Bhat NS, Singh KA, et al. Cervical spinal cord injuries without radiographic evidence of trauma: a prospective study. Spinal Cord 2013; 51(11):815–8.

81. Sun LQ, Shen Y, Li YM. Quantitative magnetic resonance imaging analysis correlates with surgical outcome of cervical spinal cord injury without radiologic evidence of trauma. Spinal Cord 2014; 52(7):541–6.

82. Boese CK, Oppermann J, Siewe J, et al. Spinal cord injury without radiologic abnormality in children: a systematic review and meta-analysis. J Trauma Acute Care Surg 2015;78(4):874–82.

83. Thorburn W. Cases on injury to the cervical region of the spinal cord. Brain 1887;(9):510–43.

84. Schneider RC, Cherry G, Pantek H. The syndrome of acute central cervical spinal cord injury; with special reference to the mechanisms involved in hyperextension injuries of cervical spine. J Neurosurg 1954;11(6):546–77.

85. Aarabi B, Hadley MN, Dhall SS, et al. Management of acute traumatic central cord syndrome (ATCCS). Neurosurgery 2013;72(Suppl 2):195–204.

86. Collignon F, Martin D, Lenelle J, et al. Acute traumatic central cord syndrome: magnetic resonance imaging and clinical observations. J Neurosurg 2002;96(1 Suppl):29–33.

87. Martin D, Schoenen J, Lenelle J, et al. MRI-pathological correlations in acute traumatic central cord syndrome: case report. Neuroradiology 1992; 34(4):262–6.

88. Quencer RM, Bunge RP, Egnor M, et al. Acute traumatic central cord syndrome: MRI-pathological correlations. Neuroradiology 1992;34(2):85–94.

89. Pappas CT, Gibson AR, Sonntag VK. Decussation of hind-limb and fore-limb fibers in the monkey corticospinal tract: relevance to cruciate paralysis. J Neurosurg 1991;75(6):935–40.

90. Levi AD, Tator CH, Bunge RP. Clinical syndromes associated with disproportionate weakness of the upper versus the lower extremities after cervical spinal cord injury. Neurosurgery 1996;38(1): 179–83 [discussion: 183–5].

91. Fonov VS, Le Troter A, Taso M, et al. Framework for integrated MRI average of the spinal cord white and gray matter: the MNI-Poly-AMU template. Neuroimage 2014;102 Pt 2:817–27.

92. Martin AR, Aleksanderek I, Cohen-Adad J, et al. Translating state-of-the-art spinal cord MRI techniques to clinical use: a systematic review of clinical studies utilizing DTI, MT, MWF, MRS, and fMRI. Neuroimage Clin 2016; 10:192–238.

93. Le Bihan D, Breton E, Lallemand D, et al. MR imaging of intravoxel incoherent motions: application to diffusion and perfusion in neurologic disorders. Radiology 1986;161(2):401–7.

94. Sagiuchi T, Tachibana S, Endo M, et al. Diffusion-weighted MRI of the cervical cord in acute spinal cord injury with type II odontoid fracture. J Comput Assist Tomogr 2002;26(4):654–6.

95. Tsuchiya K, Fujikawa A, Honya K, et al. Value of diffusion-weighted MR imaging in acute cervical cord injury as a predictor of outcome. Neuroradiology 2006;48(11):803–8.

96. Zhang JS, Huan Y. Multishot diffusion-weighted MR imaging features in acute trauma of spinal cord. Eur Radiol 2014;24(3):685–92.

97. Pouw MH, van der Vliet AM, van Kampen A, et al. Diffusion-weighted MR imaging within 24 h post-injury after traumatic spinal cord injury: a qualitative meta-analysis between T2-weighted imaging and diffusion-weighted MR imaging in 18 patients. Spinal Cord 2012;50(6):426–31.

98. Budde MD, Skinner NP. Diffusion MRI in acute nervous system injury. J Magn Reson 2018;292: 137–48.

99. Endo T, Suzuki S, Utsunomiya A, et al. Prediction of neurological recovery using apparent diffusion coefficient in cases of incomplete spinal cord injury. Neurosurgery 2011;68(2):329–36.

100. Basser PJ, Mattiello J, LeBihan D. Estimation of the effective self-diffusion tensor from the NMR spin echo. J Magn Reson B 1994;103(3):247–54.

101. Le Bihan D, Mangin JF, Poupon C, et al. Diffusion tensor imaging: concepts and applications. J Magn Reson Imaging 2001;13(4):534–46.

102. Iima M, Le Bihan D. Clinical intravoxel incoherent motion and diffusion MR imaging: past, present, and future. Radiology 2016;278(1):13–32.

103. Beaulieu C, Allen PS. Determinants of anisotropic water diffusion in nerves. Magn Reson Med 1994; 31(4):394–400.

104. Budde MD, Kim JH, Liang HF, et al. Toward accurate diagnosis of white matter pathology using diffusion tensor imaging. Magn Reson Med 2007; 57(4):688–95.

105. Budde MD, Xie M, Cross AH, et al. Axial diffusivity is the primary correlate of axonal injury in the experimental autoimmune encephalomyelitis spinal cord: a quantitative pixelwise analysis. J Neurosci 2009;29(9):2805–13.

106. Talbott JF, Nout-Lomas YS, Wendland MF, et al. Diffusion-weighted magnetic resonance imaging characterization of white matter injury produced by axon-sparing demyelination and severe contusion spinal cord injury in rats. J Neurotrauma 2016;33(10):929–42.

107. Facon D, Ozanne A, Fillard P, et al. MR diffusion tensor imaging and fiber tracking in spinal cord compression. AJNR Am J Neuroradiol 2005;26(6): 1587–94.

108. Vedantam A, Eckardt G, Wang MC, et al. Clinical correlates of high cervical fractional anisotropy in acute cervical spinal cord injury. World Neurosurg 2015;83(5):824–8.

109. Shanmuganathan K, Gullapalli RP, Zhuo J, et al. Diffusion tensor MR imaging in cervical spine trauma. AJNR Am J Neuroradiol 2008;29(4):655–9.

110. Cheran S, Shanmuganathan K, Zhuo J, et al. Correlation of MR diffusion tensor imaging parameters with ASIA motor scores in hemorrhagic and nonhemorrhagic acute spinal cord injury. J Neurotrauma 2011;28(9):1881–92.

111. Shanmuganathan K, Zhuo J, Chen HH, et al. Diffusion tensor imaging parameter obtained during acute blunt cervical spinal cord injury in predicting long-term outcome. J Neurotrauma 2017;34(21):2964–71.

112. Shen H, Tang Y, Huang L, et al. Applications of diffusion-weighted MRI in thoracic spinal cord injury without radiographic abnormality. Int Orthop 2007;31(3):375–83.

113. D'Souza MM, Choudhary A, Poonia M, et al. Diffusion tensor MR imaging in spinal cord injury. Injury 2017;48(4):880–4.

Imaging of Intraspinal Tumors

Luke N. Ledbetter, MD*, John D. Leever, MD

KEYWORDS

• Intraspinal tumors • Space-based localization • MR imaging • Intradural extramedullary space

KEY POINTS

- Localization of intraspinal masses to intramedullary, intradural extramedullary, or extradural spaces can lead to an appropriate list of tumors commonly located in each area.
- MR imaging is essential to characterize intraspinal tumors whereas CT plays a less important role.
- Intradural extramedullary space is the most commonly involved intraspinal location, and nerve sheath tumors, such as schwannomas and neurofibromas, are the most common masses to occur in this space.
- Ependymomas and astrocytomas are the most common intramedullary masses and can be differentiated based on patient age and imaging findings.
- Metastases, lymphoma, and leukemia can affect all intraspinal locations and their appearance varies based on the specific location involved.

INTRODUCTION

Spinal tumors encompass a wide range of benign and malignant masses. Although most spinal tumors originate from the osseous components of the vertebral segments, intraspinal tumors are rare, with an incidence between 1.0 and 1.5 per 100,000 individuals.[1] Spinal tumors often present with nonspecific back pain or radicular symptoms, and imaging has a key role in discovering and characterizing the mass.[1–4] Intraspinal tumors are typically characterized best on MR imaging because it provides superb soft tissue differentiation. Although osseous spinal tumors necessitate evaluation with CT for bone characterization, CT is less important in characterizing intraspinal tumors. Given the broad range of tumors affecting the spinal canal, space-based localization can be used to form a space-specific differential diagnosis. The intraspinal spaces are commonly divided into intramedullary, intradural extramedullary, and

extradural spaces. Once a tumor is localized to a space and an appropriate differential list of possible diagnoses is formed, its MR imaging features can be used to reach a most likely diagnosis. In keeping with this practice, this article is divided into intramedullary, intradural extramedullary, and extradural sections, where the most common neoplasms are described.

INTRAMEDULLARY TUMORS
Ependymoma

Ependymoma is the most common intramedullary spinal tumor in adults and second most common spinal tumor in children.[5,6] Ependymomas make up 50% to 60% of all adult spinal tumors and approximately 30% of pediatric spinal tumors.[5,7] These lesions arise from the ependymal cells lining the central canal of the cord. Ependymomas are divided into 3 categories by the World Health Organization (WHO): myxopapillary ependymomas

Disclosure Statement: Nothing to disclose.
Department of Radiology, University of Kansas Health System, 3901 Rainbow Boulevard, Mailstop 4032, Kansas City, KS 66160, USA
* Corresponding author.
E-mail address: lledbetter@kumc.edu

Radiol Clin N Am 57 (2019) 341–357
https://doi.org/10.1016/j.rcl.2018.09.007

(MPEs) and subependymomas are grade 1, standard ependymomas are grade 2, and anaplastic ependymomas are grade 3. Grade 2 ependymomas can be further divided by histology type into classic, papillary, clear cell, and tanycytic subtypes. A subtype referred to as cellular ependymoma was removed in the 2016 update to the WHO classification to central nervous system (CNS) tumors due overlap with the classic subtype.[8]

Ependymomas are most often sporadic and can occur at any age, most commonly between 40 years and 50 years of age.[9] Multiple ependymomas, together with schwannomas and meningiomas, can occur in the setting of neurofibromatosis type 2. Most ependymomas in the setting of neurofibromatosis type 2 are indolent and often are treated conservatively.[10]

Classic ependymomas of the cord are typically located in the cervical or thoracic cord.[9,11,12] These tumors occur near the middle of the cord due to the central location of the ependymal cells lining on the central canal. Ependymomas displace and compress the surrounding parenchyma, leading to a well circumscribed or encapsulated appearance with symmetric expansion of the cord. Most commonly, ependymomas demonstrate vertical extension with an average length of 4 vertebral bodies.[13] Ependymomas demonstrate enhancement and T2 hyperintense signal in relation to the adjacent cord. Cyst formation is common with ependymomas, and the cysts can be within the tumor, at the margins of the tumor, or related to an adjacent syrinx. Intratumoral cysts are often complex and contain old blood products, protein, and necrosis and peripherally enhance when encased by tumor.[14] Marginal cysts occur at the cranial or caudal margins do not exhibit peripheral enhancement. Adjacent syrinx is related to at least partial obstruction of the central canal and results in cysts with central cerebrospinal fluid (CSF) intensity, which extend beyond the length of the mass. Cystic change related to both polar cysts or syrinx may be quite large in comparison with the size of the focal mass. Hemorrhage, especially along the margin of the mass, is common for ependymomas and results in a T2 hypointense hemosiderin cap at the margins of the tumor (**Fig. 1**).[10,13–15]

Gross total resection of ependymomas is the treatment of choice and offers best overall outcomes.[16] Recurrence rates of ependymomas vary by location with higher rates of recurrence in the lower cord compared with the cervical cord.[17] Radiation therapy can be performed for incomplete resections with chemotherapy reserved for failed surgery and radiotherapy.[18]

Astrocytoma

Astrocytomas are the most common primary intramedullary spinal tumor in children and the second most common primary spinal tumor in adults.[5,19] These tumors originate from astrocyte glial cells. Most spinal astrocytomas are pilocystic (WHO grade I) or fibrillary (WHO II), with a smaller percentage of anaplastic astrocytomas (WHO grade III). Glioblastomas (WHO grade IV) are exceedingly rare and only account for 0.2% to 1.5% of spinal astrocytomas.[7] Most astrocytomas are sporadic There is an increased risk, however, with neurofibromatosis types 1 and 2. Ependymoma is much more common than astrocytomas in the setting of neurofibromatosis type 2.[20,21]

Astrocytomas most commonly occur in cervical spine or cervicothoracic junction in children, with adult tumors occurring in the thoracic cord more frequently. Spinal fibrillary astrocytomas are infiltrating tumors spreading along the normal cellular architecture of the cord as opposed to the focal masslike nature of ependymomas. Pilocytic astrocytomas are more focal and less infiltrative. The most common appearance of a spinal astrocytoma is elongated eccentric T2 hyperintense mass without well-defined borders. Astrocytomas demonstrate variable vertical extension and average approximately 4 vertebral segments in length.[22] Rare holocord involvement results in the entire cord infiltration from the medulla to the conus. A little less than half of astrocytomas present with cystic change, either intratumoral cysts or cysts related with syringohydromyelia. Spinal astrocytomas usually demonstrate moderate enhancement at any grade unlike intracranial astrocytomas. Unlike ependymomas, hemorrhage is rarely associated with astrocytomas (**Fig. 2**).[6,7,19,23]

Gross total resection for astrocytomas can be challenging given the infiltrating nature of the tumor. Given challenges and potential morbidity, surgical resection is considered based on the clinical presentation.[22] Intraoperative ultrasound can assist in characterizing solid tumor from adjacent cystic change or edema.[24]

Hemangioblastoma

Hemangioblastomas are rare vascular and histologically benign tumors of the CNS. Spinal hemangioblastomas make up between 2% and 15% of all spine tumors.[25,26] These tumors typically present in patients that are between 40 years and 50 years in age.[27] Hemangioblastomas can be sporadic or occur in the setting of von Hippel-Lindau disease; between 20% and 40% of von Hippel-Lindau patients develop hemangioblastomas.

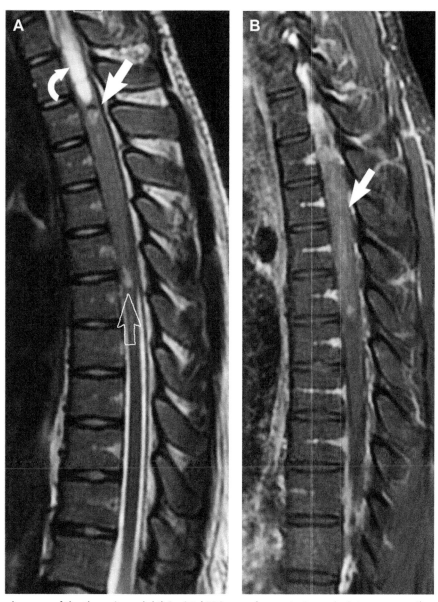

Fig. 1. Ependymoma of the thoracic cord. (*A*) Sagittal T2 image demonstrates an isointense expansile mass. Classic findings of ependymoma include a T2 hypointense hemosiderin cap (*solid white arrow*), marginal cyst (*open white arrow*), and associated syrinx (*curved white arrow*). (*B*) Sagittal postcontrast image shows heterogenous enhancement (*white arrow*) of the ependymoma.

Spinal hemangioblastomas most commonly occur in the cervical and thoracic cord with decreasing incidence in the lumbar region.[25] Sporadic hemangioblastomas typically present with a single lesion as opposed to von Hippel-Lindau patients, where multiple hemangioblastomas are frequently present. The size of the lesions is variable and most often less than 10 mm, but lesions can extend several centimeters in length. The tumors tend to be smaller than 10 mm in diameter in patients with von Hippel-Lindau disease. With

sporadic spinal hemangioblastomas, the tumors can get bigger up to 6 cm in diameter.[28] Most hemangioblastomas occur in the dorsal superficial aspect of the cord with a smaller percentage of ventral superficial lesions.[29] These lesions often approach the pial surface of the cord where arterial vessels supply the vascular mass. When small, hemangioblastomas are typically round or nodular lesions with T1 signal similar to the surrounding cord, high T2 signal, and homogeneous enhancement. Once large in size (greater than 15 mm),

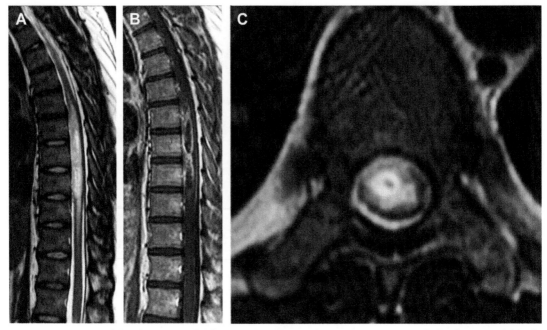

Fig. 2. Astrocytoma of the thoracic cord. (*A*) Sagittal T2 images shows a heterogeneously bright mass within the anterior cord and extending at least 4 vertebral segments. (*B*) Sagittal T1 postcontrast image demonstrates ill-defined and heterogenous enhancement. (*C*) Axial T2 images shows slightly eccentric expansile mass with ill-defined margins occupying the transverse section of the cord.

signal characteristics of the tumor are typically heterogeneous and vascular flow voids are often visualized. Cyst formation is common with hemangioblastomas resulting in a nodule in a cyst appearance. Extensive peritumoral edema and syrinx are commonly findings, described in up to 70% of patients (**Fig. 3**).[25]

Surgical resection is the treatment of choice in solitary hemangioblastomas but offers significant risk of morbidity due to the highly vascular nature of the benign tumor. Microsurgery can be safely performed with smaller tumors.[30] Preoperative angiography can delineate feeding arterial vessels, and optional embolization prior to surgery can reduce intraoperative hemorrhage.[31] Radiation therapy can be used with multiple, recurrent, or residual hemangioblastomas if symptoms necessitate.[32] Not infrequently, especially for multiple hemangioblastomas, close observation can be performed.

Ganglioglioma

Gangliogliomas are benign intramedullary tumors comprising both neuronal and glial cells. These spinal tumors are WHO grade I tumors are more common within the first 3 decades of life and occur most frequently in the cervical cord.[33] Gangliogliomas typically extend multiple vertebral segments and involve most of the cross-sectional area of

the cord. T1 and T2 signal are most likely heterogenous and eccentric within the cord. Enhancement characteristics are variable from solid masslike enhancement to heterogeneous or rim enhancement (**Fig. 4**). Intratumoral cysts are common, with gangliogliomas with associated nodular or circumferential enhancement.[33,34]

INTRADURAL EXTRAMEDULLARY TUMORS
Schwannoma

Schwannomas are histologic benign, WHO grade I, tumors of Schwann cells occurring within a nerve sheath. Schwann cells are the principal supporting glial cell for peripheral nerves. Schwannomas can occur anywhere along course of peripheral nerves but are most commonly located in the intradural extramedullary location. Schwannomas are the most common mass in the intradural extramedullary location.[1] The presenting symptoms are most commonly pain and paresthesia according to the level of the nerve root affected.[35,36] Symptoms from cord compression can occur with larger lesions. These lesions most commonly present in middle age and have no gender predilection.[36]

Schwannomas can be sporadic and solitary, related to schwannomatosis with multiple peripheral nerve schwannomas, or associated with neurofibromatosis type 2 resulting in multiple

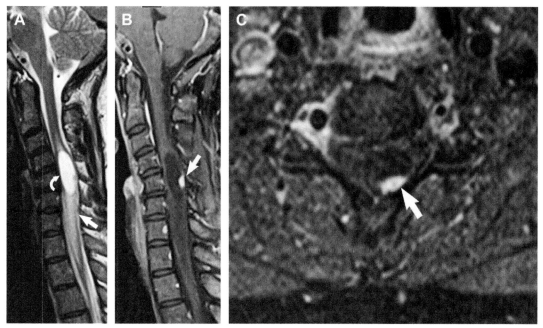

Fig. 3. Hemangioma of the cervical cord. (*A*) Sagittal T2 image demonstrates a well circumscribed cystic lesion with focal cord expansion (*curved white arrow*). There is extensive cord edema extending from the caudal margin of the cyst (*straight white arrow*). (*B*) Sagittal T1 postcontrast image with fat saturation shows the enhancing nodule along the margin of the cyst (*arrow*). (*C*) Axial T1 postcontrast image with fat saturation better shows the enhancing nodule adjacent to the pial surface of the cord (*arrow*).

schwannomas, meningiomas, and ependymomas. Their growth is typically slow, with typical volume increases between 2% and 7% per year. Occasionally, schwannomas can grow rapidly after a longer period of slow growth.[37] Schwannomas are typically eccentric to the nerve fibers. Microscopic evaluation of schwannomas demonstrates a biphasic pattern of alternating sheets of Antoni A and B tissues. Antoni A tissue represents cellular bundles of interlocking fascicles, and Antoni B tissue is recognized by less cellular and myxoid components. Internal cystic change or hemorrhage is common in larger schwannomas.

Spinal schwannomas occur at any level of the spine and are more common in the lumbar region.[35,36] Most schwannomas are small round or larger ovoid masses as they grow along the course of the nerve. They can be very small, measuring several millimeters, to very large, extending through the neural foramen into the paraspinal tissues. The masses demonstrating both an intradural and extradural component are typically dumbbell-shaped with a narrower waist at the neural foramen.[38] The neural foramen in these cases is typically expanded compared with the contralateral side with benign bony remodeling.[39] Most schwannomas are T2 hyperintense and T1 isointense to the adjacent spinal cord. The T2

intensity of the mass can vary depending on the dominate Antoni A, more cellular and less T2 bright, or Antoni B, more myxoid and more T2 bright. As discussed previously, schwannomas can undergo central cystic degeneration during growth and present with focal T2 hyperintense cystic change within the mass. Due to internal vascularity, schwannomas diffusely enhance after contrast administration (**Figs. 5** and **6**). Pattern of enhancement, however, can become heterogeneous or rim type in the setting of internal cystic change or hemorrhage.

Complete surgical removal is the treatment standard of symptomatic spinal schwannomas typically through a posterior approach.[36] Stereotactic radiation can provide safe and long-term control of spinal schwannomas when surgical resection cannot be performed.[40]

Meningioma

Meningiomas are tumors arising from arachnoid cap cells occurring in the dural layers of the thecal sac. Spinal meningioma is the second most common of intradural extramedullary mass after schwannoma.[1] Most spinal meningiomas are benign WHO grade I tumors with rare presentation of more aggressive WHO grade II or III tumors.

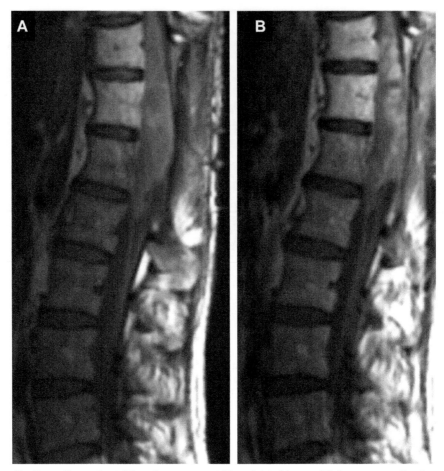

Fig. 4. Ganglioglioma. Precontrast (*A*) and postcontrast T1-weighted image (*B*) shows a ganglioglioma involving most of the inferior thoracic cord with small areas of precontrast T1 hyperintensity and eccentric enhancement greatest along the posterior cord. The heterogenous and eccentric appearance is common with gangliogliomas. (*Courtesy of* L. Shah, MD, Salt Lake City, UT.)

Most spinal meningiomas occur spontaneously but, similar to the previously described ependymomas and schwannomas, multiple meningiomas occur in the setting of neurofibromatosis type 2. Occasionally, multiple meningiomas occur together in the setting of meningiomatosis outside of neurofibromatosis type 2. Most meningiomas exhibit benign behavior, with slow growth and no invasion into the surrounding structures. Progressive growth and compression the cord can result in myelopathic symptoms of sensory or motor defects and less commonly pain.

Spinal meningiomas most commonly occur in middle-aged women, with a greater distribution of women to men, 5:1, compared with intracranial meningiomas.[41] Presentation prior to age 40 may suggest a genetic disorder, such as neurofibromatosis type 2, or more aggressive histology, such as clear cell.[41,42] Meningiomas have multiple histologic subtypes, such as transitional, fibrous, psammomatous, or mengiothelial. Clear cell histology typically affects younger patients and results in higher incidence of recurrence after treatment.[41]

The thoracic spine is the site of up to 80% all spinal meningiomas. The cervical and lumbar spine are involved much less frequently.[43] Meningiomas grow along a broad dural attachment, most commonly located along the lateral thecal sac.[44] Morphology can be focal and masslike or rarely flat en plaque extension along the dura. The dural attachment may be visualized as a tail, or oblique attachment, to the dural surface. On MR imaging, meningiomas are typically T1 isointense and T2 hyperintense in comparison to the spinal cord (**Fig. 7**). Meningiomas and their dural attachment intensely and homogenously enhance. Calcification is rare in spinal meningiomas but, when present, can decrease intensity of T2 signal.[39,45]

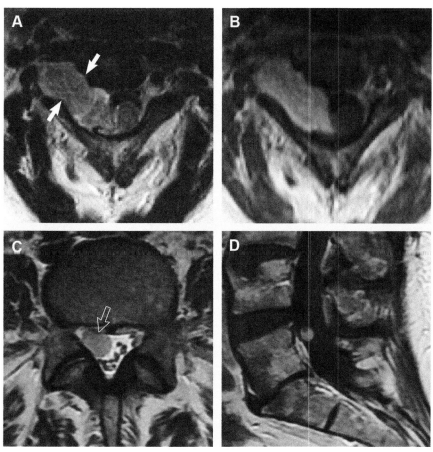

Fig. 5. Schwannoma. (A) Axial T2 image of the cervical spine shows an ovoid hyperintense schwannoma coursing along the intradural and extradural right cervical nerve root. The right neural foramen is expanded when compared with the left (*arrows*). (B) Postcontrast T1 in the same patient demonstrates homogeneous enhancement of the schwannoma. (C) Axial T2 image in a different patient with a schwannoma shows the intradural extramedullary location of a T2 hyperintense mass (*open arrow*) in comparison to the normal nerve roots. (D) Sagittal postcontrast T1 image in second patient shows typical appearance of an enhancing nodule along the cauda equina.

The mainstay of surgical treatment of symptomatic spinal meningiomas is complete surgical resection. Outcomes of resection are related to size of tumor, location, and preoperative neurologic state of patient.[46,47] Stereotactic radiation can be utilized in poor surgical candidates, incomplete resection, or recurrent tumor.[48]

Neurofibroma

Neurofibromas are peripheral nerve sheath tumors with a similar imaging appearance to schwannomas. Neurofibromas are histologically composed of neoplastic schwann cells, fibroblasts, and abundant collagen fibers and cause diffuse enlargement of the nerve root. Unlike schwannomas, neurofibromas do not have a capsule and typically have peripheral nerve fibers intermixed into the tumor.[49] Neurofibromas, similar to the other common intradural extramedullary tumors, are typically benign, WHO grade I tumors with slow growth. The majority of neurofibromas are sporadic and solitary with the remaining patients affected with neurofibromatosis type 1.[50] Neurofibromatosis type 1 is characterized by multiple neurofibromas, optic gliomas, café au lait spots, and multiple spinal abnormalities, such as lateral meningoceles.

Neurofibromas involving the spine can have several different morphologies: a focal nerve sheath mass, diffuse nerve sheath masses, or plexiform masses. Given this variability, the appearance of a neurofibroma can range from a small round or ovoid mass along the course of a spinal nerve to extensive masses along numerous peripheral nerves in multiple different anatomic spaces. MR imaging appearance of neurofibromas is typically T2 hyperintense with variable enhancement.

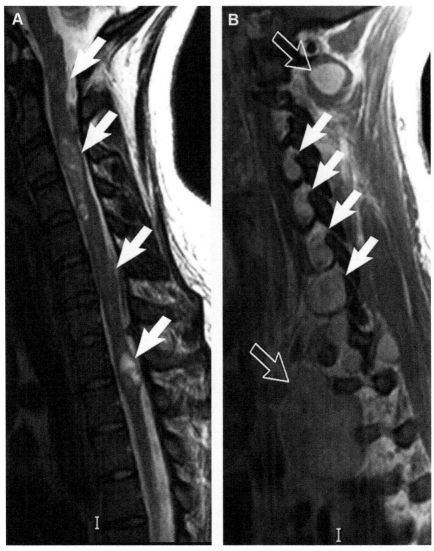

Fig. 6. Neurofibromatosis type 2. (*A*) Midline sagittal T2 image shows multiple hyperintense masses within the central cord consistent with ependymomas (*arrows*) in the setting of neurofibromatosis type 2. (*B*) Sagittal post-contrast T1 off midline in the same patient shows multiple enhancing nerve sheath masses in the neural foramina (*solid white arrows*) and paraspinal soft tissues (*open white arrows*) compatible with schwannomas.

The appearance of the target sign, central T2 hyperintensity with peripheral T2 hypointensity, is highly suggestive of a neurofibroma but not entirely specific as schwannomas can have a similar appearance (**Fig. 8**).[51] The low T2 signal is due to hemorrhage, collagen, and densely packed Schwann cells.[52] Intradural and extramedullary neurofibromas often extend through a widened neural foramen.

Close observation of neurofibromas is currently the treatment of choice. Malignant degeneration of neurofibromas are rare. In the setting of neuro-fibromatosis type 1, however, up to 6% of patients develop a malignant peripheral nerve sheath tumor (MPNST).[53,54] Surgical resection or debulking

of neurofibromas can be considered in symptom-atic patients usually related to compression of sur-rounding structures.

Schwannomas and neurofibromas are often indistinguishable radiographically. Some helpful imaging features to differentiate between the entities are listed in **Table 1**.

Myxopapillary Ependymoma

MPEs usually occur from ependymal cells at the conus medullaris or filum terminale, most commonly appearing as intradural extramedullary lesions despite an intramedullary component. MPEs are the second most common subtype of

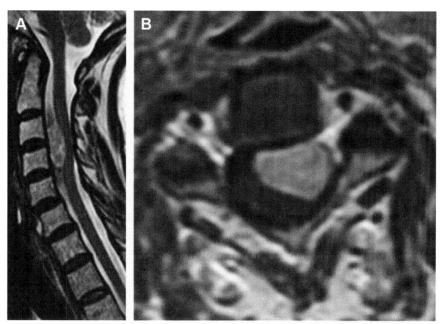

Fig. 7. Meningioma. (*A*) Sagittal T2 image demonstrates a well-circumscribed hyperintense intradural extramedullary meningioma in the anterior thecal sac. (*B*) Axial T1 postcontrast image shows broad dural contact of the enhancing meningioma with compression of the cord.

ependymoma in adults and are considered rare in children.[1,55] These are indolent tumors and often grow large before becoming symptomatic.[56] Histology demonstrates tumor cells with low mitotic

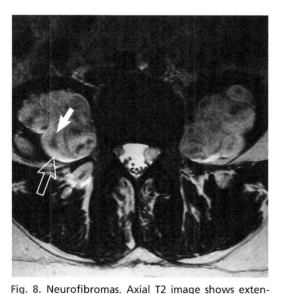

Fig. 8. Neurofibromas. Axial T2 image shows extensive hyperintense neurofibromas in both the intradural extramedullary space as well as the paravertebral soft tissues. The neurofibromas demonstrate a target appearance, with darker center (*solid arrow*) and brighter rim (*open arrow*). This patient has neurofibromatosis type 1.

activity intermixed with mucoid matrix.[49] This mucoid component results in T2 hyperintensity of the mass. Like classic ependymomas, MPEs commonly hemorrhage at the margins of the tumor, which can result in low T2 signal. MPE typically demonstrate intense enhancement in variable patterns related to degree of internal hemorrhage (**Fig. 9**). These tumors are low grade and slow growing and can expand and remodel the spinal canal or neural foramina.

Less Common Intradural Extramedullary Tumors

Several additional rare masses occur in the intradural extramedullary space of the spine. As discussed previously, MPNSTs can form from neurofibromas or schwannomas. MPNSTs occur in the same locations as benign nerve sheath tumors and can be intradural extramedullary, extradural, or paraspinal. Malignant degeneration may be suspected with increase in size or imaging characteristics of nerve sheath tumors.[57]

MR imaging features that have been described to distinguish MPNSTs from neurofibromas are increased largest dimension of the mass, presence of peripheral enhanced pattern, presence of perilesional edema-like zone, and presence of intratumoral cystic lesion.[57] Elevated fludeoxyglucose F 18 uptake on PET imaging should also increase suspicion for MPNST.[50]

Table 1
Imaging features of schwannomas and neurofibromas

	CT	MR Imaging
Schwannoma	• Foraminal enlargement • Pedicular erosion • Posterior vertebral scalloping • Thinned lamina	• Hemorrhage • Cyst formation • Fatty degeneration • Displace the nerve roots due to their asymmetric growth • T1 isointense to hypointense • Markedly T2/short tau inversion recovery hyperintense; mixed T2 signal • Intense homogeneous enhancement
Neurofibroma	• Foraminal enlargement • Pedicular erosion • Posterior vertebral scalloping • Thinned lamina	• Encase the nerve roots in a fusiform manner • T1 isointense to hypointense • Markedly T2/short tau inversion recovery hyperintense • Target sign • Peripheral enhancement

Intradural lipomas appear similar to lipomas elsewhere in the body with fat density on CT, T1 bright signal on noncontrast MR imaging, and lack of enhancement. Intradural lipomas are typically juxtamedullary and subpial in location but can rarely be intramedullary. They may be associated with dysraphic defects in lumbar spine, and patients present with neurologic deficits (ie, numbness, extremity spastic weakness, and back pain) due to cord compression in the cervical and thoracic spine. Filum fibrolipomas are small and linear fatty lesions closely associated with the filum terminale. Although typically incidental, in some individuals, it is associated with spinal dysraphism and tethered cord syndrome.

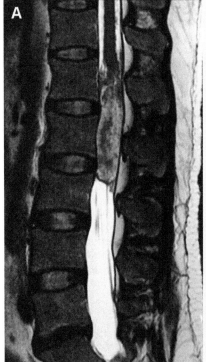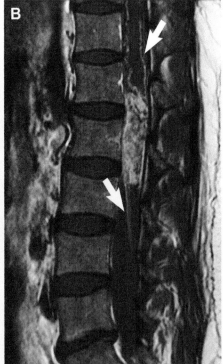

Fig. 9. MPE. (*A*) Sagittal T2 image demonstrates a well-circumscribed MPE with heterogeneous internal signal. (*B*) Sagittal T1 image postcontrast shows the MPE with heterogeneous enhancement. Linear and nodular enhancement along the distal cord and cauda equina is due to CSF spread of tumor (*arrows*).

Spinal paragangliomas are rare intradural extramedullary spinal mass lesions, most often occurring in the region of the cauda equina. These well-defined hypervascular masses demonstrate intense enhancement and can be indistinguishable from MPEs. T2-weighted images may show prominent flow voids or findings of previous hemorrhage, such as internal cystic change or dark signal from hemosiderin deposition (**Fig. 10**).

EXTRADURAL TUMORS

A majority of extradural lesions originate from the surrounding vertebral structures and secondarily extend into the epidural space, such as osseous metastatic disease, primary osseous or cartilaginous neoplasms, infectious processes, or fibrosis from previous vertebral segment surgical intervention. These lesions are discussed in other articles of this issue. Primary extradural tumors of the spine are rare, constituting approximately 4% of spinal tumors.[58]

Nonosseous Extradural Tumors

Most nonosseous tumors primary to the extradural space are nerve sheath tumors from spinal nerve roots near the neural foramen, discussed previously. Other rare nonosseous extradural tumors include neuroblastoma and angiolipoma.

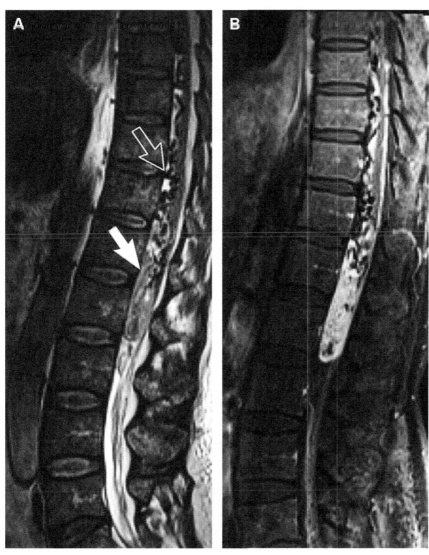

Fig. 10. Paraganglioma. (*A*) Sagittal T2 image shows a well circumscribed hyperintense paraganglioma (*solid arrow*) which appears similar to MPE. Paragangliomas often have associated enlarged flow voids (*open arrow*). (*B*) Sagittal T1 postcontrast images with fat saturation shows intense enhancement of the mass with redemonstrations of the large flow voids.

Neuroblastic tumors include neuroblastoma, ganglioneuroblastoma, and ganglioneuroma. Neuroblastic tumors are primarily pediatric diagnoses, most common in the first several years of life and rare after the age of 10 years.[59] These tumors arise from neural crest progenitor cells related to the sympathetic nervous system. Neuroblastic tumors commonly occur in the paraspinal tissue and extend into the extradural space through the neural foramina, resulting in a dumbbell-shaped appearance. Imaging demonstrates a well-defined enhancing mass with variable soft tissue characteristics (**Fig. 11**).

Angiolipomas are rare benign masses with both vascular and adipose components. Angiolipomas most frequently involve the extremities or neck and less frequently the extradural space. When involving the spine, angiolipomas are most common in the thoracic spine and typically extend up to 4 vertebral bodies in length.[60] Lipomatous components demonstrate fat density on CT and T1 hyperintensity. Vascular components show enhancement and best visualized on T1-weighted images with fat suppression. Flow voids are not typically identified in relation to angiolipomas (**Fig. 12**).

OTHER SPINAL TUMORS

Several spinal tumors, such as metastases, lymphoma, and/or leukemia, can involve all spinal spaces. The appearance of these masses varies depending on the spinal location of involvement.

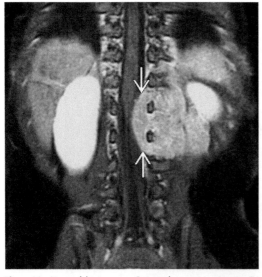

Fig. 11. Neuroblastoma. Coronal postcontrast T1 with fat saturation demonstrates homogeneously enhancing neuroblastoma involving the extradural space (*arrows*) contiguous with a large paraspinal component via extension through the neural foramina. (*Courtesy of* L. Shah, MD, Salt Lake City, UT.)

Metastasis

The spinal cord is a rare location for metastatic disease. Spinal cord metastases are most commonly from lung cancer, focally enhance, and demonstrate extensive adjacent T2 hyperintense cord edema. Asymptomatic presentation without previously identified primary tumor site is not uncommon.[61] The presence of hemorrhage or cystic change is rare with metastases and suggestive of another intramedullary tumor, such as an ependymoma. The rim sign of more intense rim of peripheral enhancement and flame sign of flamelike enhancement at rostral and caudal margins are more common with metastases compared with primary cord masses.[62] Metastases can be solitary or multiple even with an asymptomatic presentation.

Intradural extramedullary metastases include (1) leptomeningeal disease and (2) solitary intradural extramedullary lesions from non-CNS tumors.[63] The latter are rare and have a longer overall survival than leptomeningeal metastases. Leptomeningeal disease has become increasingly prevalent, because novel therapeutic interventions extend the survival of cancer patients.

Metastatic disease in this location can result from multiple routes of spread. Leptomeningeal metastatic disease results from CSF dissemination of neoplastic cells through the subarachnoid space either from CNS tumors contiguous with the subarachnoid space or through lymphovascular deposition. Hematogenous spread of metastases is most common with lung and breast cancers as well as melanoma. CNS tumors with highest risk of leptomeningeal spread include medulloblastoma, germinoma, and ependymoma. CSF cytology after lumbar puncture is poorly sensitive, is positive in as low as 40% of evaluations, and may necessitate repeat evaluation or resampling of CSF from a site closer in proximity to the abnormality.[64]

Isolated extradural metastases are rare. Extraosseous extension of metastases into the epidural space, however, is not uncommon (**Fig. 13**).

Lymphoma

Nonosseous spinal lymphoma is rare and can either represent primary disease or spread of extraspinal sources. Lymphoma can affect any area of the spinal canal, and the appearance varies based on the affected location. The extradural space is more commonly involved with nonosseous lymphoma, with decreasing frequency of involvement within the intradural extramedullary space and intramedullary cord. Non-Hodgkin

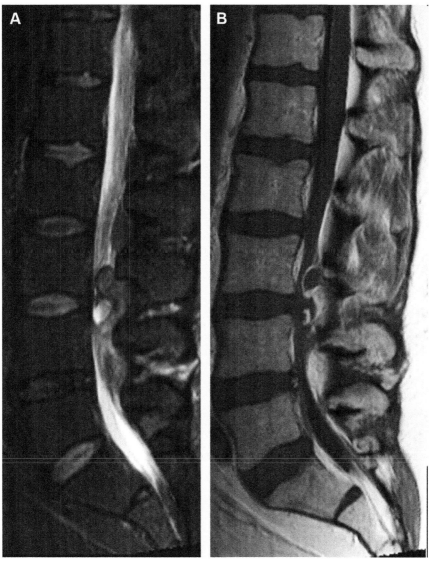

Fig. 12. Angiolipoma. (*A*) Sagittal T2 image with fat suppression demonstrates a mixed intensity poorly margin-ated posterior extradural mass with mass effect on the thecal sac. (*B*) Postcontrast T1 image demonstrates T1 bright signal throughout the extradural mass with focal cyst at the superior aspect. Fatty component show T1 hyperintensity and vascular components intensely enhance. (*Courtesy of* L. Shah, MD, Salt Lake City, UT.)

lymphoma is more common than Hodgkin disease in the spine.[65–68]

Intramedullary lymphoma most commonly in-volves the cervical cord with decreasing incidence of the thoracic and lumbar cord. Lesions are typi-cally ill defined, enhancing, T2 hyperintense to the surrounding cord, and surrounded by vasogenic edema (**Fig. 14**). Intramedullary involvement may be multifocal as well.[65]

Intradural lymphoma commonly presents as lymphomatous meningitis. Multiple small nodules or smooth continuous coating of the pial surface

of the cord and nerve roots. Leptomeningeal lym-phoma appear similar to other forms of leptome-ningeal carcinomatosis.

Extradural lymphoma is the most common non-osseous presentation of spinal lymphoma. Thoracic involvement is most common with decreasing occurrence in the lumbar and cervical epidural spaces respectively. Epidural lymphoma often extends multiple vertebral segments and frequently extends through neural foramina. MR imaging characteristics are typically T1 and T2 iso-intense to the cord with homogenous and intense

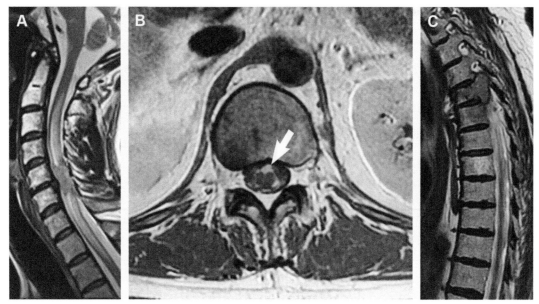

Fig. 13. .Metastases. (*A*) Intramedullary metastasis. Sagittal T2 image demonstrates an intramedullary and extramedullary metastasis in a patient with breast cancer and associated cord edema. (*B*) Intradural extramedullary metastases. Nodular enhancing metastases from an intracranial ependymoma from CSF spread of tumor coat the conus medullaris (*arrow*). (*C*) Extradural metastasis. An osseous metastasis from renal cell carcinoma extends out of the cortex of the bone into the epidural fat and neural foramen.

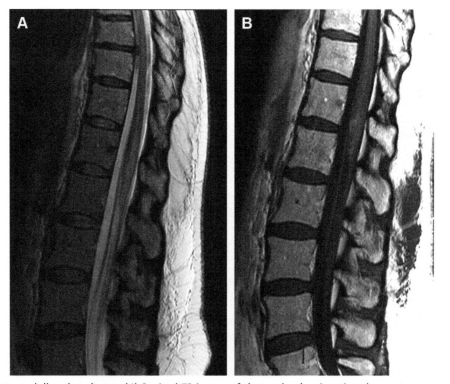

Fig. 14. Intramedullary lymphoma. (*A*) Sagittal T2 image of thoracolumbar junction demonstrates expansile T2 hyperintensities extending into the conus medullaris. (*B*) Sagittal postcontrast T1 image shows patchy ill-defined enhancement with the region of signal abnormality in a patient with angiotrophic lymphoma. (*Courtesy of* L. Shah, MD, Salt Lake City, UT.)

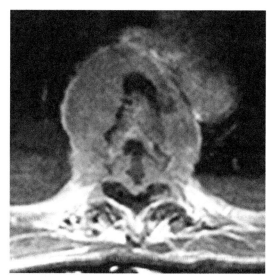

Fig. 15. Extradural lymphoma. Axial T1 postcontrast image shows epidural, osseous, and paravertebral enhancing soft tissue in a patient with non-Hodgkin lymphoma. Extradural lymphoma often involves the adjacent osseous structures.

enhancement. There may or may not be adjacent bone involvement (**Fig. 15**).

Leukemia

Nonosseous leukemia is also rare in the spinal canal. Leukemia can present in the spine as a focal granulocytic sarcomatous mass, also known as a chloroma. When present, this focal leukemic mass typically accompanies acute myeloid leukemia.[69] This most frequently occurs in the extradural space but also occurs as an intradural extramedullary mass either involving the dura or along the cauda equina nerve roots. MR imaging characteristics of granulocytic sarcomas are T1 isointense to muscle, intermediate T2 signal, and homogeneous enhancement. Patients typically have bone marrow findings of leukemic infiltrate on initial presentation of granulocytic sarcoma; however, patients in remission with development of a focal leukemic mass do not typically demonstrate marrow involvement.[63]

SUMMARY

Intraspinal tumors are not common in the general population and present with nonspecific symptoms, such as back pain, radicular symptoms, or paresthesias. Localization of an intraspinal mass to the intramedullary, intradural extramedullary, or extradural space together with MR imaging characterization can often lead to a diagnosis. Benign intradural extramedullary nerve sheath tumors, such as schwannoma and neurofibroma,

together with meningiomas make up a majority of intraspinal tumors. Ependymomas are the most common intramedullary tumor in adults, with astrocytomas more common in the pediatric population. Intraspinal metastases, lymphoma, and leukemia can occur in any intraspinal location.

REFERENCES

1. Weber C, Gulati S, Jakola AS, et al. Incidence rates and surgery of primary intraspinal tumors in the era of modern neuroimaging: a national population-based study. Spine 2014;39(16):E967–73.
2. Engelhard HH, Villano JL, Porter KR, et al. Clinical presentation, histology, and treatment in 430 patients with primary tumors of the spinal cord, spinal meninges, or cauda equina. J Neurosurg Spine 2010;13(1):67–77.
3. Wald JT. Imaging of spine neoplasm. Radiol Clin North Am 2012;50(4):749–76.
4. Mechtler LL, Nandigam K. Spinal cord tumors: new views and future directions. Neurol Clin 2013;31(1):241–68.
5. Duong LM, McCarthy BJ, McLendon RE, et al. Descriptive epidemiology of malignant and nonmalignant primary spinal cord, spinal meninges, and cauda equina tumors, United States, 2004-2007. Cancer 2012;118(17):4220–7.
6. Van Goethem JWM, van den Hauwe L, Özsarlak Ö, et al. Spinal tumors. Eur J Radiol 2004;50(2):159–76.
7. Huisman TA. Pediatric tumors of the spine. Cancer Imaging 2009;9(Spec No A):S45–8.
8. Louis DN, Perry A, Reifenberger G, et al. The 2016 World Health Organization classification of tumors of the central nervous system: a summary. Acta Neuropathol 2016;131(6):803–20.
9. Oh MC, Kim JM, Kaur G, et al. Prognosis by tumor location in adults with spinal ependymomas. J Neurosurg Spine 2013;18(3):226–35.
10. Plotkin SR, O'Donnell CC, Curry WT, et al. Spinal ependymomas in neurofibromatosis Type 2: a retrospective analysis of 55 patients. J Neurosurg Spine 2011;14(4):543–7.
11. Klekamp J. Spinal ependymomas. Part 1: intramedullary ependymomas. Neurosurg Focus 2015;39(2):E6.
12. Gilbert MR, Ruda R, Soffietti R. Ependymomas in adults. Curr Neurol Neurosci Rep 2010;10(3):240–7.
13. Sun B, Wang C, Wang J, et al. MRI features of intramedullary spinal cord ependymomas. J Neuroimaging 2003;13(4):346–51.
14. Kahan H, Sklar EM, Post MJ, et al. MR characteristics of histopathologic subtypes of spinal ependymoma. AJNR Am J Neuroradiol 1996;17(1):143–50.
15. Yuh EL, Barkovich AJ, Gupta N. Imaging of ependymomas: MRI and CT. Childs Nerv Syst 2009;25(10):1203–13.

16. Tarapore PE, Modera P, Naujokas A, et al. Pathology of spinal ependymomas. Neurosurgery 2013;73(2): 247–55.

17. Oh MC, Tarapore PE, Kim JM, et al. Spinal ependymomas: benefits of extent of resection for different histological grades. J Clin Neurosci 2013;20(10): 1390–7.

18. Wahab SH, Simpson JR, Michalski JM, et al. Long term outcome with post-operative radiation therapy for spinal canal ependymoma. J Neurooncol 2007; 83(1):85–9.

19. Smith AB, Soderlund KA, Rushing EJ, et al. Radiologic-pathologic correlation of pediatric and adolescent spinal neoplasms: part 1, intramedullary spinal neoplasms. AJR Am J Roentgenol 2012;198(1): 34–43.

20. Arun D, Gutmann DH. Recent advances in neurofibromatosis type 1. Curr Opin Neurol 2004;17(2): 101–5.

21. Asthagiri AR, Parry DM, Butman JA, et al. Neurofibromatosis type 2. Lancet 2009;373(9679):1974–86.

22. Babu R, Karikari IO, Owens TR, et al. Spinal cord astrocytomas. Spine 2014;39(7):533–40.

23. Rossi A, Gandolfo C, Morana G, et al. Tumors of the spine in children. Neuroimaging Clin N Am 2007; 17(1):17–35.

24. Zhou H, Miller D, Schulte DM, et al. Intraoperative ultrasound assistance in treatment of intradural spinal tumours. Clin Neurol Neurosurg 2011;113(7): 531–7.

25. Deng X, Wang K, Wu L, et al. Intraspinal hemangioblastomas: analysis of 92 cases in a single institution: clinical article. J Neurosurg Spine 2014;21(2): 260–9.

26. Miller DJ, McCutcheon IE. Hemangioblastomas and other uncommon intramedullary tumors. J Neurooncol 2000;47(3):253–70.

27. Westwick HJ, Giguère J-F, Shamji MF. Incidence and prognosis of spinal hemangioblastoma: a surveillance epidemiology and end results study. Neuroepidemiology 2016;46(1):14–23.

28. Vassiliou V, Papamichael D, Polyviou P, et al. Intramedullary spinal cord metastasis in a patient with colon cancer: a case report. J Gastrointest Cancer 2012;43:370–2.

29. Chu BC, Terae S, Hida K, et al. MR findings in spinal hemangioblastoma: correlation with symptoms and with angiographic and surgical findings. AJNR Am J Neuroradiol 2001;22(1):206–17.

30. Sun HÌ, Özduman K, Usseli MÌ, et al. Sporadic spinal hemangioblastomas can be effectively treated by microsurgery alone. World Neurosurg 2014;82(5): 836–47.

31. Wilson MA, Cooke DL, Ghodke B, et al. Retrospective analysis of preoperative embolization of spinal tumors. AJNR Am J Neuroradiol 2010;31(4):656–60.

32. Bridges KJ, Jaboin JJ, Kubicky CD, et al. Stereotactic radiosurgery versus surgical resection for spinal hemangioblastoma: a systematic review. Clin Neurol Neurosurg 2017;154:59–66.

33. Gessi M, Dörner E, Dreschmann V, et al. Intramedullary gangliogliomas: histopathologic and molecular features of 25 cases. Hum Pathol 2016;49: 107–13.

34. Oppenheimer D, Johnson M, Judkins A. Ganglioglioma of the spinal cord. J Clin Imaging Sci 2015; 5(1):53–5.

35. Jinnai T, Koyama T. Clinical characteristics of spinal nerve sheath tumors: analysis of 149 cases. Neurosurgery 2005;56(3):510–5 [discussion: 510–5].

36. Lenzi J, Anichini G, Landi A, et al. Spinal nerves schwannomas: experience on 367 cases—historic overview on how clinical, radiological, and surgical practices have changed over a course of 60 years. Neurol Res Int 2017;2017(1):1–12.

37. Ando K, Imagama S, Ito Z, et al. How do spinal schwannomas progress? The natural progression of spinal schwannomas on MRI. J Neurosurg Spine 2016;24(1):155–9.

38. Kobayashi K, Imagama S, Ando K, et al. Contrast MRI findings for spinal schwannoma as predictors of tumor proliferation and motor status. Spine 2017;42(3):E150–5.

39. Liu WC, Choi G, Lee S-H, et al. Radiological findings of spinal schwannomas and meningiomas: focus on discrimination of two disease entities. Eur Radiol 2009;19(11):2707–15.

40. Sachdev S, Dodd RL, Chang SD, et al. Stereotactic radiosurgery yields long-term control for benign intradural, extramedullary spinal tumors. Neurosurgery 2011;69(3):533–9.

41. Barresi V, Alafaci C, Caffo M, et al. Clinicopathological characteristics, hormone receptor status and matrix metallo-proteinase-9 (MMP-9) immunohistochemical expression in spinal meningiomas. Pathol Res Pract 2012;208(6):350–5.

42. Maiuri F, Del Basso De Caro ML, de Divitiis O, et al. Spinal meningiomas: age-related features. Clin Neurol Neurosurg 2011;113(1):34–8.

43. Ravindra VM, Schmidt MH. Management of spinal meningiomas. Neurosurg Clin N Am 2016;27(2): 195–205.

44. Maiti TK, Bir SC, Patra DP, et al. Spinal meningiomas: clinicoradiological factors predicting recurrence and functional outcome. Neurosurg Focus 2016;41(2):E6–10.

45. De Verdelhan O, Haegelen C, Carsin-Nicol B, et al. MR imaging features of spinal schwannomas and meningiomas. J Neuroradiol 2005;32(1):42–9.

46. Nakamura M, Tsuji O, Fujiyoshi K, et al. Long-term surgical outcomes of spinal meningiomas. Spine 2012;37(10):E617–23.

47. Riad H, Knafo S, Segnarbieux F, et al. Spinal menin-giomas: surgical outcome and literature review. Neurochirurgie 2013;59(1):30–4.

48. Noh SH, Kim KH, Shin DA, et al. Treatment out-comes of 17 patients with atypical spinal meningi-oma, including 4 with metastases: a retrospective observational study. Spine J 2018. https://doi.org/10.1016/j.spinee.2018.06.006.

49. Soderlund KA, Smith AB, Rushing EJ, et al. Radio-logic-pathologic correlation of pediatric and adoles-cent spinal neoplasms: part 2, intradural extramedullary spinal neoplasms. AJR Am J Roent-genol 2012;198(1):44–51.

50. Ferner RE, O'Doherty MJ. Neurofibroma and schwannoma. Curr Opin Neurol 2002;15(6):679–84.

51. Bhargava R, Parham DM, Lasater OE, et al. MR im-aging differentiation of benign and malignant pe-ripheral nerve sheath tumors: use of the target sign. Pediatr Radiol 1997;27(2):124–9.

52. Bloomer CW, Ackerman A, Bhatia AG. Imaging for spine tumors and new applications. Top Magn Re-son Imaging 2006;17(2):69–87.

53. Khong P-L, Goh WHS, Wong VCN, et al. MR imaging of spinal tumors in children with neurofibromatosis 1. AJR Am J Roentgenol 2003;180(2):413–7.

54. Ruggieri M, Polizzi A, Spalice A, et al. The natural history of spinal neurofibromatosis: a critical review of clinical and genetic features. Clin Genet 2014; 87(5):401–10.

55. Lucchesi KM, Grant R, Kahle KT, et al. Primary spi-nal myxopapillary ependymoma in the pediatric population: a study from the Surveillance, Epidemi-ology, and End Results (SEER) database. J Neurooncol 2016;130(1):133–40.

56. Klekamp J. Spinal ependymomas. Part 2: ependy-momas of the filum terminale. Neurosurg Focus 2015;39(2):E7.

57. Wasa J, Nishida Y, Tsukushi S, et al. MRI features in the differentiation of malignant peripheral nerve sheath tumors and neurofibromas. AJR Am J Roent-genol 2010;194(6):1568–74.

58. Kelley SP, Ashford RU, Rao AS, et al. Primary bone tumours of the spine: a 42-year survey from the Leeds Regional Bone Tumour Registry. Eur Spine J 2007;16:405–9.

59. Trahair T, Sorrentino S, Russell SJ, et al. Spinal canal involvement in neuroblastoma. J Pediatr 2017;188: 294–8.

60. Wang FF, Wang S, Xue WH, et al. Epidural spinal an-giolipoma: a case series. BMC Res Notes 2017; 10(1):128.

61. Rykken JB, Diehn FE, Hunt CH, et al. Intramedullary spinal cord metastases: MRI and relevant clinical features from a 13-year institutional case series. AJNR Am J Neuroradiol 2013;34(10):2043–9.

62. Rykken JB, Diehn FE, Hunt CH, et al. Rim and flame signs: postgadolinium MRI findings specific for non-CNS intramedullary spinal cord metastases. AJNR Am J Neuroradiol 2013;34(4):908–15.

63. Knafo S, Pallud J, Le Rhun E, et al. Intradural extra-medullary spinal metastases of non-neurogenic origin. Neurosurgery 2013;73(6):923–32.

64. Bae YS, Cheong J-W, Chang WS, et al. Diagnostic accuracy of cerebrospinal fluid (CSF) cytology in metastatic tumors: an analysis of consecutive CSF samples. Korean J Pathol 2013;47(6):563–7.

65. Flanagan EP, O'Neill BP, Porter AB, et al. Primary in-tramedullary spinal cord lymphoma. Neurology 2011;77(8):784–91.

66. Flanagan EP, O'Neill BP, Habermann TM, et al. Sec-ondary intramedullary spinal cord non-Hodgkin's lymphoma. J Neurooncol 2011;107(3):575–80.

67. Taylor JW, Flanagan EP, O'Neill BP, et al. Primary leptomeningeal lymphoma: International Primary CNS Lymphoma Collaborative Group report. Neurology 2013;81(19):1690–6.

68. Le Xiong, Liao L-M, Ding J-W, et al. Clinicopatho-logic characteristics and prognostic factors for pri-mary spinal epidural lymphoma: report on 36 Chinese patients and review of the literature. BMC Cancer 2017;17(1):131.

69. Yilmaz AF, Saydam G, Sahin F, et al. Granulocytic sarcoma: a systematic review. Am J Blood Res 2013;3(4):265–70.

Spinal Marrow Imaging
Clues to Disease

Richard L. Leake, MD*, Megan K. Mills, MD, Christopher J. Hanrahan, MD, PhD

KEYWORDS

• Marrow replacement • Spinal marrow • Spine pathology

KEY POINTS

- The adult spine is made up of predominantly fatty marrow with T1 hyperintensity, T2 hyperintensity, and hypointensity on fat-saturated or short-tau inversion recovery sequences.
- Diffuse marrow replacement may be the result of cellular deposition or depletion, such as in multiple myeloma or osteoporosis, respectively.
- Focal marrow replacement can occur with benign entities, such as intraosseous hemangioma, disk degeneration, or fracture. Malignant focal marrow replacement is most commonly seen in the setting of metastatic disease.

INTRODUCTION

Spinal bone marrow is often an afterthought when it comes to evaluation of spine MR imaging. Interpretation focuses on degenerative disk disease, facet arthropathy, and avoidance of missing important extradural or intradural pathology that may result in significant neurologic compromise. This article reviews the expected appearance and maturation of spinal bone marrow, the pathologic appearance of spinal marrow, and the differential diagnosis of marrow abnormalities with the goal of making the reader more comfortable with spinal marrow imaging evaluation. Although this article focuses primarily on the MR imaging characteristics of spinal marrow disease processes, radiographic and computed tomography (CT) evaluation are important adjuncts to MR imaging and in certain instances may even provide improved disease characterization.

MR IMAGING PROTOCOLS

Routine MR imaging sequences used everyday practice provide ample spinal marrow evaluation. Most routine protocols include sagittal T1-weighted, T2-weighted, and short-tau inversion recovery (STIR) sequences, with some practices replacing the sagittal T1-weighted with a T1 fluid-attenuated inversion recovery (T1 FLAIR) sequence.[1] The use of T1-weighted or T1 FLAIR sequences is currently based on practice preference. The T1 FLAIR sequence is favored in the literature for its distinct depiction of cord pathology and higher contrast within spinal marrow.[2] The STIR sequence is very sensitive to evaluate spinal marrow for edema from contusion/fracture or degeneration or from cellular marrow changes related to neoplasm or treatment (chemotherapy or radiation).

Other nontraditional sequences can provide additional help in the assessment of marrow abnormalities and include diffusion-weighted imaging (DWI) and chemical shift, or phase-imaging. Continuing advancements in MR imaging technology have enabled improved DWI imaging in the spine with reduced artifacts.[3] Clinically, DWI can help distinguish degenerative disk disease from osteomyelitis based on the pattern of diffusion restriction.[4] Chemical shift imaging is a simple

Disclosure Statement: Authors have no commercial or financial conflicts of interest to disclose.
Department of Radiology and Imaging Sciences, University of Utah, 30 North 1900 East #1A071, Salt Lake City, UT 84132, USA
* Corresponding author.
E-mail address: Richard.Leake@hsc.utah.edu

Radiol Clin N Am 57 (2019) 359–375
https://doi.org/10.1016/j.rcl.2018.09.008
0033-8389/19/© 2018 Elsevier Inc. All rights reserved.

addition to routine sequences and has little time penalty.[5] Chemical shift imaging includes in-phase images, where the signal from water and fat within the same voxel are additive, and out-of-phase images, where the signal between fat and water cancels out. Any voxel containing both water and fat will have little signal on out-of-phase images (dark), whereas a voxel with only fat or only water will be bright on the out-of-phase image. This is helpful for distinguishing pathology, particularly if a lesion has no grossly apparent internal fat. In this scenario, if there is a greater than 20% signal decrease when comparing the in-phase image with the out-of-phase image, the spinal marrow lesion is overwhelmingly benign.[6]

NORMAL MARROW

To understand the normal spinal MR imaging appearance, it is helpful to remember the main constituents of bone marrow. The major components include fat and water, which provide adequate MR imaging contrast to recognize normal from abnormal marrow. The content of fat is determined by the maturation of bone marrow. At birth, the bone marrow is highly cellular or so-called red marrow, containing only 40% macroscopic fat. With aging, there is conversion to fatty marrow, so-called yellow marrow, containing 80% fat.[7] In the extremities, this occurs in a distal to proximal fashion with persistence of cellular marrow in the proximal appendicular skeleton into adulthood. In the spinal marrow, fully cellular marrow is present at birth and conversion to fatty marrow occurs adjacent to the basivertebral plexus, usually between adolescence and age 40.[8] After age 40, conversion to fatty marrow through the remainder of the vertebral body begins. This process occurs through 1 of 3 patterns: (1) micronodular, (2) macronodular, or (3) peripheral followed by a nodular pattern.[8] In the elderly, a higher proportion of fat is present within the spinal marrow.[8]

SPINAL MARROW PATHOLOGY

Pathologic marrow can be either cellular proliferation/infiltration or cellular depletion. Because a strength of spinal MR imaging is depicting the contrast between fat and water, pathology is recognized by changes in these fundamental components of spinal marrow. Proliferative marrow processes result in increased cellular elements and, hence, increased water content, whereas depletive processes decrease cellular content and increase fat within the marrow.

Proliferative Pathologic Marrow

Abnormal marrow is primarily identified by the decrease in T1 signal compared with surrounding normal fat, such that the signal is equal to or less than the signal of the adjacent disk or paraspinal musculature. If the area of concern/lesion is of lower signal intensity than that of muscle/disk, it also typically has increased STIR signal. This can range from the obvious in which there are multiple lesions in the bone marrow, or clear extension of disease through the vertebral body cortex to more subtle abnormalities. In areas in which the signal meets the previous criteria but is subtle, chemical shift imaging can be helpful. In the case of pathologic marrow, the chemical shift imaging demonstrates persistent bright signal on the out-of-phase images when pathologic or cellular marrow is present, whereas benign entities, such as red marrow, would show greater than 20% signal dropout on out-of-phase images.[6] Contrast enhancement can be helpful in some cases but is not necessary to confirm pathologic marrow. More importantly, contrast can help identify paraspinal or epidural extension of disease.[9]

Bone Marrow Depletion

In contrast to proliferation, marrow-depletive processes increase the amount of fat within the marrow and include iatrogenic causes, such as radiation, as well as metabolic abnormalities, such as osteomalacia or osteoporosis. By reducing cellular/water content, these processes demonstrate increased fat in the spinal marrow and, thus, increased T1 signal. In the case of radiation, fatty changes are confined to the radiation field/port. With metabolic or poor nutritional states, the process is more diffuse in the marrow.

Benign Diffuse Marrow Replacement

Osteoporosis
Osteoporosis is a metabolic disease of bone characterized by decreased bone mass and altered microarchitecture, which leads to increased fragility and risk of fracture.[10] As the bone undergoes the changes of osteoporosis, the cellular marrow contents are replaced with intramedullary fat. T1-weighted, non–fat-saturated (FS) sequences demonstrate heterogeneous, predominantly hyperintense signal from the fatty marrow replacement (**Fig. 1**). T2-weighted, non-FS sequences (such as fast spin echo and turbo spin echo) typically demonstrate heterogeneous signal similar to the T1-weighted sequences, but this can vary from person to person. With FS or STIR sequences, the fat content of the marrow is

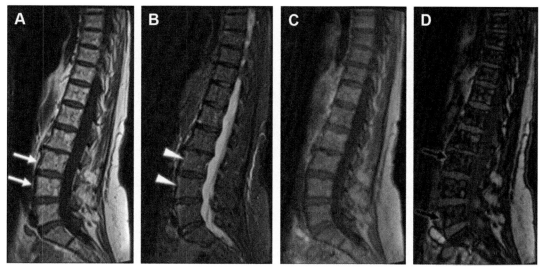

Fig. 1. MR imaging of osteoporosis, DEXA proven. (A) Sagittal T1-weighted image of the lumbar spine demonstrates heterogeneous, predominantly hyperintense marrow signal (*white arrows*). (B) Sagittal STIR image demonstrates heterogeneous, predominantly hypointense marrow signal (*white arrowheads*). Sagittal T1 in (C) and (D) out-of-phase sequences demonstrate heterogeneous marrow signal with loss of signal on the out-of-phase sequence (*black arrows*) secondary to fatty marrow.

predominantly hypointense when compared with normal marrow or skeletal muscle.[11,12] Chemical shift imaging also demonstrates heterogeneous marrow signal in osteoporosis with drop out of signal on the out-of-phase sequences due to the differences in precession of fat and water.[13]

Myelofibrosis

Myelofibrosis is a chronic myeloproliferative disorder of hematopoietic stem cells characterized by reactive bone marrow fibrosis secondary to abnormal cytokine secretion. It is associated with polycythemia vera, essential thrombocytopenia, chemotherapy, radiation therapy, multiple myeloma, leukemia, or metastatic disease.[14] The primary form of myelofibrosis is known as myelofibrosis with myeloid metaplasia or idiopathic myelofibrosis. Angiogenesis, osteosclerosis, and extramedullary hematopoiesis are common findings in idiopathic and secondary myelofibrosis.[15] MR imaging in primary and secondary myelofibrosis shows hypointense T1 and T2 marrow signal on non--at-suppressed sequences (**Fig. 2**). On fat-suppressed and postcontrast T1-weighted sequences, the bone marrow can demonstrate isointense to mildly hyperintense signal relative to the adjacent intervertebral disk and skeletal muscle.[16]

Mastocytosis

Systemic mastocytosis is a rare group of disorders characterized by abnormal mast cell proliferation throughout the body. Mastocytosis can

occur with or without other hematologic disorders, myeloproliferative neoplasms, myelodysplastic syndrome, or lymphoma and leukemia.[17] Bone marrow involvement is seen in up to 90% of patients with systemic mastocytosis. The disease is characterized by fibroblastic activity and granulomatous reaction secondary to increased cytokine secretion. This results in trabecular destruction with lytic lesions and osteoporosis or new bone formation leading to osteosclerosis.[18] MR imaging in patients with systemic mastocytosis is nonspecific and can demonstrate homogeneous or heterogeneous marrow signal intensity, typically with hypointense T1 and T2 signal (**Fig. 3**). In cases of less-extensive marrow infiltration and fibroblast proliferation, the T2 and STIR signal can be hyperintense compared with muscle.[17,18]

Gaucher disease

Gaucher disease is an autosomal recessive lysosomal storage disorder characterized by decreased activity of glucocerebrosidase (acid β-glucosidase), a lysosomal hydrolase, with resultant accumulation of glucocerebroside-laden macrophages in the liver, spleen, and bone.[19] Skeletal abnormalities are seen in most of these patients and can be debilitating. Bone marrow changes in Gaucher disease are secondary to infiltration and replacement of the fatty marrow by glucocerebrosidase-laden macrophages, or Gaucher cells.[20] MR imaging shows replacement of the normal hyperintense T1

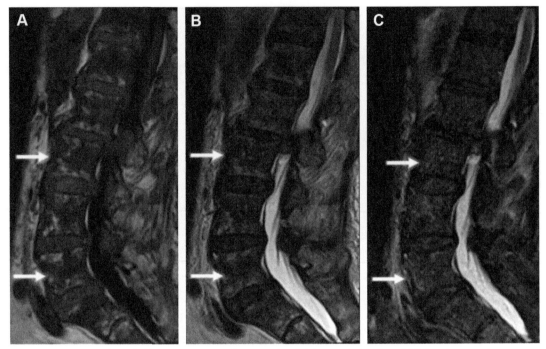

Fig. 2. MR imaging of myelofibrosis. (*A*) Sagittal T1-weighted, (*B*) T2-weighted, and (*C*) STIR images demonstrate diffuse heterogeneous, predominantly hypointense marrow signal on all sequences (*arrows*).

fatty marrow signal with hypointense T1/T2 signal (**Fig. 4**).[19] Endplate osteonecrosis is commonly seen in patients with Gaucher disease. In patients with active pain related to Gaucher disease, T2 and STIR sequences can demonstrate focal areas of T2/STIR hyperintense signal, which may reflect

an active disease process, bone crisis, fracture, or infection.[12]

Hemosiderosis
Hemosiderosis is caused by excess cellular deposition of iron. This can be due to chronic blood

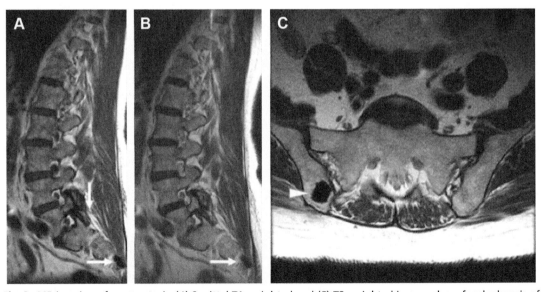

Fig. 3. MR imaging of mastocytosis. (*A*) Sagittal T1-weighted and (*B*) T2-weighted images show focal sclerosis of the S3 vertebral body (*arrow*). (*C*) Axial T2-weighted images shows focal sclerosis of the right iliac bone (*arrowhead*).

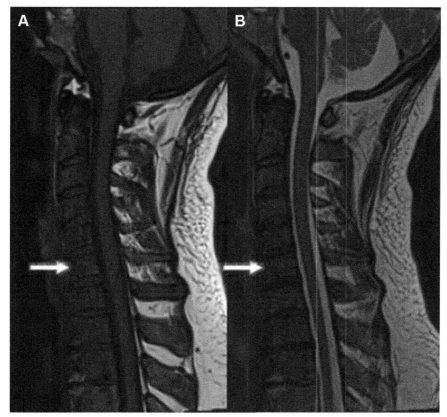

Fig. 4. MR imaging of Gaucher disease. (*A*) Sagittal T1-weighted and (*B*) T2-weighted images demonstrate diffuse hypointense marrow signal (*arrows*) secondary to replacement of fatty marrow by Gaucher cells.

transfusions, chronic hemolysis in patients with diseases such as sickle cell disease or thalassemia, or metabolic disorders in chronic inflammatory diseases.[21] The magnetic susceptibility of hemosiderin results in hypointense T1 signal, which can be similar to cortical bone (**Fig. 5**).[22]

MALIGNANT DIFFUSE MARROW REPLACEMENT
Multiple Myeloma

Multiple myeloma is a heterogeneous group of malignant plasma cell neoplasms characterized

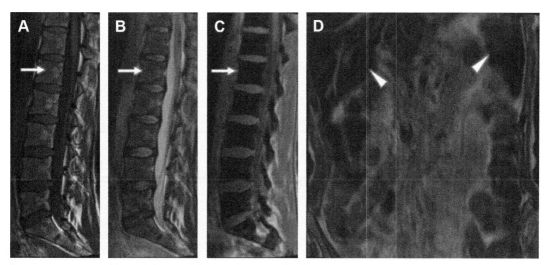

Fig. 5. MR imaging of hemosiderosis. (*A*) Sagittal T1-weighted, (*B*) T2-weighted, and (*C*) STIR images of the lumbar spine demonstrate hypointense marrow signal (*arrows*) secondary to hemosiderin deposition. (*D*) Coronal T2-weighted image demonstrates hypointense signal in the liver and spleen (*arrowheads*) secondary to iron deposition, which can help distinguish from myelofibrosis.

by uncontrolled proliferation of clonal plasma cells in the bone marrow. Multiple myeloma accounts for approximately 10% of hematologic malignancies.[23] Patients with multiple myeloma typically present with hypointense T1 bone marrow lesions due to replacement by neoplastic plasma cells. On fluid-sensitive MR imaging sequences, such as FS T2 and STIR, myelomatous lesions are typically hyperintense due to their high cellularity and water content (Figs. 6 and 7). Five different imaging patterns have been described in patients with multiple myeloma (Table 1).[24,25]

Multiple myeloma has a varied MR imaging posttreatment appearance. T1-weighted sequences demonstrate progressive replacement of the infiltrated marrow by red marrow followed by yellow, fatty marrow. Decrease in size and/or disappearance of lesions indicates treatment response.[26]

Lymphoma/Leukemia

Lymphoma and leukemia comprise a heterogeneous group of white blood cell malignancies. Leukemia occurs primarily in the bone marrow and blood, whereas lymphoma occurs primarily in lymph nodes and other tissues. MR imaging of spinal marrow in leukemia typically shows hypointense T1 signal (Fig. 8).[27] Bone marrow involvement in lymphoma can be placed in 2 categories: primary bone lymphoma, which is rare, and systemic lymphoma with skeletal involvement.[28] Bone marrow involvement is identified in approximately 20% to 40% of patients with non-Hodgkin lymphoma, but is identified in only approximately 5% of newly diagnosed Hodgkin lymphoma.[29] Lymphoma in the marrow can present as lytic, sclerotic, or mixed lytic-sclerotic lesions. MR imaging shows multifocal or diffuse marrow infiltration with isointense to hypointense T1 signal and hyperintense STIR signal (Fig. 9).[28] Lymphoma in

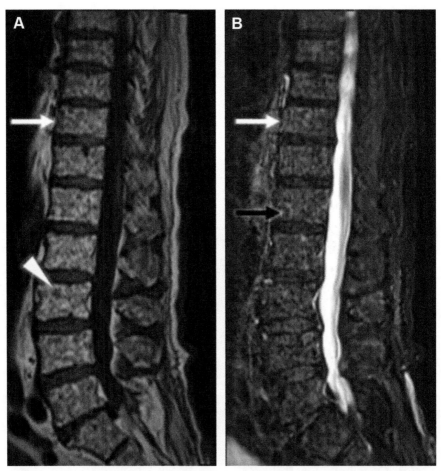

Fig. 6. MR imaging of multiple myeloma with "variegated" or "salt-and-pepper" pattern. (A) Sagittal T1-weighted and (B) STIR images demonstrate diffuse heterogeneous, patchy marrow (white arrows) with focal, small T1 hypointense (white arrowhead) and STIR hyperintense (black arrow) lesions.

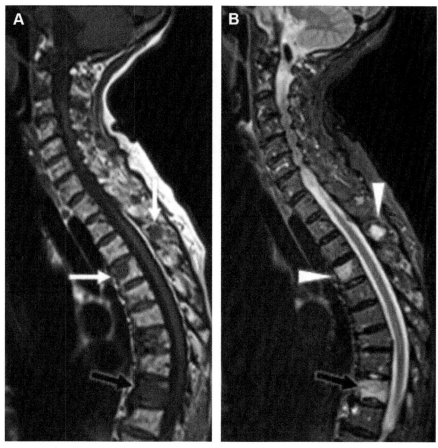

Fig. 7. MR imaging of multiple myeloma. (*A*) Sagittal T1-weighted and (*B*) STIR images demonstrate multiple T1 hypointense (*white arrow*) and STIR hyperintense (*arrowheads*) lesions within the cervical and thoracic spine with complete marrow replacement in the T9 vertebral body (*black arrows*).

Table 1
Imaging patterns of multiple myeloma

Imaging Pattern	MR Findings
Normal marrow signal	Does not exclude multiple myeloma
Focal infiltration	Focal hypointense T1 signal Focal hyperintense T2/STIR signal
Diffuse bone marrow infiltration	Homogeneous hypointense T1 signal Homogeneous hyperintense T2/STIR signal
Combined focal and diffuse infiltration	Diffuse hypointense T1 signal Interspersed focal hyperintense T2/STIR lesions
"Salt-and-pepper" infiltration	Patchy, inhomogeneous T1 and T2 signal

the spinal marrow also can have epidural extension.[12]

BENIGN FOCAL SPINAL MARROW ABNORMALITIES
Hemangioma

Spinal intraosseous hemangiomas are one of the most frequently encountered lesions in marrow containing structures. They are estimated to be present in 27% of lumbar spine MR imaging examinations and approximately one-third of hemangiomas are multifocal.[30] Lesions are most frequently encountered in the vertebral bodies but can extend into the posterior elements. Enlarged vascular spaces and proliferation of fatty stroma within hemangiomas result in characteristic T1 and T2 hyperintense signal that follows fat (**Figs. 10 and 11**), with loss of signal on STIR or FS sequences, and avid contrast enhancement due. Vertebral body hemangiomas have also been described as having a "polka-dot" or "corduroy"

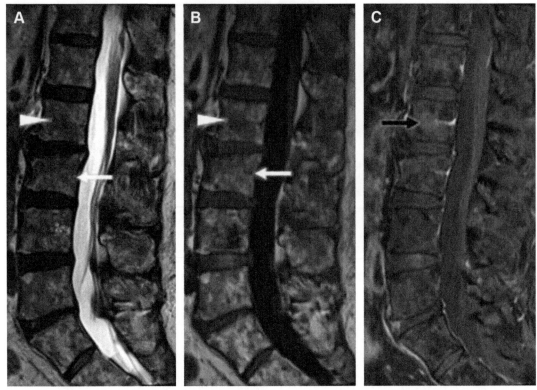

Fig. 8. MR imaging of leukemia. (*A*) Sagittal T1-weighted, (*B*) T2-weighted, (*C*) T1-weighted FS postcontrast images show heterogeneous marrow signal (*white arrows*) with focal T1/T2 hypointense lesion (*white arrowheads*) in the L2 vertebral body with mild enhancement (*black arrow*).

appearance most apparent on radiographs and CT due to the coarsened trabecula seen on end in the axial plane or in profile on sagittal or coronal projections. CT may play a central role in diagnosis

of an "atypical" hemangioma. Atypical hemangiomas have increased vascular spaces and decreased fat content compared with their typical counterparts, resulting in an "atypical" appearance

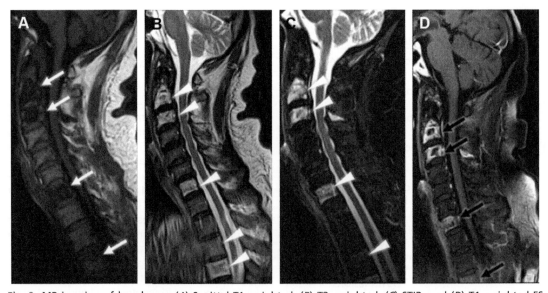

Fig. 9. MR imaging of lymphoma. (*A*) Sagittal T1-weighted, (*B*) T2-weighted, (*C*) STIR, and (*D*) T1-weighted FS postcontrast images show T1 hypointense (*white arrows*), T2/STIR hyperintense (*white arrowheads*), enhancing lesions (*black arrows*) in multiple vertebral bodies.

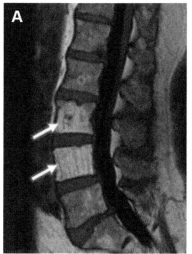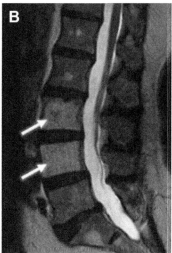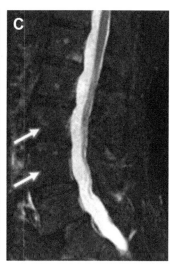

Fig. 10. MR imaging of multiple typical vertebral body hemangiomas. (A) Sagittal T1-weighted MR imaging shows multiple hyperintense lesions replacing nearly the entirety of the vertebral body marrow (arrows). (B) The same marrow-replacing lesions are hyperintense on sagittal T2-weighted MR imaging (arrows). (C) STIR-weighted MR imaging at the same level shows hypointense signal within these lesions (arrows) and imaging characteristics identical to the subcutaneous fat.

on MR imaging, often with T1 hypointense and STIR hyperintense signal. MR imaging features of hemangiomas can vary, but their "polka-dot" or "corduroy" CT appearance is typically preserved.[31]

Most vertebral body hemangiomas are asymptomatic, although locally aggressive variants exist.[31] Although histologically similar, aggressive variant hemangiomas may show rapid growth and extension into the adjacent epidural space or soft tissues.[31] Aggressive hemangiomas may mimic neoplastic disease processes, including primary osseous malignancy and metastatic disease. Lesion growth during pregnancy is an established phenomenon.[32] Hemangioma growth can result in spinal cord or nerve root compression, in which case, intervention may be warranted with vertebroplasty, embolization, or surgical decompression.[33,34]

Disk Degeneration

Intervertebral disk degeneration is a frequent cause of low back pain, which is one of the most common reasons for patients to seek medical care. In addition to changes in the intervertebral disk (eg, low T2 signal and loss of disk height), reactive changes also occur in the adjacent vertebral body endplates and marrow. Degenerative endplate pathophysiology follows a characteristic imaging pattern, described by Modic and colleagues[35] as 3 types. Type 1 changes are T1 hypointense and T2 hyperintense due to edema in the adjacent marrow, often seen in patients with active back pain. Type 2 changes are T1 and T2 hyperintense, reflective of fatty marrow proliferation due to chronic ischemic change. Type 3 changes are

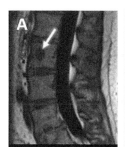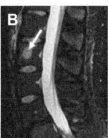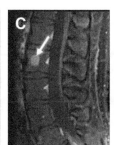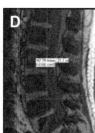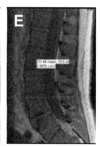

Fig. 11. "Atypical" hemangioma. (A–C) T1, STIR, and T1 postcontrast sagittal sequences through the lumbar spine show an enhancing lesion (arrows) with T1 hypointensity and T2 hyperintensity. This lesion does not follow the imaging characteristics of a typical hemangioma. Loss of signal within this lesion on opposed-phase T1-weighted sequence (D) compared with the unopposed phase (E) suggests the lesions is a hypocellular "atypical" hemangioma.

T1 and T2 hypointense due to sclerosis of the end plates (**Fig. 12**).[35] Identifying the type of Modic changes is less important than being able to distinguish marrow signal changes due to disk degeneration from other pathologies. Endplate marrow signal changes centered about the disk and the presence of adjacent diseased intervertebral disks aid in diagnosis. However, marrow signal changes due to disk degeneration and signal changes due to infection may have overlap. Distinguishing features are further discussed in the section on vertebral marrow infection.

Fracture

Vertebral body fractures result in marrow signal changes due to cortical, trabecular, and marrow injury. Both osteoporotic compression fractures and traumatic fractures have similar marrow signal changes, which mimic the characteristics of fractures elsewhere in the body, including T1 hypointense and STIR hyperintense signal, often in a linear distribution (**Fig. 13**).[36]

Distinguishing a benign from a pathologic compression fracture can be challenging, as marrow signal changes of acute fracture can be superimposed on existing marrow pathology. Findings that suggest benign fractures include multiple contiguous levels of involvement, linear marrow signal abnormality at the site of fracture with otherwise normal surrounding marrow, and the presence of fracture retropulsion. Multifocal marrow lesions, convex posterior vertebral body

cortex, involvement of the adjacent soft tissues, and marrow signal abnormality of both pedicles suggest pathologic fracture (**Fig. 14**).[12,37]

Infection

Spinal infection typically spreads from the vertebral endplates to the adjacent disks, marrow spaces, and soft tissues. Endplates are susceptible to intravascular seeding of a bloodborne pathogens due to the rich vascular supply. The lumbar spine is the most common location of spinal infection, usually sparing the posterior elements. *Staphylococcus aureus* is the most common pathogen. Recent intervention/instrumentation may increase the risk of direct inoculation, and immunocompromised patients are at greatest risk for acquiring and spreading infection via the circulation.[38]

Early imaging findings of infection include endplate erosion and edema. Infection spreads outward from the endplates to the adjacent intervertebral disk and marrow, and into the adjacent soft tissues. If unchecked, transspatial spread into the epidural and even intradural spaces is possible.[38]

MR imaging provides the greatest sensitivity in detecting findings of diskitis/osteomyelitis. MR imaging findings of infection in the spinal marrow are similar to infectious marrow changes elsewhere in the body. Increased signal on fluid-sensitive sequences is consistent with sites of edema, which may predominant early in the disease process.

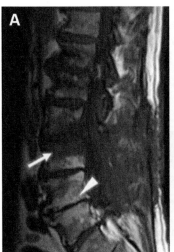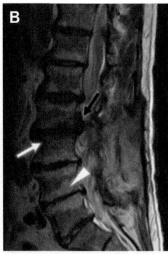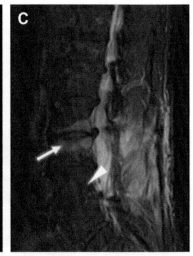

Fig. 12. Degenerative marrow changes. (*A*) Sagittal T1-weighted image with both Modic type 1 (*arrow*) and type 2 (*arrowhead*) changes. Note the marrow edema associated with type 1 changes and fatty replacement associated with type 2 changes. (*B*) Modic type 1 (*white arrow*) and type 2 (*arrowhead*) changes on T2-weighted sequences. Disk disease with large disk extrusion (*black arrow*) and adjacent acute Modic type 1 endplate changes. (*C*) Sagittal STIR sequence at the same level with hyperintense type 1 Modic changes (*arrow*) and hypointense type 2 Modic changes (*arrowhead*).

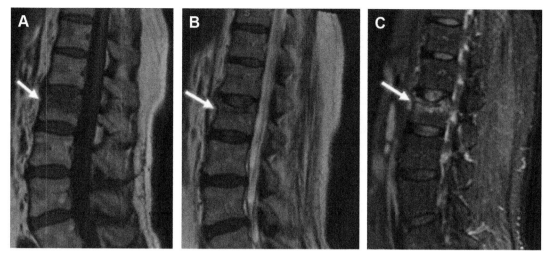

Fig. 13. Vertebral body compression fracture in an osteopenic patient. (A) T1-weighted, (B) T2-weighted, and (C) STIR sagittal images demonstrate linear signal abnormality (*arrow*) at the site of vertebral body fracture and surrounding marrow edema.

Postcontrast T1-weighted sequences may further outline areas of active osseous and soft tissue infection (**Fig. 15**).[39] Distinguishing infectious endplate changes from Modic type 1 degenerative endplate changes can be a diagnostic challenge. The presence of paraspinal inflammation, disk enhancement, fluid signal within the disk, and erosion of the endplates have been found to be the most sensitive findings of disk infection on standard MR imaging sequences.[40] Specialized MR imaging sequences, such as DWI, can aid in distinguishing degenerative endplate changes from infection. In cases of diskitis/osteomyelitis, a pattern of *diffuse* increased signal on DWI in the affected vertebral bodies can be seen.[41] Alternatively, type 1 degenerative endplate changes result in a more *linear* pattern of increased diffusion, described as the "claw sign," in which increased DWI signal is present at the interface between fibrovascular tissue and normal marrow.[4]

Fungal infection often has a more indolent course and may not follow the same pattern of disease progression that is seen with bacterial diskitis/osteomyelitis. Fungal pathogens, including tuberculosis, often spread in the spine via a subligamentous route resulting in noncontiguous involvement and even potential sparing of disk spaces.[39] In cases in which imaging findings are equivocal or if isolation of a pathogen is required for targeted antibiotic treatment, biopsy may be indicated. Despite the often-florid imaging findings of active spine infection, percutaneous biopsy yields positive results in fewer than 50% of cases.[42]

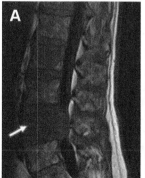
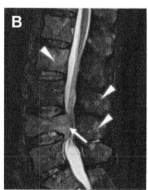
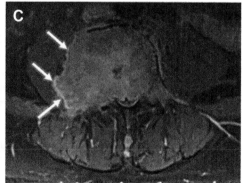

Fig. 14. Pathologic compression fracture in a patient with multifocal osseous metastases. (A) Sagittal T1-weighted image with diffuse replacement (*arrow*) of the normal hyperintense fatty marrow and depression of the superior endplate. (B) Sagittal T2-weighted image shows hyperintense signal within the lesion and convex bowing of the posterior cortex (*arrow*). Multiple additional T2 hyperintense lesions are present in the vertebral bodies and posterior elements (*arrowheads*). (C) Axial postcontrast T1-weighted image through the fractured vertebral body shows soft tissue extension of tumor (*arrows*).

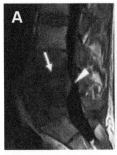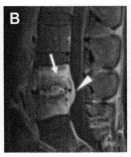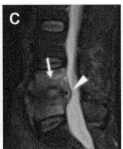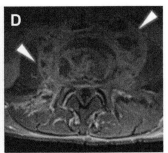

Fig. 15. MR imaging of diskitis/osteomyelitis. (*A*) Sagittal T1-weighted MR imaging with confluent replacement of the normal T1 marrow signal (*arrow*). The infected disk material extends into the ventral epidural space with mass effect on the thecal sac (*arrowhead*). (*B*) Sagittal postcontrast FS T1-weighted image in the same patient shows extensive abnormal enhancement within the disk, the marrow (*arrow*), and the adjacent epidural soft tissues (*arrowhead*). (*C*) Sagittal STIR image shows edema throughout the marrow (*arrow*), the intervertebral disk, and the adjacent epidural soft tissues (*arrowhead*). (*D*) Axial postcontrast FS T1-weighted image demonstrates the extensive soft tissue changes of infection. Note the complex, heterogeneous, and enhancing infected paraspinal soft tissues (*arrowheads*) with multiple nonenhancing foci consistent with developing abscesses.

Paget Disease

Paget disease results from dysregulation of osteoclastic and osteoblastic activity. This disease process is considered a tumorlike entity due to the resulting disordered bone growth and remodeling. Although the precise etiology is unknown, Paget disease is thought to be multifactorial, with both environmental and genetic influences. Paget disease is seen almost exclusively in the adult population, rarely affecting patients younger than 50 years.[43]

Up to 75% of patients with Paget disease have involvement of the spine with the same disordered appearance of the vertebral bodies and posterior elements seen elsewhere in the body. Paget disease progresses through 3 phases that have varying radiographic features. The early or active phase during which osteolytic changes predominate, a mixed lytic and sclerotic phase, and a late phase in which sclerotic bone changes are seen. Bone resorption during the lytic phase can have aggressive imaging features, and as the disease progresses, the cortices and trabecula become increasingly sclerotic resulting in a disordered imaging appearance with overall bone enlargement in late phases.[38] During the mixed phase, vertebral involvement has been described as having a "picture frame" appearance due to the relatively lytic-appearing marrow space and thickened sclerosis of the surrounding vertebral body cortex. In late phases, the vertebral bodies becoming increasingly sclerotic centrally and can have an "ivory vertebral body" appearance.[38]

MR imaging findings vary based on the phase of the disease. Heterogeneous T1 and T2 signal changes can be seen in both early and late phases. Similarly, enhancement is variable and often heterogeneous (**Fig. 16**). In the late phase of the disease, involved vertebral bodies contain more marrow fat than uninvolved sites.[44] If there is loss of the hyperintense marrow fat, especially in the late phase of the disease, this may suggest sarcomatous degeneration or complication, such as pathologic fracture.[45,46]

Paget disease can mimic metastatic disease and multiple myeloma, particularly in the lytic phase. Both entities can have increased uptake on bone scan, limiting the usefulness of molecular imaging. Sclerotic osseous metastatic disease and myelofibrosis demonstrate similar imaging features of late-phase Paget disease. When faced with lytic or sclerotic vertebral body lesions of uncertain etiology, the presence of osseous enlargement and trabecular thickening suggest a diagnosis of Paget disease.[38]

Ankylosing Spondylitis

The spine is frequently involved in ankylosing spondylitis and MR imaging marrow change may be the earliest and sometimes only imaging changes to suggest the disease. Inflammatory changes can be present at ligamentous insertion sites, including the corners of the vertebral body endplates, in the central endplates, or within synovial joints, such as the facet and sacroiliac articulations. Sites of active marrow inflammation will have hyperintense T2 and hypointense T1 signal, but it is often the distribution of disease that is characteristic of this disease process.[47]

Romanus lesions are an early finding in ankylosing spondylitis and are characterized by inflammatory changes at the corners of the vertebral bodies at the annulus fibrosis attachment. MR imaging signal changes of Romanus lesions depend

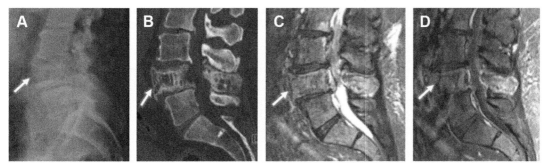

Fig. 16. Paget disease involving the L4 vertebral body with both lytic and sclerotic changes. (*A*) Lateral radiograph and (*B*) sagittal CT show enlargement of the vertebral body, thickened trabecula, and characteristic "picture frame" appearance (*arrows*). (*C*) Sagittal STIR and (*D*) sagittal postcontrast FS T1-weighted images in the same patient show the heterogeneous marrow signal abnormality and heterogeneous enhancement (*arrows*). The thickened trabecula and overall osseous enlargement are also appreciable.

on the temporality of lesions and can evolve from sites of active inflammation with high T2/STIR signal, to more chronic sites of fatty infiltration with T1 hyperintensity, and end-stage sclerosis with hypointense T1 and T2 signal.[48] Andersson lesions are marrow signal changes at the central endplates due to inflammatory changes of the intervertebral disk.[49] Additional sites of enthesitis with inflammatory changes in the marrow include the interspinous ligament insertion on the spinous process and sacrospinal ligament insertion on the iliac spines (**Fig. 17**).[38] Ankylosing spondylitis progresses to syndesmophyte formation and eventual ankylosis at sites of chronic inflammation.[50] Once ankylosis is present, even minor trauma can result in devastating spine insult, and these patients should be evaluated with CT and MR imaging to evaluate for osseous and soft tissue injury.[38,51]

MALIGNANT FOCAL SPINAL MARROW ABNORMALITIES
Metastatic Disease

Metastatic disease is by far the most common tumor encountered in the spine.[52] Metastatic involvement of the osseous structures is frequent, following only the lung and liver in prevalence. Like metastases elsewhere in the body, cells from a primary malignancy spread via the lymphatics and vasculature. Metastatic lesions in the spine are most frequently encountered in the vertebral bodies due to their rich vascular supply, but some types of neoplasm, such as hepatocellular carcinoma, show a predilection for the posterior elements.[53]

Metastases vary in appearance depending on the type of primary neoplasm, and may be lytic, sclerotic, or mixed in their radiographic and CT

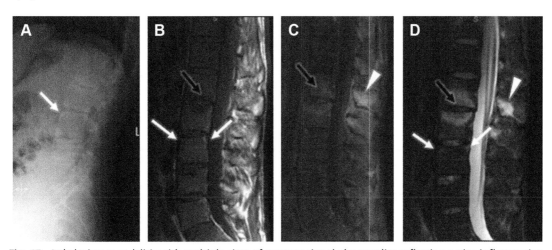

Fig. 17. Ankylosing spondylitis with multiple sites of marrow signal abnormality reflecting active inflammation. (*A*) Radiograph with sclerotic "shiny corners" of the endplates (*white arrow*). (*B–D*) Sagittal T1-weighted, postcontrast FS T1-weighted, and STIR images show Romanus lesions at the insertion sites of the annulus fibrosis (*white arrows*) as well as Andersson lesions (*black arrows*). Edema and inflammation are also present at the insertion of the interspinous ligaments (*arrowhead*).

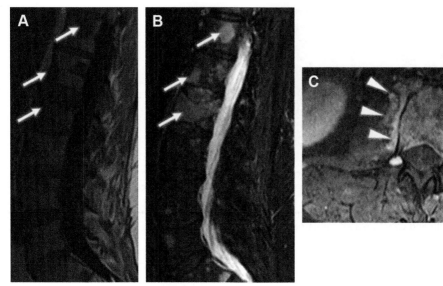

Fig. 18. MR imaging of the typical features of metastatic disease with multifocal involvement of the vertebral bodies in the thoracolumbar spine. (*A*) Sagittal T1-weighted image of the thoracolumbar spine shows multiple hypointense lesions (*arrows*) that are darker than the adjacent disk. (*B*) Sagittal STIR sequence shows these lesions to be hyperintense. (*C*) Axial postcontrast FS T1 image shows the avid enhancement (*arrow*) and soft tissue extension (*arrowheads*) of the tumor, which is characteristic of metastatic disease.

appearance. Most lytic and mixed vertebral metastases demonstrate hypointense to isointense signal on T1-weighted sequences and hyperintense signal on T2-weighted/STIR sequences due to increased cellularity of the neoplasm (**Fig. 18**).[54] Densely sclerotic metastasis may have hypointense to isointense signal on both T1-weighted and T2-weighted sequences.[55] The T1 signal of a neoplastic lesion is typically lower than that of the adjacent disk.[12]

In cases in which standard MR imaging findings are equivocal, chemical shift MR imaging may aid in problem solving. Metastases do not typically lose signal on out-phase sequences and the vast majority of lesions show some degree of contrast enhancement. Densely sclerotic lesions or certain types of gastrointestinal tract neoplasms, may have absent enhancement.[53] Attenuation measurements on CT may be helpful to distinguish osteoblastic metastases from benign lesions, such as enostoses.[56] Some focal vertebral marrow lesions cannot be confidently identified as benign or malignant and require biopsy for definitive diagnosis.

SUMMARY

MR imaging of the spine can be useful to distinguish diffuse and focal as well as benign from malignant disease processes. Understanding the common imaging characteristics of the spine on T1-weighted, T2-weighted, STIR, and more advanced imaging sequences is key to proper diagnosis and management of spinal pathology. Clues for differentiating diffuse and focal marrow-replacing entities can be found in **Boxes 1** and **2**.

Box 1
MR imaging clues to diffuse marrow replacement

Heterogeneous T1/T2 non–fat-saturated (FS) hyperintense and T2 FS/short-tau inversion recovery (STIR) hypointense:

- Osteoporosis

Hypointense T1 and T2:

- Myelofibrosis
- Mastocytosis
- Gaucher disease
- Hemosiderosis
- Leukemia

Hypointense T1 and hyperintense STIR:

- Multiple myeloma

Isointense to hypointense T1 and hyperintense STIR:

- Lymphoma

7. Vogler JB, Murphy WA. Bone marrow imaging. Radiology 1988;168(3):679–93.
8. Ricci C, Cova M, Kang YS, et al. Normal age-related patterns of cellular and fatty bone marrow distribution in the axial skeleton: MR imaging study. Radiology 1990;177(1):83–8.
9. Shah LM, Salzman KL. Imaging of spinal metastatic disease. Int J Surg Oncol 2011;2011:769753.
10. Kanis JA, Melton J, Christiansen C, et al. The diagnosis of osteoporosis. J Bone Miner Res 1994;9(8): 1137–41.
11. Griffith JF, Yeung KW, Antonio GE, et al. Vertebral marrow fat content and diffusion and perfusion indexes in women with underlying bone marrow density; MR evaluation. Radiology 2006;241(3): 831–8.
12. Hanrahan CJ, Shah LM. MRI of spinal bone marrow: part 2, T1-weighted imaging-based diagnosis differential diagnosis. AJR Am J Roentgenol 2011;197(6): 1309–21.
13. Gokalp G, Mutlu S, Yazici Z, et al. Evaluation of vertebral bone marrow fat content by chemical-shift MRI in osteoporosis. Skeletal Radiol 2011; 40(5):577–85.
14. Sale GE, Deeg J, Porter BA. Regression of myelofibrosis and osteosclerosis following hematopoietic cell transplantation assessed by magnetic resonance imaging and histologic grading. Biol Blood Marrow Transplant 2006;12(12):1285–94.
15. Diamond T, Smith A, Schnier R, et al. Syndrome of myelofibrosis and osteosclerosis: a series of case reports and review of the literature. Bone 2002; 30(3):498–501.
16. Amano Y, Onda M, Amano M, et al. Magnetic resonance imaging of myelofibrosis STIR and gadolinium-enhanced MR images. Clin Imaging 1997;21(4):264–8.
17. Roca M, Mota J, Giraldo P, et al. Systemic mastocytosis: MRI of bone marrow involvement. Eur Radiol 1999;9(6):1094–7.
18. Fritz J, Fishman EK, Carino JA, et al. Advanced imaging of skeletal manifestations of systemic mastocytosis. Skeletal Radiol 2012;41(8):887–97.
19. Poll LW, Koch JA, vom Dahl S, et al. Magnetic resonance imaging of bone marrow changes in Gaucher disease during enzyme replacement therapy: first German long-term results. Skeletal Radiol 2001; 30(9):496–503.
20. Roca M, Mota J, Alfonso P, et al. S-MRI score: a simple method for assessing bone marrow involvement in Gaucher disease. Eur J Radiol 2007;62(1):132–7.
21. Vande Berg BC, Malghem J, Lecouvet FE, et al. Classification and detection of bone marrow lesions with magnetic resonance imaging. Skeletal Radiol 1998;27(10):529–45.
22. Levin TL, Sheth SS, Comerci SC, et al. MR marrow signs of iron overload in transfusion-dependent

Box 2

MR imaging clues to focal marrow replacement

Hyperintense T1/T2-non-FS, hypointense STIR and FS:

- Intraosseous hemangioma

Hypointense T1 and STIR hyperintense, often linear:

- Fracture

Confluent hypointense T1, Hyperintense T2/STIR, enhancing:

- Osteomyelitis-diskitis
- Modic type-1 degenerative changes

Heterogeneous T1/T2, variable enhancement, thickened cortices and trabecula:

- Paget disease

Hypointense T1, hyperintense T2/STIR vertebral body corners:

- Ankylosing spondylitis

Hypointense to isointense T1 and hyperintense T2/STIR:

- Metastases

REFERENCES

1. Erdem LO, Erdem CZ, Acikgoz B, et al. Degenerative disc disease of the lumbar spine: a prospective comparison of fast T1-weighted fluid-attenuation inversion recovery and T1-weighted turbo spin echo MR imaging. Eur J Radiol 2005;55(2):277–82.
2. Melhem ER, Israel DA, Eustace S, et al. MR of the spine with a fast T1-weighted fluid-attenuated inversion recovery sequence. AJNR Am J Neuroradiol 1997;18(3):447–54.
3. Chilla GS, Tan CH, Xu C, et al. Diffusion weighted magnetic resonance imaging and its recent trend-a survey. Quant Imaging Med Surg 2015;5(3): 407–22.
4. Patel KB, Poplawski MM, Pawha PS, et al. Diffusion-weighted MRI "claw sign" improves differentiation of infectious from degenerative Modic type 1 signal changes of the spine. AJNR Am J Neuroradiol 2014;35(8):1647–52.
5. Disler DG, McCauley TR, Ratner LM, et al. In-phase and out-of-phase MR imaging of bone marrow: prediction of neoplasia based on the detection of coexistant fat and water. AJR Am J Roentgenol 1997; 169(5):1439–47.
6. Zajick DC, Morrison WB, Schweitzer ME, et al. Benign and malignant processes: normal values and differentiation with chemical shift MR imaging in vertebral marrow. Radiology 2005;237(2):590–6.

patients with sickle cell disease. Pediatr Radiol 1995;25(8):614–9.

23. Baur-Melnyk A, Buhmann S, Becker C, et al. Whole-body MRI versus whole-body MDCT for staging of multiple myeloma. AJR Am J Roentgenol 2008; 190(4):1097–104.

24. Dutoit JC, Verstrete KL. Whole-body MRI dynamic contrast-enhanced MRI and diffusion-weighted imaging for the staging of multiple myeloma. Skeletal Radiol 2017;46(6):733–50.

25. Baur-Melnyk A, Bushman S, Durr HR, et al. Role of MRI for the diagnosis and prognosis of multiple myeloma. Eur J Radiol 2005;55(1):56–63.

26. Hanrahan CJ, Christensnen CR, Crim JR. Current concepts in the evaluation of multiple myeloma with MR imaging and FDG PET/CT. Radiographics 2010;30(1):127–42.

27. Lecouvet FE, Vande Berg BC, Michaux L, et al. Chronic lymphocytic leukemia: changes in bone marrow composition and distribution assessed with quantitative MRI. J Magn Reson Imaging 1998; 8(3):733–9.

28. Mugera C, Suh KJ, Huisman TAGM, et al. Sclerotic lesions of the spine: MRI assessment. J Magn Reson Imaging 2013;38(6):1310–24.

29. Nobauer I, Uffmann M. Differential diagnosis of focal and diffuse neoplastic disease of bone marrow in MRI. Eur J Radiol 2005;55(1):2–32.

30. Barzin M, Maleki I. Incidence of vertebral hemangioma on spinal magnetic resonance imaging in Northern Iran. Pak J Biol Sci 2009;12(6): 542–4.

31. Gaudino S, Martucci M, Colantonio R, et al. A systematic approach to vertebral hemangioma. Skeletal Radiol 2015;44(1):25–36.

32. Gupta M, Navak R, Singh H, et al. Pregnancy related symptomatic vertebral hemangioma. Ann Indian Acad Neurol 2014;17(1):120–2.

33. Acosta FL, Sanai N, Chi JH, et al. Comprehensive management of symptomatic and aggressive vertebral hemangiomas. Neurosurg Clin N Am 2008; 19(1):17–29.

34. Pinto DS, Hoisala VR, Gupta P, et al. Aggressive vertebral body hemangioma causing compressive myelopathy—two case reports. J Orthop Case Rep 2017;7(2):7–10.

35. Modic MT, Steinberg PM, Ross JS, et al. Degenerative disk disease: assessment of changes in vertebral body marrow with MR imaging. Radiology 1988;166:193–9.

36. Baker LL, Goodman SB, Perkash I, et al. Benign versus pathologic compression fractures of vertebral bodies: assessment with conventional spin-echo, chemical-shift, and STIR MR imaging. Radiology 1990;174(2):495–502.

37. Jung HS, Jee WH, McCauley TR, et al. Discrimination of metastatic from acute osteoporotic compression spinal fractures with MR imaging. Radiographics 2003;23:179–87.

38. Manaster BJ. Diagnostic imaging: musculoskeletal non-traumatic diseases. 2nd edition. Salt Lake City (UT): Elsevier; 2017.

39. Hong SH, Choi JY, Lee JW, et al. MR imaging assessment of the spine: infection or an imitation? Radiographics 2009;29:599–612.

40. Ledermann HP, Schweitzer ME, Morrison WB, et al. MR imaging findings in spinal infections: rules or myths? Radiology 2003;228:506–14.

41. Eguchi Y, Ohtori S, Yamashita M, et al. Diffusion of magnetic resonance imaging to differentiate degenerative from infectious endplate abnormalities in the lumbar spine. Spine 2011;36(3):E198–202.

42. McNamara AL, Dickerson EC, Gomez-Hassan DM, et al. Yield of image-guided needle biopsy for infectious discitis: a systematic review and meta-analysis. AJNR Am J Neuroradiol 2017;38(10):2021–7.

43. Galson DL, Roodman GD. Pathobiology of Paget's disease of bone. J Bone Metab 2014;21(2):85–98.

44. Vande Berg BC, Malghem J, Lecouvet FE, et al. Magnetic resonance appearance of uncomplicated Paget's disease of bone. Semin Musculoskelet Radiol 2001;5(1):69–77.

45. Forest M, De Pinieux G, Knuutila S. Secondary osteosarcomas. In: Fletcher CDM, Unni KK, Mertens F, editors. World Health Organization classification of tumours: pathology and genetics of tumours of soft tissue and bone. Lyon (France): IARC Press; 2002. p. 277–9.

46. Sundaram M, Khanna G, El-Khoury GY. T1-weighted MR imaging for distinguishing large osteolysis of Paget's disease from sarcomatous degeneration. Skeletal Radiol 2001;30(7):378–83.

47. Lacout A, Rousselin B, Pelage JP. CT and MRI of spine and sacroiliac involvement in spondyloarthropathy. AJR Am J Roentgenol 2008;191: 1016–23.

48. Romanus R, Yden S. Destructive and ossifying spondylitic changes in rheumatoid ankylosing spondylitis (pelvo-spondylitis ossificans). Acta Orthop Scand 1952;22(2):88–9.

49. Bron JL, de Vries MK, Snieders MN, et al. Discovertebral (Andersson) lesions of the spine in ankylosing spondylitis revisited. Clin Rheumatol 2009; 28(8):883–92.

50. Maksymowych WP, Chiowchanwisawakit P, Clare T, et al. Inflammatory lesions of the spine on magnetic resonance imaging predict the development of new syndesmophytes in ankylosing spondylitis: evidence of a relationship between inflammation and new bone formation. Arthritis Rheum 2009;60(1):93–102.

51. Campagna R, Pessis E, Feydy A, et al. Fractures of the ankylosed spine: MDCT and MRI with emphasis on individual anatomic spinal structures. AJR Am J Roentgenol 2009;192:987–95.

52. Perrin RG, Laxton AW. Metastatic spine disease: epidemiology, pathophysiology, and evaluation of patients. Neurosurg Clin N AM 2004;15(4): 365–73.

53. An C, Lee YH, Kim S, et al. Characteristic MRI findings of spinal metastases from various primary cancers: retrospective study of pathologically-confirmed cases. J Korean Soc Magn Reson Med 2013;17(1):8–18.

54. Daffner RH, Lupetin AR, Dash N, et al. MRI in the detection of malignant infiltration of bone marrow. AJR Am J Roentgenol 1986;146:353–8.

55. Ross JS, Moore KR, Borg B, et al. Diagnostic imaging: spine, vol. 2. Salt Lake City (UT): Amirsys; 2010.

56. Ulano A, Bredella MA, Burke P, et al. Distinguishing untreated osteoblastic metastases from enostoses using CT attenuation measurements. AJR Am J Roentgenol 2016;207(2):362–8.

Spine Oncology
Imaging and Intervention

Wende N. Gibbs, MD, MA[a],*, Kambiz Nael, MD[b], Amish H. Doshi, MD[b], Lawrence N. Tanenbaum, MD[c]

KEYWORDS

- Spine • Metastatic disease • Diffusion-weighted imaging
- Dynamic contrast-enhanced MR imaging • Spinal instability neoplastic score
- Epidural spinal cord compression scale • Kyphoplasty • Ablation

KEY POINTS

- Osseous metastases are the most common spine tumor, and increasingly prevalent as advances in oncology are allowing patients to live longer with their disease.
- Evidence-based treatment algorithms derive the majority of their data from imaging studies and reports; the radiologist should provide this information in the language of the treatment team.
- In cases of osseous metastatic disease, the radiologist should report the Spinal Instability Neoplastic Score (SINS) and Epidural Spinal Cord Compression (ESCC) grade to ensure clear communication and timely, appropriate patient care.
- Advanced imaging techniques, such as diffusion-weighted and dynamic contrast-enhanced MR imaging, are increasingly used for diagnosis and posttreatment problem solving.
- Radiologists have a growing role in the treatment of metastatic disease, performing cement augmentation for stabilization and tumor ablation for pain palliation and tumor control.

Spinal metastases are increasingly common: the population is aging, treatments are improving, and patients with cancer are living longer with their disease. Despite rapid, remarkable advances in the understanding and treatment of cancer, metastases, and especially those of the spinal column, are the most complex and potentially dangerous conditions for these individuals. Biomechanical failure of the spinal column with pathologic fracture or epidural extension of disease can produce substantial morbidity and mortality. Osseous metastatic disease is by far the most common tumor of the spine, and imaging is central to detection and diagnosis. All radiologists will encounter subtle and advanced cases of metastatic disease in the emergency, outpatient, and inpatient settings. Appropriate imaging, relevant reporting, and multidisciplinary treatment of osseous metastatic disease is the focus of this review.

Osseous spinal metastases are ideally treated by a coordinated team of surgeons, radiation and medical oncologists, and radiologists. Radiologists have always provided valuable information for diagnosis and posttreatment assessment. Increasingly, radiologists are adding value in sophisticated treatment planning protocols and as integral members of the treatment team by performing percutaneous interventions for pain palliation, stabilization, and in some cases, tumor

Disclosure Statement: W.N. Gibbs and L.N. Tanenbaum have no relevant disclosures. K. Nael: Olea Medical Advisory Board; Siemens Research Consultant. A.H. Doshi: Merit Medical Speaker's Bureau.
[a] Department of Radiology, Keck School of Medicine at the University of Southern California, 1520 San Pablo Street, LL1451, Los Angeles, CA 90033, USA; [b] Department of Radiology, Icahn School of Medicine at Mount Sinai, 1176 5th Avenue, MC Level, New York, NY 10029, USA; [c] RadNet, 5 Columbus Circle 9th Floor, New York, NY 10019, USA
* Corresponding author.
E-mail address: Wende.Gibbs@med.usc.edu

Radiol Clin N Am 57 (2019) 377–395
https://doi.org/10.1016/j.rcl.2018.10.002
0033-8389/19/© 2018 Elsevier Inc. All rights reserved.

control. Communication and collaboration with our surgical and oncology colleagues will ensure that radiologists remain relevant and vital in the care of these patients.

CONVENTIONAL, NUCLEAR, AND ADVANCED IMAGING
Conventional Imaging

MR imaging is the modality of choice for the assessment of spine tumors, maximizing sensitivity, specificity, and spatial localization. The superior soft tissue characterization and differentiation between normal and pathologic tissues allows for earlier detection of pathology in comparison with other modalities. MR imaging is adept at accurate anatomic localization, description of solid and cystic components, and assessment of edema, as well as involvement of the epidural space, cord compression, and cord signal abnormality. Other modalities can provide complementary information. Computed tomography (CT) is used to assess osseous integrity and tumor matrix. If there is a contraindication to MR imaging, CT myelography can add information about thecal sac impingement, cord compression, and intradural disease. Nuclear bone scintigraphy, a standard imaging method to screen for osseous metastasis, is sensitive to the reactive new bone formation that results from tumor involvement. [18F]-FDG PET/CT highlights the increased glucose metabolism in tumor cells, allowing for early detection of marrow involvement, as well as assessment of treatment response.

MR imaging

MR imaging is the most sensitive technique for the detection and characterization of osseous metastases: evaluation with T1-weighted, T2-weighted, and short T1 inversion recovery (STIR) sequences is more than 98% sensitive and specific for osteolytic and osteoblastic spinal metastases.[1] Marrow infiltration is detected well before trabecular or cortical destruction are seen on CT scans or radiographs. STIR sequences are the most sensitive sequence because of the high contrast between hyperintense tumor and suppressed marrow fat signal intensity. Low T1 signal in the majority of metastases becomes isointense to marrow after the administration of contrast; therefore, fat suppression is necessary for detection on contrast-enhanced images. Contrast-enhanced Dixon fat water separation imaging can provide even greater lesion conspicuity through increased background suppression on opposed phase images, which cancel signal from marrow water

and fat, and fat-only images, in which lesions appear dark against the normal hyperintense marrow fat.[2] Sclerotic metastases are hypointense on T1- and T2-weighted images, and may have little or no enhancement after contrast administration (Fig. 1). Contrast is useful for the detection of metastatic infiltration of marrow, but vital for characterization of epidural and paraspinal tumor extension.

After surgery, MR imaging is used to assess the extent of tumor resection and, if subsequent radiation or chemotherapy is planned, performed before additional therapy. Early postoperative imaging is necessary to establish an accurate baseline, because enhancing inflammation and neovascularity may develop within 24 hours. Susceptibility artifact from metallic hardware may be reduced by using thinner slices, smaller voxels, and longer echo train length. Fast/turbo spin echo T2-weighted sequences are preferred over gradient recalled echo sequences, which lack radiofrequency refocusing pulses. The frequency encoding gradient should be oriented parallel to screw long axis (the anteroposterior direction). In the presence of spinal hardware, a 1.5 T field strength may be preferred over 3 T.[3] However, with sufficient knowledge and careful attention to sequence parameters, 3 T can be optimized to produce equal if not superior images.[4]

Computed tomography

CT is useful for characterizing cortical and trabecular bone, new bone formation, osseous destruction by aggressive malignancies, or smooth remodeling in the case of indolent processes. In addition, CT is useful for planning and performing image-guided biopsy or percutaneous ablation. Conventional CT scanning is less useful for detecting marrow infiltration (Fig. 2).

However, advances in dual energy CT (DECT) show promise in this setting. In one recent study, use of a virtual noncalcium technique to detect pathologic marrow infiltration in multiple myeloma produced excellent diagnostic performance using both visual and region of interest-based analysis.[5] Other new techniques, such as temporal subtraction, obtained with serial CT scans and use of nonrigid registration, may increase efficiency and reader confidence in detecting new or changing metastatic lesions on follow-up examinations.[6]

CT myelography can characterize cord compression and the degree of myelographic block in patients with contraindication to MR, spinal hardware, or in some cases in which MR imaging findings are unclear (Fig. 3). This

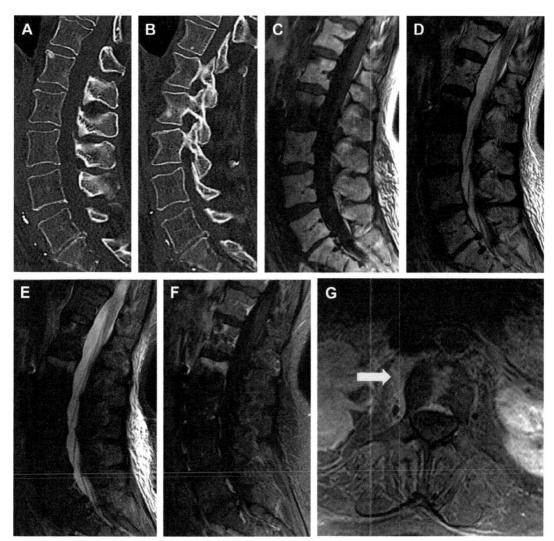

Fig. 1. Sclerotic metastases in a man with history of bladder adenocarcinoma. Two sagittal images from a computed tomography study of the abdomen and pelvis (A, B) show small, sclerotic foci in the L1 and L2 vertebral bodies. These were considered to be nonspecific in this patient, who did not have known metastatic disease. On MR imaging, the sclerotic foci are hypointense on T1 (C), T2 (D) and STIR (E) and do not enhance (F). However, there is substantial edema and enhancement surrounding the sclerotic components, and paraspinal extension of tumor (arrow) seen on the axial fat-saturated postcontrast image (G).

technique is frequently used in treatment planning for stereotactic body radiotherapy (SBRT), especially when susceptibility artifact from hardware degrades image quality. Monochromatic/monoenergetic datasets reconstructed from DECT can substantially decrease beam hardening artifact and improve visualization of hardware and local structures. The optimal energy level depends on the tissue or material of interest: 110 keV is the ideal energy level for the instrumented spine.[4] An additional method of reducing metal-related artifact is use of projection-based metal artifact reduction algorithms. This technique uses detection and segmentation of data corresponding with metal, followed by the removal and interpolation of corrupted data, which is iteratively reconstructed to generate a corrected image.[7] A complementary approach to combating metal artifact is the development of new surgical materials, such as carbon fiber-based pedicle screws and fixation rods, which have strength equal to titanium, but are nearly radiolucent, allowing for improved visualization of local structures and more accurate radiotherapy dose planning.[8]

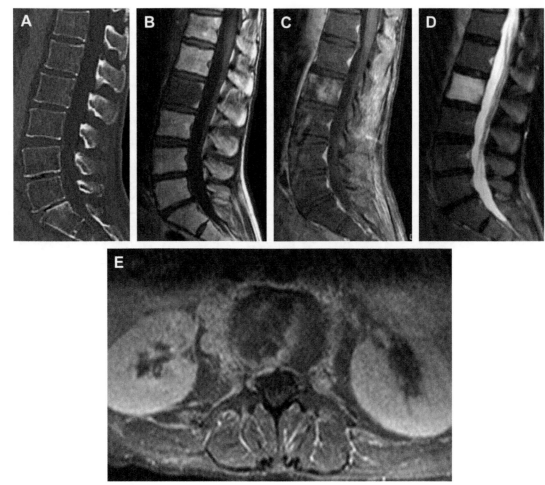

Fig. 2. Superiority of MR imaging in the evaluation of marrow processes. This 64-year-old woman with a history of rectal cancer presented with back pain. Aside from degenerative disc disease, no abnormality is seen on CT (*A*). Given her history of cancer, MR was performed. Note the near-complete infiltration of the L2 vertebral body, well seen on T1 (*B*), fat-saturated postcontrast (*C*), and STIR (*D*) images. The axial fat-saturated postcontrast image (*E*) shows paraspinal soft tissue extension of disease.

Nuclear Medicine

Technetium-99m bone scintigraphy is a useful screening method for osseous metastases, with tracer accumulation in reactive new bone. Although this modality aids in detecting the osteoblastic activity of many tumor types, uptake is nonspecific and can result from trauma, infection, and arthropathy. The presence of multiple lesions is suggestive of a metastatic etiology in a patient with known cancer, but for a single lesion, the specificity is only 50%.[9] False-negative results can also occur with diffuse accumulation of tracer throughout the skeleton—a super scan—most commonly associated with prostate carcinoma. In this case, the widespread abnormality may be mistaken for a normal study. Sensitivity and specificity depend on primary tumor histology. In the case of prostate cancer, the most common

histology to result in spine metastases, the sensitivity is 70% and the specificity is 57%. The addition of single photon emission CT (SPECT) raises the sensitivity to 92% and specificity to 82%.[10]

[18F]-FDG PET/CT plays a valuable role in cancer staging and monitoring, combining functional information about the metabolic activity of a tumor (and its metastases) and associated anatomic information. The diagnostic usefulness of PET depends on the histology and composition of the lesion: the sensitivity for lytic lesions is substantially higher than for blastic lesions, which often have low FDG uptake. PET/CT can aid in the differentiation of benign osteoporotic compression fractures from malignant vertebral fractures, a common conundrum in elderly patients with cancer.[11,12] In the posttreatment

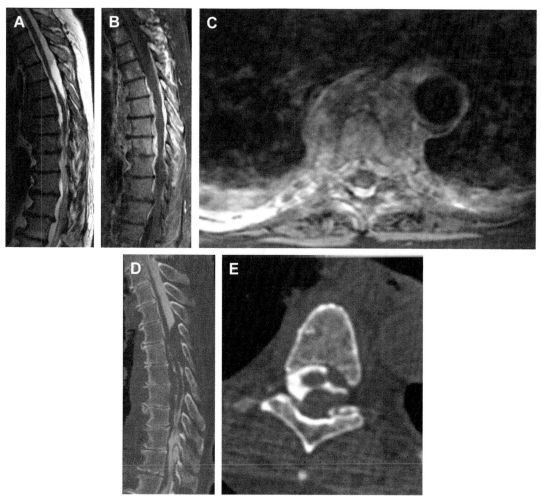

Fig. 3. Added value of myelography in assessment of cord compression. T2 (*A*) and fat-saturated postcontrast (*B*, *C*) images of a patient with metastatic anaplastic angiosarcoma present an incomplete, confusing picture of the processes occurring within the spinal canal. The T2 hyperintense collections and enhancement have different configurations. Myelography (*D*, *E*) is required to determine the degree of cord compression and characterize epidural disease and loculated fluid collections.

setting, PET/CT can potentially discriminate between metabolically active blastic metastases and sclerotic, inactive, treated disease (**Fig. 4**).[13] In the presence of spinal hardware, PET/CT may be superior to MR imaging if images are degraded by susceptibility artifact. [18F]-FDG PET/MR is a promising development for evaluation of patients with cancer, with absence of ionizing radiation, superior soft tissue resolution, and a wider range of sequences, including contrast-enhanced and diffusion-weighted imaging. In spine oncology, clinical impact will likely be greatest for marrow disease and soft tissue extension of tumor.

Na[18F] PET/CT is evolving as an important modality for evaluation of osseous metastatic disease, with greater sensitivity and specificity than conventional bone scintigraphy. Uptake of Na[18F] is twice that of Tc-99MDP, because it binds minimally to serum proteins, allowing for rapid single pass extraction and clearance from the soft tissues. Greater bone uptake results in improved resolution. Blood flow is the rate-limiting step, similar to bone scintigraphy. The diagnostic usefulness relies on histology. In the setting of prostate cancer, Na[18F] PET/CT has shown near perfect sensitivity and specificity.[10] A recently described combined examination with both Na[18F]-PET/CT and [18F]-FDG PET/CT would allow for single session staging of osseous and soft tissue disease components.[14]

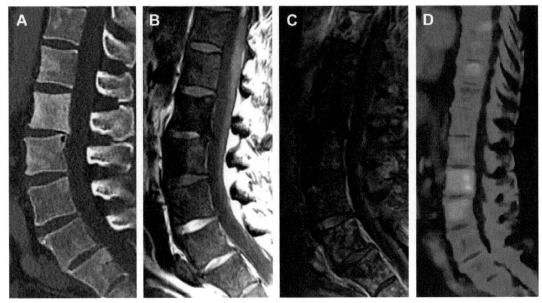

Fig. 4. Usefulness of [18F]-FDG PET/CT in the evaluation of posttreatment sclerotic lesions. Imaging was prompted by increasing prostate-specific antigen levels and back pain in this patient with previously treated prostate cancer. No prior imaging was available for comparison. The sagittal CT image (*A*) demonstrates numerous sclerotic lesions. The T1 precontrast (*B*) and fat-saturated postcontrast (*C*) images are indeterminate: a lack of enhancement does not exclude active tumor when metastases are sclerotic. (The apparent enhancement of T12 is artifactual.) The PET/CT (*D*) demonstrates metabolically active disease in multiple lumbar and thoracic vertebral bodies.

Advanced Imaging

Diffusion-weighted imaging

Diffusion-weighted imaging (DWI) characterizes the tissue-specific molecular diffusion of protons. In tissues with high cell densities, such as neoplasms, a larger number of intracellular and intercellular membranes act as diffusion barriers. DWI has been used for the assessment and characterization of osseous spinal pathology with mixed results.[15–20] Qualitative and quantitative assessments are useful for the diagnosis and staging of some tumor types.

For example, MR imaging is the most accurate imaging method for the detection of early bone marrow infiltration in multiple myeloma[21,22] (**Fig. 5**) and DWI, in particular, adds information about tumor cellularity.[23,24] The diffusion signal of myeloma lesions can vary during the course of disease but, in general, the lesions have an increased signal when active and a decrease in signal in response to successful treatment.[24]

DWI can be applied to the important issue of treatment response evaluation. Conventional MR imaging sequences are sensitive for marrow pathology, but not specific in this setting because of the variable signal intensity changes after radiation and chemotherapy.[25] The addition of DWI to conventional sequences improves sensitivity and conspicuity of even small osseous and soft tissue lesions.[26] A subjective decrease in signal[25] or quantitative assessment of apparent diffusion coefficient values may prove useful in the posttreatment setting because an increase in the diffusion coefficient indicates a favorable treatment response[19,27] (**Fig. 6**).

Dynamic contrast-enhanced MRI

Dynamic contrast-enhanced (DCE) MRI has shown promise in differentiating benign from malignant marrow processes and evaluating tumor response to radiation therapy. Tumors require angiogenesis to sustain rapid growth. The immature vessels have wider endothelial junctions than normal vessels, allowing contrast to leak from the vascular space into the interstitial space, and then diffuse back into the vascular space for clearance.

DCE data can be processed semiquantitatively using dynamic changes during passage of the contrast bolus that are depicted as time–intensity curves. In this scenario, perfusion values such as peak enhancement, wash-in, and wash-out can be obtained. Myeloma and metastatic lesions often have curves with rapid wash-in (with or without wash-out), whereas posttreatment changes demonstrate slow wash-in with a

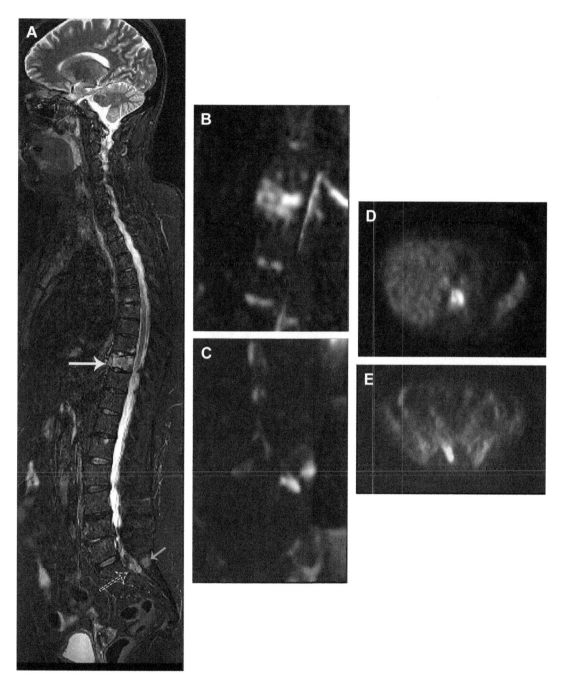

Fig. 5. A 53-year-old woman with relapsed multiple myeloma based on serum markers. Sagittal short T1 inversion recovery (STIR) images (*A*) from the entire spine show a hyperintense lesion involving T9 vertebral body and another lesion in the S1 posterior element and epidural space (*arrows*). These lesions are easily visualized on diffusion-weighted imaging (*B*, *C*). Corresponding axial PET images (*D*, *E*) performed on the same day show increased metabolic activity, suggesting active myeloma. This finding was confirmed by histopathologic examination after biopsy of the sacral lesion.

persistent or plateau course of enhancement[28–30] (**Fig. 7**).

The absolute quantification of DCE data can be performed using mathematical modeling that depicts changes in tissue contrast concentrations instead of signal intensity changes over time.[31] In this scenario, perfusion values such as permeability (K_{trans}) and plasma volume (V_p) have shown promising results in the evaluation of posttreatment changes.[32,33]

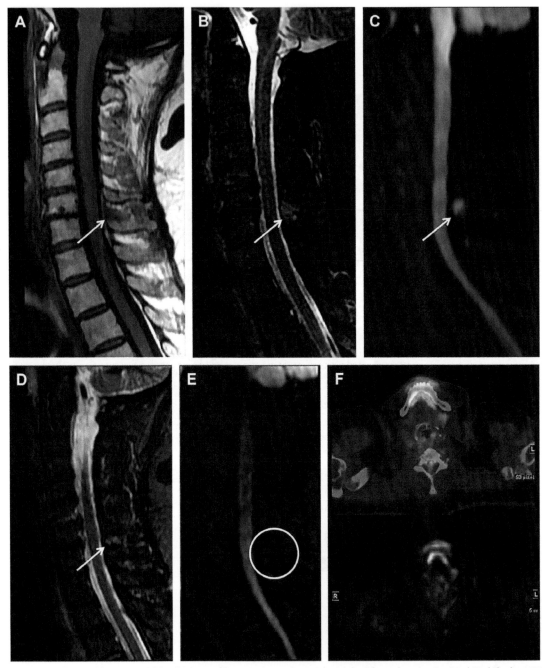

Fig. 6. A 58-year-old woman with a history of lung cancer who presented with neck pain. Sagittal T1 (*A*), short T1 inversion recovery (STIR) (*B*), and diffusion-weighted imaging (DWI) (*C*) demonstrate a T1 hypointense, STIR hyperintense lesion (*arrow*) in the spinous process of C7, which is also hyperintense and easily seen on DWI. Follow-up MR imaging (*D, E*) obtained 3 months after radiation treatment shows decreased STIR signal (*arrow* in *D*). DWI shows complete resolution of diffusion signal, favoring treatment response (*circle* in *E*). This finding was confirmed by a same-day PET scan, which shows no metabolic activity (*F*).

The application of DCE in the spine has shown utility in differentiating different tumor types and grades, benign from malignant vertebral fractures, and treatment-related marrow changes from recurrent disease.[34,35]

Small studies have shown that changes in perfusion parameters after radiotherapy, especially plasma volume (V_p), likely reflect diminished vascularity in successfully treated lesions.[32,33,36]

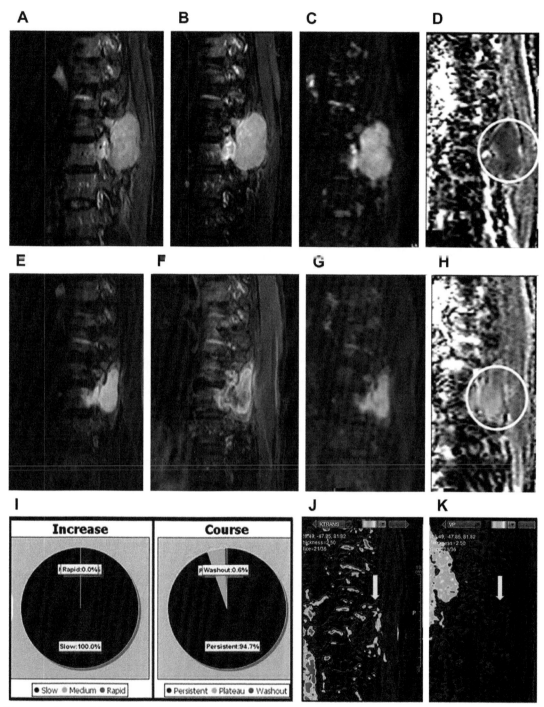

Fig. 7. A 76-year-old man with a history of hepatocellular carcinoma presented with a large metastasis involving the T11 and T12 vertebral bodies. Sagittal T1 postcontrast (*A*), short T1 inversion recovery (*B*), diffusion-weighted imaging (*C*), and apparent diffusion coefficient maps (*D*) are shown from pretreatment MR imaging and 2 months after radiation and chemotherapy treatment (*E–H*). (Circles in H and K highlight tumor on the pre and post treatment ADC maps.) There is decrease in size and enhancement of the mass. There is an increase in apparent diffusion coefficient values (from 1370 to 2200 × 10^{-6} mm 2/s) within the residual mass suggesting treatment response. Semiquantitative assessment of the signal–time dynamic curve (*I*) demonstrates 100% slow wash-in and predominant plateau (persistent) dynamic course favoring posttreatment changes. The permeability (K_{trans}) (*J*) and plasma-volume (V_p) (*K*) maps from dynamic contrast-enhanced MR imaging show modest values of K_{trans} (0.05 min^{-1}) and no increased V_p values within the treated tumor bed (*arrows*).

The combination of DWI and DCE applied to the difficult problem of differentiating treatment change from residual or recurrent tumor is promising, and refinement of this technique will be valuable for the early identification of poor responders, allowing modification of treatment and improved patient outcomes (**Fig. 8**).

ASSESSMENT AND TREATMENT

Spinal metastases are considered more complex and important than other osseous metastases, given their potential impact on neural structures. They often produce significant pain, loss of function, and poor performance status depending on the location and extent of disease. Forty percent to 80% of patients with cancer will develop spinal metastatic disease and, of these, approximately 10% to 20% will develop spinal cord compression.[37,38]

The goals of treatment include pain palliation, local durable pain control, maintenance or recovery of neurologic function and ambulation, mechanical stability, and improved quality of life.

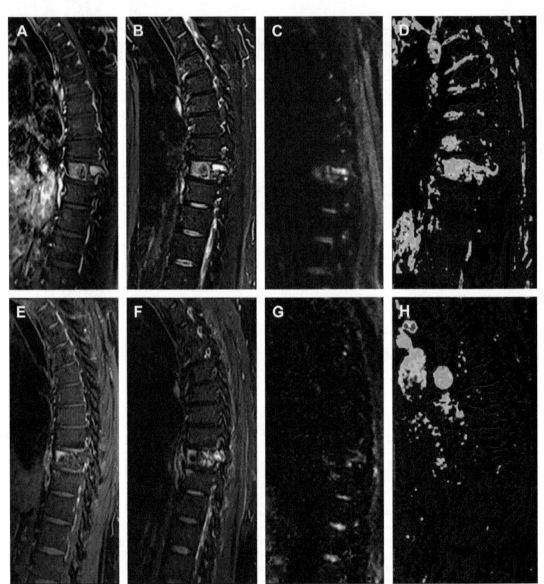

Fig. 8. A 61-year-old man with a history of renal cell carcinoma metastasis to the T9 vertebral body. Sagittal T1 post-contrast (*A*), short T1 inversion recovery (STIR) (*B*), and diffusion-weighted imaging (*C*), as well as a plasma-volume (V_p) map from dynamic contrast-enhanced studies (*D*) are shown from pretreatment MR imaging and 3 months after radiation treatment (*E–H*). After treatment the enhancement and STIR hyperintensity have decreased. There is a substantial decrease in diffusion signal and V_p, suggesting a favorable treatment response.

The principle methods of treatment include surgery and radiation therapy. Radiotherapy is often the initial treatment modality. Surgical treatment may involve decompression alone or include stabilization. Immunotherapy, chemotherapy, radionuclides, and hormones may also play a role in treatment. Percutaneous cement augmentation and tumor ablation are increasingly used interventions for patients with painful metastases without cord compression.

History and Recent Advances

Traditionally, osseous spinal metastases were treated with extensive surgeries with en bloc resections that resulted in substantial morbidity and provided poor long-term tumor control. Alternatively, conventional external beam radiotherapy (cEBRT) was used for pain and tumor control in the subset of cancers responsive to this treatment (Table 1). For this reason, patients with less than 3 months to live were usually not considered good candidates for aggressive surgical or radiation treatment.

In the last 2 decades, we have seen tremendous advances in oncology, with new discoveries in tumor biology facilitating the development of novel treatments, such as immunotherapies and chemotherapies based on tumor genetic subtypes. In spinal oncology, the development and increasing use of SBRT and spine stereotactic radiosurgery (SRS), as well as new surgical techniques and tools allow for less invasive, more effective treatment. There is an increasing role for radiologists in the treatment of these patients using percutaneous cement augmentation for stabilization and thermal ablation for pain palliation and local tumor control. In combination, these factors have resulted in patients living longer with their cancer and metastatic disease. In the past, the presence of spine metastases was considered a palliative condition, but now, in some cases, this is considered a chronic condition to be managed for years rather than months. Given the increasing number of patients with metastatic disease and the central role of the radiologist in diagnosis and in some cases treatment, it is vital to understand the most current management options.

Radiation Therapy and Surgery

Conventional external beam radiotherapy is typically delivered using 2 opposed beams with near full-dose radiation across the entire width of the patient. For this reason, doses must be kept low, within tolerance of the most sensitive structures, such as the spinal cord. In contrast, SBRT/SRS is a highly conformal therapy using multiple beams or arcs focused on the tumor target with a steep dose fall-off, allowing for a high, ablative dose in 1 to 5 fractions. Tumors that were moderately sensitive or not sensitive to cEBRT are sensitive to SBRT/SRS, with very high rates of tumor control. Goals of radiation therapy include pain palliation, prevention of local disease progression, and arrest or reversal of neurologic compromise by tumor. The advent of SBRT/SRS has made radiotherapy the first line treatment for osseous spinal metastases in most cases. Indications for surgical treatment include spinal instability and deformity, progressive neurologic deficits, cord or nerve root compression by epidural disease or retropulsed bone, or treatment of metastases for which radiotherapy cannot safely be delivered. The term separation surgery refers to a minimal tumor resection to separate the tumor margin from the spinal cord to permit optimal SBRT/SRS dosing to the bulk of the tumor.

Evidence-Based Treatment Algorithms

The advances in oncology and the growing desirability of evidence-based treatments have resulted in development of management algorithms that allow a personalized approach to each patient. These frameworks guide discussion in multidisciplinary management, suggesting treatment options based on the most current literature and options. The most commonly used frameworks are NOMS[39] and LMNOP,[40] which take into account the patient's neurologic status, oncologic status, spinal stability, and overall physical condition. These aspects of the patient's disease status are used to guide systemic and radiation therapy and surgery and nonsurgical spinal stabilization. The neurologic status includes the degree of spinal cord compression, myelopathy, and radiculopathy.

Table 1
Radiosensitivity to cEBRT

Very Sensitive	Moderately Sensitive	Not Sensitive
• Lymphoma	• Breast	• Colon
• Myeloma	• Prostate	• Renal cell
• Small cell lung cancer	• Thyroid	• Melanoma
		• Sarcoma
		• Squamous cell lung cancer

The oncologic status considers tumor histology, chemosensitivity, hormonal sensitivity, and radiosensitivity. Spinal stability is of utmost importance, because an unstable spine must be treated urgently, typically before or concurrent with oncologic treatment. Systemic status includes comorbidities and considers the patients ability to tolerate surgery.

The Radiologist's Role in Assessment

Approximately 50% of the data required for input into the evidence-based frameworks is derived from imaging studies. For this reason, radiologists should be familiar with the current grading scales and language used by the treatment team, to provide efficient, effective communication. The two most important scales for the radiologist to report are the Spinal Instability Neoplastic Score (SINS) and the epidural spinal cord compression scale (ESCC).

The Spinal Instability Neoplastic Score

Mechanical instability is an indication for surgical stabilization or percutaneous cement augmentation, regardless of neurologic or oncologic assessments. The determination is almost completely image based, giving the radiologist a primary role in triaging patients with an unstable spine to surgical consultation. Timely triage is vital to prevent the catastrophic consequences of spinal failure in the setting of metastatic disease: severe pain, loss of function, or paralysis.

In 2010, the Spine Oncology Study Group created a classification system with easily assigned radiographic and patient factors: the SINS grading system[41] (Table 2). SINS grades spinal stability by adding together five radiographic and one clinical component to create a total score ranging from 0 to 18. The five radiologic features include location of the metastasis in the spine, spinal alignment, lesion quality (lytic, sclerotic, or mixed), the degree of vertebral body involvement and collapse, and involvement of the posterior elements (Fig. 9). A unique characteristic of oncologic instability is the presence of movement-related pain.[41,42] Therefore, the assessment of mechanical back pain is necessary to provide a complete SINS score. The radiologist may not have this information, but can still report the remaining parameters for final grading by the treatment team. A high SINS score, 13 to 18, indicates the need for urgent surgical intervention. The indeterminate category, a score of 7 to 12, should prompt surgical consultation as quickly as possible. A score of 1 to 6 suggests that the spine is stable and that planning can

Table 2 Spinal Instability Neoplastic Score (SINS)	
Category	Points Assigned
Location	
Junctional spine (occiput-C2, C7-T2, T11-L1, L5-S1)	3
Mobile spine (C3-6, L2-4)	2
Semirigid spine (T3-10)	1
Rigid spine (S2-5)	0
Alignment	
Subluxation or translation	4
New kyphosis or scoliosis	2
Normal alignment	0
Vertebral body involvement	
>50% collapse	3
<50% collapse	2
No collapse, but >50% involved	1
None	0
Posterior element involvement	
Bilateral	3
Unilateral	1
None	0
Lesion quality	
Lytic	2
Mixed	1
Blastic	0
Pain	
Yes, mechanical	3
Occasional nonmechanical	1
None	0

be carried out with less concern for spinal stabilization.

The Epidural Spinal Cord Compression Scale

Neurologic considerations focus primarily on the degree of spinal cord compression. The 6-point ESCC is used in conjunction with clinical assessment of myelopathy and/or radiculopathy for treatment decisions[39,43] (Box 1). Grading is performed on axial T2-weighted images at the site of most severe compression. If the spine is stable, radiation is considered for the initial treatment of low-grade compression (ESCC grades 0, 1a, 1b, 1c) (Fig. 10). High-grade compression (grades 2 and 3) requires initial minimal surgical decompression of the epidural space, unless the tumor is highly radiosensitive or the patient cannot tolerate surgery[39] (Fig. 11).

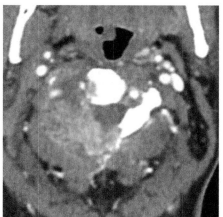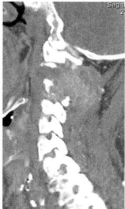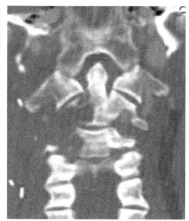

Fig. 9. A 37-year-old man with metastatic thyroid cancer. MR imaging is typically required to accurately calculate a Spinal Instability Neoplastic Score (SINS) score, but occasionally computed tomography (CT) can be used. The SINS score for this case is calculated as follows: location in the junctional spine (3 points), alignment is preserved (0 points), no collapse, but greater than 50% body involvement (1 point), bilateral posterior element involvement (3 points), lesion quality is lytic (2 points), and we receive report of mechanical neck pain (3 points). The SINS score is 12. This score is at the upper limit of the indeterminate category; we recommend a prompt surgical consultation.

The Radiologist's Role in Treatment

The pain produced by osseous spinal metastases is complex and challenging to treat. Biologic pain related to periosteal stretch and other local tumor factors in the marrow microenvironment is more common at night, unrelieved with change in position, and best treated with steroids or radiation. Mechanical back pain caused by oncologic instability is a result of tumor infiltration of the vertebral body and posterior elements, with pathologic fracture or microfracture. This type of pain is worse with axial loading and relieved by recumbency. Mechanical pain is treated with surgical or percutaneous stabilization. Patients are often debilitated and at a greater risk for surgical morbidity. High surgical complication rates with resultant decreased quality of life are especially undesirable in patients with a limited life expectancy. For this reason, minimally invasive procedures are popular options for this population. The radiologist can play an integral role in treatment in this area by performing percutaneous vertebral cement augmentation and ablation.

Percutaneous cement augmentation, vertebroplasty and kyphoplasty, is now among the most commonly used treatments in spinal oncology for pain palliation.[44] The structural integrity of bone is carefully regulated through the actions of osteoclasts and osteoblasts. This balance is disrupted by both cancer and cancer treatment. In patients with spinal metastases, treatment with steroids, androgen deprivation in patients with prostate cancer, and aromatase inhibitors used for breast cancer may contribute to osteopenia. Radiation therapy decreases the ability of vertebral marrow to withstand axial loads and may cause osteonecrosis. Pathologic fractures may occur under normal physiologic stress. Stabilization with percutaneous cement augmentation provides a high rate of pain relief and improved quality of life

---

Box 1
Epidural Spinal Cord Compression Scale (ESCC)

Low grade

- Grade 0: osseous disease only
- Grade 1a: epidural involvement without thecal sac deformation
- Grade 1b: thecal sac deformation without cord contact
- Grade 1c: thecal sac deformation with cord contact

High grade

- Grade 2: cord compression with preservation of some CSF
- Grade 3: cord compression with complete effacement of CSF

Abbreviation: CSF, cerebrospinal fluid.
Data from Bilsky MH, Laufer I, Fourney DR, et al. Reliability analysis of the epidural spinal cord compression scale. J Neurosurg Spine 2010;13(3):324–8.

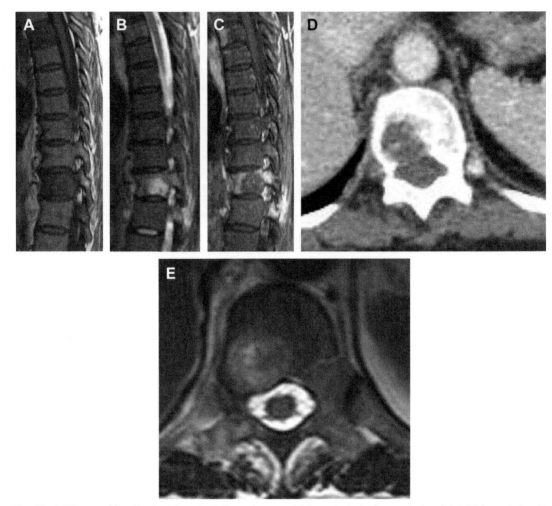

Fig. 10. A 32-year-old patient with metastatic melanoma. This metastasis demonstrates faint T1 hyperintensity (*A*). The lesion is hyperintense on STIR (*B*). The lesion is nonenhancing (*C*), but the marrow around lesion does enhance. On the axial computed tomography image (*D*) the lesion is shown to be lytic. On the axial T2 image (*E*) at the level of greatest compression, we see that the lesion is confined to the bone: the epidural spinal cord compression scale is grade 0.

(**Fig. 12**). Despite this, the procedure is only slowly gaining acceptance, given a historically higher rate of procedure-related complications, including increased rate of cement leakage compared with patients with osteoporotic compression fractures.[45]

Percutaneous ablative therapy is another treatment used to treat the pain of osseous metastases, and in some cases, provide local tumor control.[46] Ablation is used as an adjunct or alternative therapy in patients without epidural disease producing high-grade cord compression. Energy-based ablation destroys tumor through either thermal (heat or cold) or nonthermal mechanisms. Radiofrequency ablation uses thermal energy to produce coagulation necrosis of the tumor as well as destruction of pain-sensitive nerve fibers (**Fig. 13**). Microwave ablation is a subtype of radiofrequency ablation, although with distinct device and applicator differences. Microwaves radiate through tissue with high impedance to electric current, such as bone, allowing them to continuously generate heat in a greater volume of tissue surrounding the application. As a result, ablation zones are larger, hotter, and produced faster compared with radiofrequency current.[47] Cryoablation destroys tissue by the application of freezing temperature. This technique involves coaxial placement of a probe with pressurized circulating argon that rapidly cools producing a temperature decrease to approximately -100°C

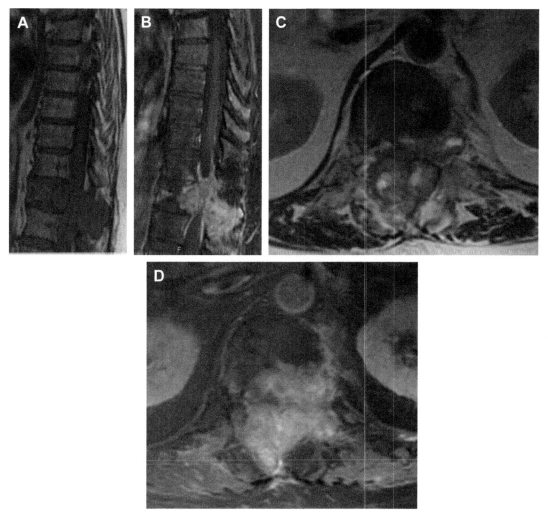

Fig. 11. A 64-year-old woman with metastatic squamous cell carcinoma. Precontrast and postcontrast images (*A*, *B*, *D*) show high-grade cord compression at T12 from a pathologic fracture, epidural extension of disease, and a tumor extending ventrally from the posterior elements. The Epidural Spinal Cord Compression (ESCC) is measured at the level of greatest compression on the axial T2-weighted image (*C*). This is ESCC grade 3: cord compression with complete effacement of the cerebrospinal fluid. This condition requires surgical resection of tumor from the epidural space to create a free margin around the spinal cord before stereotactic body radiotherapy can be considered.

within seconds. Cryoablation is predominantly used for tumors with an extraosseous soft tissue component because the ablated volume is visible on CT images. Ablation is typically followed by cement augmentation to prevent potential instability.

Imaging is performed 6 to 8 weeks after ablation treatment to allow for a decrease in procedure-related inflammation. The ablation cavity is composed of central coagulation necrosis surrounded by a rim of hemorrhagic congestion and granulation tissue. There should be no enhancement within the treatment cavity. T1 hyperintensity and mild T2 hyperintensity may be present.[48]

Comparison with preablation images is required to assess the adequacy of the treatment (Fig. 14). Residual or recurrent tumor will be T2 hyperintense and enhancing at the margin of the ablation cavity. This pattern occurs most commonly at the posterior vertebral body and pedicles, sites not always amenable to aggressive ablation secondary to proximity to the spinal cord and nerve roots. Vascular fibrosis relating to treatment may have a similar appearance, complicating definitive diagnosis. Fibrosis should not be FDG avid; therefore, [18F]-FDG PET/CT scanning may be useful for further evaluation in difficult cases.

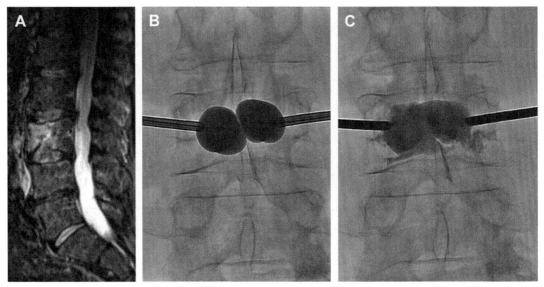

Fig. 12. A 70-year-old patient with multiple myeloma producing severe lumbar pain. STIR (*A*) demonstrates hyperintense signal in the L3 vertebral body corresponding with a pathologic compression fracture. The neuroradiologist performed balloon kyphoplasty with cement augmentation for pain control and fracture stabilization. Fluoroscopic images show a bipedicular approach with kyphoplasty balloon inflation (*B*) and subsequent fill of the created cavity with cement (*C*).

SUMMARY

Osseous spinal metastatic disease is increasingly common, as patients are living longer with their cancer. The emergence of multidisciplinary treatment teams and evidence-based management algorithms requires radiologists to understand the most current treatment options and tools. The majority of data used in the treatment frameworks are derived from imaging and radiology reports. These factors highlight the need for reporting of these classification and grading scales used in treatment algorithms, especially the SINS and ESCC scales. Radiologists are also increasingly called upon to treat these patients, with percutaneous interventions for spine stabilization, pain palliation, and tumor control. Close communication and

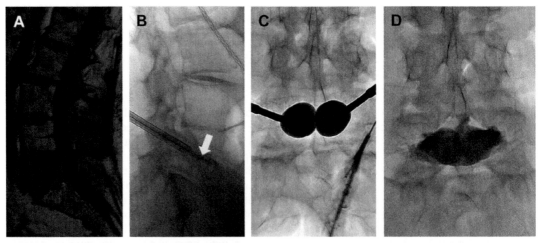

Fig. 13. A 66-year-old woman with metastatic lung carcinoma with severe lumbar pain was found to have a metastasis and pathologic compression fracture, well seen here on the T1-weighted MR image (*A*). The neuroradiologist performed radiofrequency (RF) ablation and balloon kyphoplasty for pain control, local tumor control, and fracture stabilization. RF probes (*B, yellow arrow*) were inserted before cavity creation with balloons (*C*) and subsequent injection of cement (*D*).

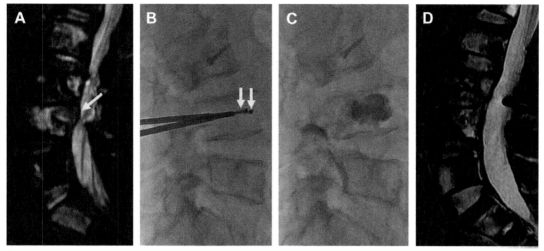

Fig. 14. A 63-year-old patient with hepatocellular carcinoma metastases causing severe pain, localized to the L4 vertebral body. The preoperative MR image of the spine demonstrates diffuse marrow involvement with epidural disease (*yellow arrow*) at L4 (*A*). The neuroradiologist performed radiofrequency (RF) ablation with cement augmentation (*B, C*). (Arrows in (*B*) indicated the tip of the RF probe.) The patient reported immediate, substantial pain relief. MR imaging performed 8 weeks after RF ablation and cement augmentation (*D*) shows decrease in epidural and marrow disease at L4.

collaboration with our surgical and oncology colleagues will ensure the continued relevance and increased role of radiology in the care of patients with spine metastases.

REFERENCES

1. Buhmann-kirchhoff S, Becker C, Duerr HR, et al. Detection of osseous metastases of the spine: comparison of high resolution multi-detector-CT with MRI. Eur J Radiol 2009;69(3):567–73.

2. Zhadanov SI, Doshi AH, Pawha PS, et al. Contrast-enhanced Dixon fat-water separation imaging of the spine: added value of fat, in-phase and opposed-phase imaging in marrow lesion detection. J Comput Assist Tomogr 2016;40(6):985–90.

3. Stradiotti P, Curti A, Castellazzi G, et al. Metal-related artifacts in instrumented spine. Techniques for reducing artifacts in CT and MRI: state of the art. Eur Spine J 2009;18(Suppl 1):102–8.

4. McLellan AM, Daniel S, Corcuera-solano I, et al. Optimized imaging of the postoperative spine. Neuroimaging Clin N Am 2014;24(2):349–64.

5. Kosmala A, Weng AM, Heidemeier A, et al. Multiple myeloma and dual-energy CT: diagnostic accuracy of virtual noncalcium technique for detection of bone marrow infiltration of the spine and pelvis. Radiology 2018;286(1):205–13.

6. Sakamoto R, Yakami M, Fujimoto K, et al. Temporal subtraction of serial CT images with large deformation diffeomorphic metric mapping in the identification of bone metastases. Radiology 2017;285(2):629–39.

7. Katsura M, Sato J, Akahane M, et al. Current and novel techniques for metal artifact reduction at CT: practical guide for radiologists. Radiographics 2018;38(2):450–61.

8. Choi D, Bilsky M, Fehlings M, et al. Spine oncology-metastatic spine tumors. Neurosurgery 2017;80(3S):S131–7.

9. Shah LM, Salzman KL. Imaging of spinal metastatic disease. Int J Surg Oncol 2011;2011:769753.

10. Even-Sapir E, Metser U, Mishani E, et al. The detection of bone metastases in patients with high-risk prostate cancer: 99mTc-MDP Planar bone scintigraphy, single- and multi-field-of-view SPECT, 18F-fluoride PET, and 18F-fluoride PET/CT. J Nucl Med 2006;47(2):287–97.

11. Baur-melnyk A. Malignant versus benign vertebral collapse: are new imaging techniques useful? Cancer Imaging 2009;9:S49–51.

12. Cho WI, Chang UK. Comparison of MR imaging and FDG-PET/CT in the differential diagnosis of benign and malignant vertebral compression fractures. J Neurosurg Spine 2011;14(2):177–83.

13. Mahajan A, Azad GK, Cook GJ. PET imaging of skeletal metastases and its role in personalizing further management. PET Clin 2016;11(3):305–18.

14. Mick CG, James T, Hill JD, et al. Molecular imaging in oncology: (18)F-sodium fluoride PET imaging of osseous metastatic disease. AJR Am J Roentgenol 2014;203(2):263–71.

15. Baur A, Stäbler A, Brüning R, et al. Diffusion-weighted MR imaging of bone marrow:

differentiation of benign versus pathologic compression fractures. Radiology 1998;207(2):349–56.

16. Castillo M, Arbelaez A, Smith JK, et al. Diffusion-weighted MR imaging offers no advantage over routine noncontrast MR imaging in the detection of vertebral metastases. AJNR Am J Neuroradiol 2000;21(5):948–53.

17. Baur A, Huber A, Ertl-wagner B, et al. Diagnostic value of increased diffusion weighting of a steady-state free precession sequence for differentiating acute benign osteoporotic fractures from pathologic vertebral compression fractures. AJNR Am J Neuroradiol 2001;22(2):366–72.

18. Thawait SK, Marcus MA, Morrison WB, et al. Research synthesis: what is the diagnostic performance of magnetic resonance imaging to discriminate benign from malignant vertebral compression fractures? Systematic review and meta-analysis. Spine 2012;37(12):E736–44.

19. Tanenbaum LN. Clinical applications of diffusion imaging in the spine. Magn Reson Imaging Clin N Am 2013;21(2):299–320.

20. Sung JK, Jee WH, Jung JY, et al. Differentiation of acute osteoporotic and malignant compression fractures of the spine: use of additive qualitative and quantitative axial diffusion-weighted MR imaging to conventional MR imaging at 3.0 T. Radiology 2014;271(2):488–98.

21. Hillengass J, Landgren O. Challenges and opportunities of novel imaging techniques in monoclonal plasma cell disorders: imaging "early myeloma". Leuk Lymphoma 2013;54:1355–63.

22. Rajkumar SV, Dimopoulos MA, Palumbo A, et al. International Myeloma Working Group updated criteria for the diagnosis of multiple myeloma. Lancet Oncol 2014;15(12):e538–48.

23. Caers J, Withofs N, Hillengass J, et al. The role of positron emission tomography-computed tomography and magnetic resonance imaging in diagnosis and follow up of multiple myeloma. Haematologica 2014;99(4):629–37.

24. Dutoit JC, Verstraete KL. MRI in multiple myeloma: a pictorial review of diagnostic and post-treatment findings. Insights Imaging 2016;7(4):553–69.

25. Byun WM, Shin SO, Chang Y, et al. Diffusion-weighted MR imaging of metastatic disease of the spine: assessment of response to therapy. AJNR Am J Neuroradiol 2002;23(6):906–12.

26. Padhani AR, Koh DM, Collins DJ. Whole-body diffusion-weighted MR imaging in cancer: current status and research directions. Radiology 2011;261(3):700–18.

27. Herneth AM, Philipp MO, Naude J, et al. Vertebral metastases: assessment with apparent diffusion coefficient. Radiology 2002;225(3):889–94.

28. Verstraete KL, Van der woude HJ, Hogendoorn PC, et al. Dynamic contrast-enhanced MR imaging of musculoskeletal tumors: basic principles and clinical applications. J Magn Reson Imaging 1996;6(2):311–21.

29. Dutoit JC, Vanderkerken MA, Verstraete KL. Value of whole body MRI and dynamic contrast enhanced MRI in the diagnosis, follow-up and evaluation of disease activity and extent in multiple myeloma. Eur J Radiol 2013;82(9):1444–52.

30. Lavini C, De jonge MC, Van de sande MG, et al. Pixel-by-pixel analysis of DCE MRI curve patterns and an illustration of its application to the imaging of the musculoskeletal system. Magn Reson Imaging 2007;25(5):604–12.

31. Tofts PS. Modeling tracer kinetics in dynamic Gd-DTPA MR imaging. J Magn Reson Imaging 1997;7(1):91–101.

32. Chu S, Karimi S, Peck KK, et al. Measurement of blood perfusion in spinal metastases with dynamic contrast-enhanced magnetic resonance imaging: evaluation of tumor response to radiation therapy. Spine 2013;38(22):E1418–24.

33. Lis E, Saha A, Peck KK, et al. Dynamic contrast-enhanced magnetic resonance imaging of osseous spine metastasis before and 1 hour after high-dose image-guided radiation therapy. Neurosurg Focus 2017;42(1):1–13.

34. Lang N, Su MY, Yu HJ, et al. Differentiation of myeloma and metastatic cancer in the spine using dynamic contrast-enhanced MRI. Magn Reson Imaging 2013;31(8):1285–91.

35. Cao Y. The promise of dynamic contrast-enhanced imaging in radiation therapy. Semin Radiat Oncol 2011;21(2):147–56.

36. Kumar KA, Peck KK, Karimi S, et al. A pilot study evaluating the use of dynamic contrast-enhanced perfusion MRI to predict local recurrence after radiosurgery on spinal metastases. Technol Cancer Res Treat 2017. 1533034617705715. [Epub ahead of print].

37. Barzilai O, Laufer I, Yamada Y, et al. Integrating evidence-based medicine for treatment of spinal metastases into a decision framework: neurologic, oncologic, mechanicals stability, and systemic disease. J Clin Oncol 2017;35(21):2419–27.

38. Kaloostian PE, Yurter A, Zadnik PL, et al. Current paradigms for metastatic spinal disease: an evidence-based review. Ann Surg Oncol 2014;21(1):248–62.

39. Laufer I, Rubin DG, Lis E, et al. The NOMS framework: approach to the treatment of spinal metastatic tumors. Oncologist 2013;18(6):744–51.

40. Paton GR, Frangou E, Fourney DR. Contemporary treatment strategy for spinal metastasis: the "LMNOP" system. Can J Neurol Sci 2011;38:396–403.

41. Fisher CG, DiPaola CP, Ryken TC, et al. A novel classification system for spinal instability in neoplastic disease: an evidence-based approach and expert consensus from the Spine Oncology Study Group. Spine 2010;35:E1221–9.

42. Fisher CG, Versteeg AL, Schouten R, et al. Reliability of the spinal instability neoplastic scale among radiologists: an assessment of instability secondary to spinal metastases. AJR Am J Roentgenol 2014; 203(4):869–74.

43. Bilsky MH, Laufer I, Fourney DR, et al. Reliability analysis of the epidural spinal cord compression scale. J Neurosurg Spine 2010;13(3):324–8.

44. Gerszten PC. Spine metastases: from radiotherapy, surgery, to radiosurgery. Neurosurgery 2014; 61(Suppl 1):16–25.

45. Georgy BA. Vertebroplasty technique in metastatic disease. Neuroimaging Clin N Am 2010;20(2): 169–77.

46. Dupuy DE, Liu D, Hartfeil D, et al. Percutaneous radiofrequency ablation of painful osseous metastases: a multicenter American College of Radiology Imaging Network trial. Cancer 2010;116(4):989–97.

47. Hinshaw JL, Lubner MG, Ziemlewicz TJ, et al. Percutaneous tumor ablation tools: microwave, radiofrequency, or cryoablation–what should you use and why. Radiographics 2014;34(5):1344–62.

48. Wallace AN, Greenwood TJ, Jennings JW. Use of imaging in the management of metastatic spine disease with percutaneous ablation and vertebral augmentation. AJR Am J Roentgenol 2015;205(2): 434–41.

Imaging of Acute Low Back Pain

Scott M. Johnson, MD, Lubdha M. Shah, MD*

KEYWORDS

- Acute low back pain • Epidural hematoma • Spinal cord infarct • Discitis osteomyelitis
- Pathologic fracture • Spinal metastases • Acute disc herniation

KEY POINTS

- It is important to remember vascular anatomy when considering causes of cord ischemia.
- Information from various imaging sequences and different modalities can be helpful to distinguish between spinal infection and its mimics.
- There are imaging features to help differentiate between osteoporotic versus pathologic fracture.
- Cauda equina syndrome is typically due to disc pathology.

ACUTE LOW BACK PAIN

Low back pain (LBP) is prevalent, with an estimated point prevalence of 11.9% and a 1-month prevalence of 23.2%.[1] It is the fifth most common cause of doctor visits in the United States, and approximately 3% of emergency department visits are for LBP.[2] Imaging of uncomplicated acute LBP, defined as symptoms lasting less than 6 weeks in duration, has not been shown to add value to patient care and is not recommended.[3] Moreover, it may be harmful because it contributes to unnecessary tests and procedures and a diminished sense of the patient's well-being.[4] Some have estimated that reducing inappropriate imaging of LBP has a potential savings of $300 million annually.[5]

Sometimes acute LBP is associated with concerning symptoms or history that may represent something more ominous underlying the pain. Such "red flags" include symptoms suggesting infection, malignancy, trauma, or other acute process (Box 1). In the setting of these "red flags," acute LBP warrants further work-up through imaging.

When developing a differential diagnosis for a lesion identified on an imaging study, it is important to consider the age, sex, and clinical history as well as the imaging features of the lesion. One classic mnemonic device to ensure that one is considering all possible causes is VINDICATE (Table 1). By going through the list of possible categories and excluding those that do not apply, one can develop a focused differential diagnosis when faced with an imaging study on a patient with acute LBP.

VASCULAR
Epidural Hematoma

Epidural hematoma (EH) may cause acute neck or back pain. Hemorrhage into the epidural space is typically seen in the setting of a fracture, but other causes include recent surgery or procedure, coagulopathy, anticoagulation (Fig. 1), or vascular lesions such as arteriovenous malformation (AVM).[6] Anticoagulant use has been linked to 17–30% of EHs.[7] Up to 40% to 50% demonstrate no identifiable risk factors for the hemorrhage.[7–10] Some investigators have postulated that spontaneous EH develop from rupture of epidural veins, epidural arteries, or a vascular malformation.[8] By exerting mass effect on the cord and nerve roots, EHs can produce devastating neurologic deficits,

Disclosure Statement: The authors have no disclosures.
Department of Radiology and Imaging Sciences, University of Utah, 30 North 1900 East, Room 1A71, Salt Lake City, UT 84132, USA
* Corresponding author.
E-mail address: lubdha.shah@hsc.utah.edu

Radiol Clin N Am 57 (2019) 397–413
https://doi.org/10.1016/j.rcl.2018.10.001

such as progressive paraparesis and bowel/bladder dysfunction, in addition to acute LBP. Therefore, early imaging evaluation to guide possible intervention is critical when a patient presents with concerning symptoms, such as acute myelopathy or cauda equina syndrome.

The upper thoracic spine is the most common site of spontaneous EHs. Often, they are dorsally located in the spinal canal and usually span multiple vertebral levels craniocaudally.

Acute EHs will be hyperdense on computed tomography (CT) (**Fig. 2**) but can be difficult to delineate. MR imaging, on the other hand, provides superb soft tissue, and the appearance of the EH will depend on the acuity of the hemorrhage. Within 24 hours of symptom onset, the EH seems isointense to the spinal cord parenchyma on T1-weighted images and hyperintense on T2-weighted images. After 24 hours, the hematoma often seems hyperintense on both T1- and T2-weighted images (**Fig. 3**), and there may be scattered foci of hypointensity.[11,12] Chronic EHs become hypointense on both T1- and T2-weighted images. Fat suppression sequences may be used to distinguish hematoma from

Table 1 Helpful mnemonic for developing a differential diagnosis	
V	Vascular
I	Infectious
N	Neoplastic
D	Degenerative
I	Iatrogenic
C	Congenital
A	Autoimmune
T	Trauma
E	Environmental

epidural fat.[13] Contrast is not necessary, but if used, active bleeding into the EH may reveal a central area of enhancement.[13] Peripheral enhancement is thought to reflect hyperemia of the dura or hypertrophic meninges.[7,13]

Spinal Cord Infarction

Spinal cord infarction is a diagnostic consideration in a patient presenting with acute LBP and with rapid onset of progressing neurologic deficits.

As discussed in other articles in this issue, spinal cord ischemia is rare due to the several vascular anastomoses supplying the spinal cord. The conus medullaris and the thoracolumbar enlargement are commonly affected sites with spinal cord ischemia.[14] Causes include aortic pathology, such as dissection, vasculitis, or aortoiliac surgical complication[15,16]; trauma; thromboembolic disease; fibrocartilaginous embolism[17]; systemic hypotension from cardiac arrest; or iatrogenic causes such as contrast injection toxicity or inadvertent intravascular injection of epidural steroid.[18]

An acute infarction of the spinal cord may have no MR imaging findings initially (**Box 2**). Diffusion restriction in the ischemic spinal cord on diffusion-weighted imaging (DWI) may not be immediately apparent in the hyperacute phase,

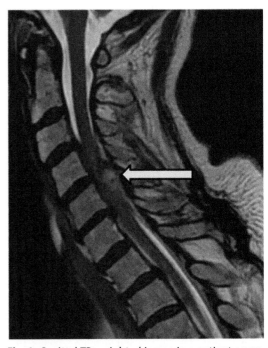

Fig. 1. Sagittal T2-weighted image in a patient on anticoagulation, presenting with spontaneous epidural hematoma in the dorsal epidural space (*yellow arrow*). Note the hyperintensity in relation to the cord parenchyma and irregular areas of hypointensity.

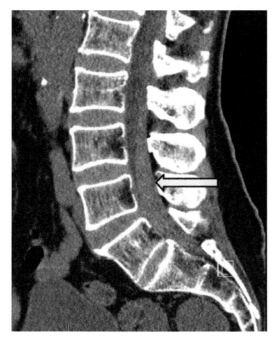

Fig. 2. Noncontrast enhanced CT sagittal reformat. Patient presenting with spontaneous epidural hematoma in the dorsal epidural space. Note the relative hyperdensity (*yellow arrow*) compared with the adjacent cerebrospinal fluid (CSF) within the thecal sac.

with one series only showing a demarcated DWI abnormality in 12 of 22 patients imaged within the first day of symptom onset[19,20] (**Fig. 4**). There is also mild swelling of the cord in the acute phase. Classically, T2 hyperintensity will develop in the frontal horns of the gray matter (**Fig. 5**), sometimes

> **Box 2**
> **Spinal cord infarct evolution**
>
> - May have no findings hyperacutely
> - Diffusion restriction and swelling in first few hours
> - T2 hyperintensity in frontal horn of gray matter (owl's eyes)
> - Enhancement in subacute stage (5 days to 3 weeks)
> - Myelomalacia and gliosis (atrophy and T2 hyperintensity) in chronic stage

referred to as the "owl's eye" pattern, although only about 50% of patients will demonstrate this within the first 24 hours. Enhancement develops in the subacute stage[21] (**Fig. 6**), typically spanning about 5 days to 3 weeks, and is due to breakdown of the blood-cord barrier. Abnormal signal in the marrow of the adjacent vertebral body due to accompanying osseous infarction can also be seen on occasion.[22]

Spinal Vascular Malformations

A spinal dural arteriovenous fistula (dAVF) can manifest as acute LBP, often with progressive lower extremity weakness and sensory loss.[6,23] This vascular lesion results from a fistula formation between a radiculomeningeal artery and a draining radicular vein. A decreased AV pressure gradient develops with increased pressure transmitted to the perimedullary veins. There may be consequent

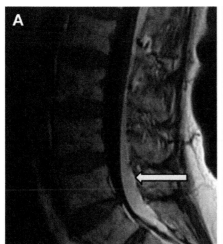
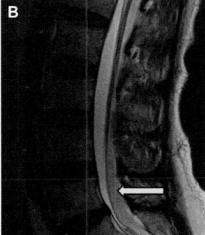

Fig. 3. (*A*) Sagittal T1-weighted MR imaging without contrast of the same patient shows the intrinsic T1 hyperintensity of the epidural hematoma. (*B*) Sagittal T2-weighted MR imaging in the same patient demonstrates relatively hyperintense signal within the hematoma (*yellow arrow*) compared with the cord and nerve roots. The hematoma is slightly hypointense compared with the subcutaneous fat and CSF.

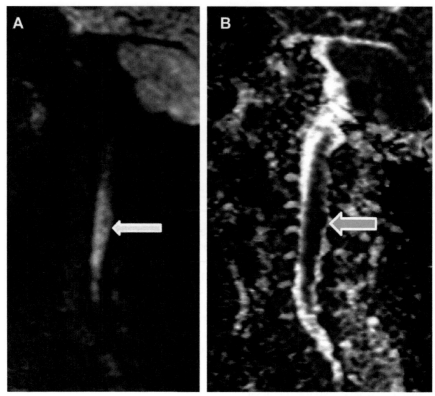

Fig. 4. Sagittal diffusion tensor imaging (*A*) shows high signal within the cervical spinal cord (*yellow arrow*). Sagittal apparent diffusion coefficient (ADC) (*B*) shows corresponding low signal (*blue arrow*), suggesting true diffusion restriction secondary to infarct.

venous engorgement with venous congestion and decreased spinal cord perfusion.

MR imaging will show a mildly enlarged, edematous cord with subtle T1 hypointensity and T2/short tau inversion recovery (STIR) hyperintensity (**Fig. 7**). T2-weighted imaging may reveal a

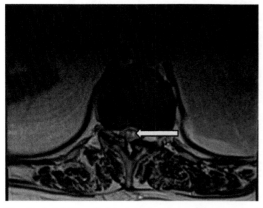

Fig. 5. Axial T2-weighted image in another patient with spinal cord infarct demonstrates T2 hyperintensity within the frontal horns of the gray matter (*yellow arrow*).

hypointense rim, which may be from deoxyhemoglobin within the congested capillaries. Postcontrast images may show patchy, ill-defined intramedullary enhancement and enhancing, tortuous veins along the cord surface, usually dorsally (**Fig. 8**). Up to 80% of these lesions are seen between the levels of T6 and L2.[6]

There are 3 other general types of shunting spinal AVMs, characterized by different feeding vessels, drainage, and volume of blood shunted.[24,25] Like dAVFs, spinal AVMs can present with acute LBP, which is a more common presentation with AVMs as compared with spinal dAVFs,[26,27] and often due to subarachnoid hemorrhage. Glomus-type AVMs (type 2) are direct communications between arteries and veins within the cord parenchyma without an intervening capillary bed or normal parenchyma. Juvenile-type AVMs (type 3) tend to be larger with normal interspersed parenchyma and may have extramedullary components. Perimedullary fistulas (type 4) result from direct intradural extramedullary fistula between the anterior or posterior spinal artery and a draining vein. The most common type to present with

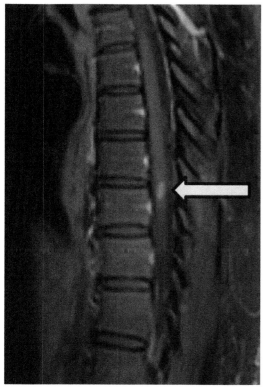

Fig. 6. Sagittal T1-weighted postcontrast fat-saturated image demonstrates enhancement in a focal area of ischemic injury in the thoracic spinal cord (*yellow arrow*). Enhancement is typically seen in the subacute stage.

subarachnoid is the glomus-type AVM, with an estimated 4% annual hemorrhage rate, and as high as 10% annual hemorrhage rate in AVMs that have bled previously.[28]

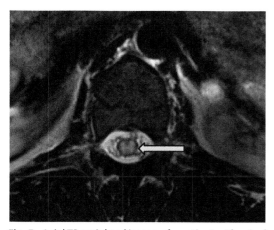

Fig. 7. Axial T2-weighted image of a patient with spinal dAVF shows mild swelling of the cord with central T2 hyperintensity (*yellow arrow*). The thin rim of hypointensity along the periphery of the cord is thought to be due to deoxyhemoglobin within congested capillaries.

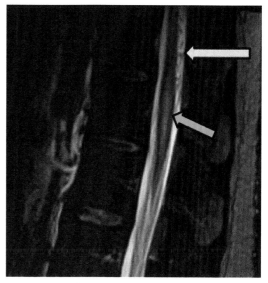

Fig. 8. Sagittal STIR images demonstrate tortuous veins along the dorsal aspect of the cord (*yellow arrow*). Also note the hyperintense STIR signal within the conus medullaris (*blue arrow*).

On MR imaging, spinal AVM may show an intramedullary or superficial lesion composed of flow voids and mixed T1 and T2 signal due to edema and blood products (**Fig. 9**).

INFECTIOUS
Discitis-Osteomyelitis

Discitis-osteomyelitis (DOM) is a fairly common source of acute LBP and can result from numerous pathways[29]: direct inoculation from a recent procedure, spread of contiguous infectious site (such as psoas abscess), hematogenous spread from a distant site of infection (identified in up to 25% of cases), or ascending infection of the urinary tract, where elevated intraabdominal pressure can allow urogenital bacteria access to the valveless paravertebral venous plexus. Intravenous (IV) drug use and immunocompromised status (eg, chronic steroid use, diabetes mellitus, cancer and its various therapies, and older age) are well-known risk factors for DOM. Although most patients with DOM may demonstrate leukocytosis and elevated C-reactive protein and/or erythrocyte sedimentation rate,[30] immunocompromised patients may not have compelling laboratory evidence of acute infection. Atypical infections such as mycobacteria or parasites may also show a lack of leukocytosis.[31]

The pain associated with DOM is typically constant and is not relieved by rest. It is usually not mechanical, that is, unrelated to movement or

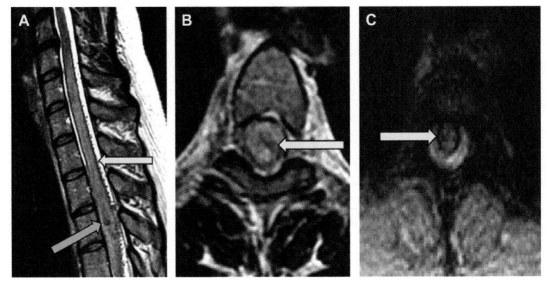

Fig. 9. (*A*) Sagittal T2-weighted image of the thoracic spine demonstrates tortuous veins along the dorsal aspect of the cord (*yellow arrow*). There is a nidus within the cord parenchyma (*blue arrow*). (*B*) Axial T1-weighted post-contrast image through the level of the nidus (*yellow arrow*). (*C*) Axial gradient-echo image through the cord demonstrates a rim of hypointensity (*yellow arrow*), which is thought to represent hemorrhage and/or deoxyhemoglobin within congested capillaries.

positioning. DOM is often accompanied by other classic signs of infection such as fever, chills, malaise, or night sweats. Staphylococcus aureus is the most common organism identified, accounting for 55% to 90% of cases where an organism is identified.[32,33]

The lumbar spine is most often involved, accounting for about 50% of cases. The thoracic spine is the next most frequent, accounting for about 35% of cases. In adults, the anterior subchondral endplate is often the start of infection of hematogenous origin because of its generous arterial blood supply. The infection usually spreads through the medullary spaces of vertebral body. A helpful clue to early DOM is the involvement of the psoas muscles as they originate from the anteromedial lumbar discs, adjacent endplates, and the transverse processes. Enhancement and T2 hyperintensity in the psoas muscle can serve as early imaging findings of DOM (**Fig. 10**), described as the "psoas sign."[34] The infectious process will eventually spread to involve the disc space and adjacent vertebral body endplate with accompanying cortical destruction. CT is helpful to demonstrate the endplate cortical destruction. MR imaging is sensitive to the marrow edema in the endplates, which is seen as T1 hypointensity and T2/STIR hyperintensity.[35] Intradiscal T2/STIR hyperintensity may also be seen; this has a sensitivity of 93.2%[36] (**Fig. 11**). The bone marrow will usually enhance on postcontrast T1 images, with

variable enhancement of the disc space.[36] Disc enhancement has a sensitivity of 95.4% and enhancing paraspinal or epidural soft tissue has a sensitivity of 97.7%.[36]

An important differential diagnosis for DOM is the fibrovascular phase of discogenic endplate degenerative change[37] (**Table 2**), which will demonstrate T2/STIR hyperintensity and linear enhancement. Some key differentiating factors that favor a degenerative process over an

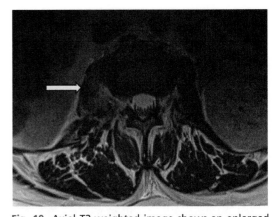

Fig. 10. Axial T2-weighted image shows an enlarged right psoas muscle with relative T2 hyperintensity (*yellow arrow*) compared with the left psoas muscle. The "psoas sign" can help differentiate DOM from degenerative changes. This patient was found to have adjacent discitis-osteomyelitis.

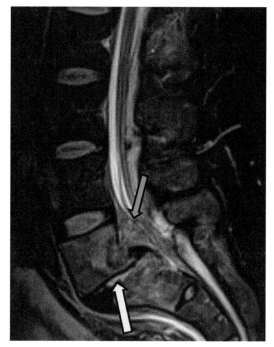

Fig. 11. Sagittal STIR image in a patient with discitis-osteomyelitis. Note the hyperintense signal within the disc space (*yellow arrow*) as well as the hyperintense signal within the endplates parallel to the disc space. Also note the ventral epidural abscess (*blue arrow*).

infectious one include intradiscal T2 hypointensity with loss of disc height, no surrounding soft tissue involvement,[38] and presence of vacuum disc phenomenon. DWI may show hyperintense diffusion

signal with corresponding elevated apparent diffusion coefficient (ADC) values in the vertebral bodies with infected discs compared with normal or degenerative vertebrae and discs.[39] A DWI "claw sign," which is a well-marginated linear hyperintensity at the boundary between normal and vascularized marrow on DWI sequence (**Fig. 12**), favors degenerative disease over infection[40] but should be considered in context with the clinical picture and findings on other conventional sequences.

Spinal neuroarthropathy (SNA), or Charcot spine, is a progressive destructive arthropathy that occurs after loss of neuroprotective sensation and proprioceptive reflexes. Patients present with symptoms of back pain despite anesthesia to the affected area, loss of stature while sitting, spinal deformity and instability, and audible noises originating from the spine with active or passive movement. SNA can mimic DOM on imaging; however, there are imaging clues to SNA. These include involvement of both anterior and posterior elements at the thoracolumbar and lumbosacral junctions, vacuum phenomenon within the disk (indicating excessive motion), malalignment, and paraspinal soft-tissue masses or fluid collections containing bone debris[41] (**Fig. 13**).

Facet Joint Septic Arthritis

Infection of a facet joint can be another infectious cause of acute LBP. As with DOM, the most common culprit is staphylococcus.[32,42] The same predisposing factors for DOM also apply to facet joint septic arthritis, including immunocompromised

Table 2		
Comparison of imaging findings in DOM and degenerative change		
	Discitis-Osteomyelitis	Degenerative Endplate Change
T1-weighted MR imaging	Irregular hypointensity along adjacent endplates May involve whole vertebral body if advanced	Linear hypointensity along endplate
T2-weighted MR imaging	Irregular hyperintensity of marrow May involve whole vertebral body if advanced Hyperintense disc space	Linear hyperintensity along endplate Usually hypointense disc space, loss of disc height
Postcontrast T1-weighted MR imaging	Variable disc space enhancement Diffuse marrow enhancement	No disc space enhancement +/−Linear enhancement along endplate
DWI	Diffuse hyperintensity in vertebral bodies	+/−Linear hyperintensity—"claw sign"
CT	Erosion of endplates	Subchondral cysts, vacuum disc, sclerosis

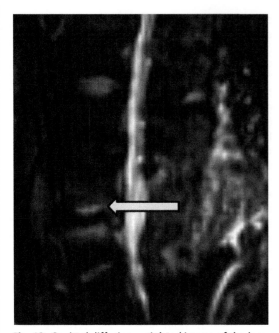

Fig. 12. Sagittal diffusion-weighted image of the lumbar spine in a patient with inflammatory phase degenerative changes. Note the hyperintensity running parallel to the endplates (*yellow arrow*), known as the "claw sign". This finding favors degenerative changes over discitis-osteomyelitis.

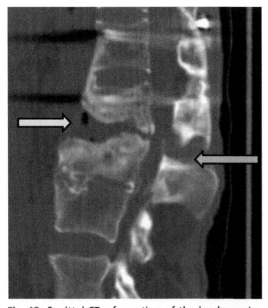

Fig. 13. Sagittal CT reformation of the lumbar spine shows changes of spinal neuroarthropathy or Charcot spine. Vacuum disc phenomenon (*yellow arrow*) and involvement of the posterior elements (*blue arrow*) help differentiate this from discitis-osteomyelitis.

state, IV drug use, and bacteremia. Although facet joint infection can occur through both hematogenous and nonhematogenous routes, the nonhematogenous route of spread is more common.[42,43] Direct extension from cutaneous or other soft tissue infection, as well as iatrogenic cause from a percutaneous procedure, can all lead to septic arthritis of a facet joint. The focal LBP tends to be unilateral, although spread through the retrodural space of Okada to the contralateral facet joint[44] may result in bilateral LBP.

MR imaging will demonstrate an enhancing, expanded joint capsule on postcontrast T1-weighted images. T2-weighted and STIR sequences will show inflammatory edema in the surrounding soft tissues (**Fig. 14A**). DWI sequences may be useful for identifying purulent collections both within the joint and the adjacent epidural space (**Fig. 14B**).[45] Advanced cases with cortical erosion may be seen on MR imaging, but CT is more sensitive for earlier osseous destructive changes (**Fig. 14C**).

Spinal Leptomeningitis

Infection of the spinal leptomeninges can present with acute LBP. It typically originates from hematogenous spread from a remote site of infection or cerebrospinal fluid (CSF) dissemination of infection elsewhere in the neural axis.[46] Back pain can be accompanied by paresthesias or sphincter dysfunction. Systemic symptoms are typically present, such as fever, malaise, and irritability.

MR imaging is the modality of choice for evaluation. T2-weighted images may demonstrate clumped nerve roots, distorted spinal cord contour, ill-defined intramedullary hyperintensity, and loculations in the subarachnoid space. Although precontrast T1-weighted images may show slight increased signal intensity of the cord and thickening of the dura, post-contrast T1-weighted images are more informative. Enhanced imaged can reveal linear or nodular enhancement of the dura and nerve roots (**Fig. 15**). Spinal meningitis can progress to chronic arachnoid septations and adhesions with altered CSF dynamics and syrinx formation.

NEOPLASTIC
Metastatic Disease

Although the differential diagnosis of acute LBP is broad, new-onset back pain in a patient with cancer commonly has a tumor-related cause.[47,48] The predominant symptom in patients with spinal metastases is pain, which can be of 3 types: constant localized pain, radicular pain, and axial pain.[49] The

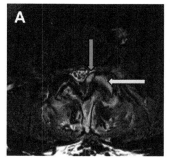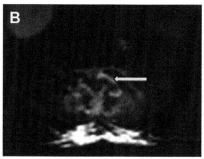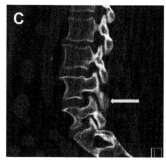

Fig. 14. (A) Axial T2-weighted fat-saturated image demonstrates widening of the left facet joint with fluid (*yellow arrow*). Also, note the adjacent epidural fluid collection (*blue arrow*). There is edema within the posterior elements and the surrounding paraspinal musculature. (B) Axial DWI image of the same patient through the same level shows hyperintense signal within the facet extending into the epidural collection (*yellow arrow*). Corresponding ADC hypointense signal confirmed the diffusion restriction (not shown). The patient had a pyogenic septic arthritis of this facet joint. (C) Sagittal CT reformation of the lumbar spine in the same patient shows demineralization and loss of cortex of the inferior left articular facet. The patient was found to have septic arthritis and osteomyelitis of that facet joint.

expanding tumor can cause periosteal "stretching" leading to constant localized pain and compression of nerve roots leading to radicular pain. Axial pain is frequently associated with pathologic vertebral body fracture and spinal instability secondary to destruction of its posterior portion.

Metastatic osseous lesions (including lymphoproliferative disorders) are the most common tumor in the adult spine,[50] more common than primary malignant bone tumors. The most common malignant neoplasms to metastasize to the spine are breast, prostate, and lung cancers. The

vertebrae are the most common site of occurrence, accounting for approximately one-third of osseous metastases.[51] The posterior half of the vertebral body is usually infiltrated first, with the anterior body, lamina, and pedicles becoming involved later.[52] Approximately 98% of spinal metastases are extradural, of which 80% involve the posterior spinal elements often leading to instability, deformity, and pain.[53,54]

Metastatic bone tumors can seem lytic, sclerotic, or mixed on radiography and CT (Figs. 16 and 17). CT provides superior evaluation of the

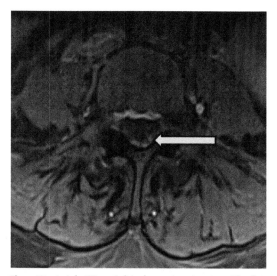

Fig. 15. Axial T1-weighted postcontrast with fat-saturated image shows enhancement of the cauda equina nerve roots (*yellow arrow*) in a patient with known meningitis. The patient was found to have laboratory evidence and clinical symptoms of spinal meningitis.

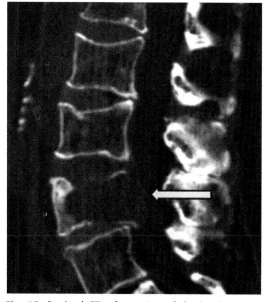

Fig. 16. Sagittal CT reformation of the lumbar spine demonstrates a lytic vertebral body metastasis with faint extra-osseous spread into the epidural space, compressing the thecal sac (*yellow arrow*).

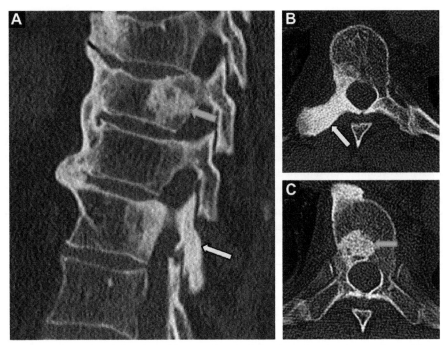

Fig. 17. Sagittal CT reformation (*A*) and axial images (*B, C*) of the thoracic spine in a patient with prostate cancer demonstrates a sclerotic metastasis in the vertebral body (*yellow arrow*) and posterior elements (*blue arrow*).

cortical integrity and delineation of lesion margins. This osseous definition is a useful complement to the soft tissue assessment seen by MR imaging. Comparing marrow signal to the disc spaces at 1.5 T on T1-weighted images has a 94% sensitivity and 98% specificity[55] for detecting an abnormality. On T1-weighted images, metastatic lesions are typically hypercellular and will therefore seem abnormally dark compared with the relatively bright signal of normal vertebral fatty marrow (**Fig. 18**).

Key imaging features to evaluate in the spinal metastatic lesions are the extent of epidural disease and the associated thecal sac and neural foraminal narrowing, paraspinal spread, and pathologic fracture (discussed later). A distinguishing feature of metastatic disease involving adjacent vertebral bodies is that malignancy in the spine usually spares the disc space, unlike discitis-osteomyelitis (**Fig. 19**).

Osseous metastatic disease can progress to epidural spinal cord compression, which may be the first manifestation of cancer in up to one-fourth of patients.[56] After back pain develops, there may be rapid neurologic deterioration with paraplegia, loss of lower extremity sensation, and/or incontinence.

Leptomeningeal carcinomatosis, spread of tumor cells through the subarachnoid space, can

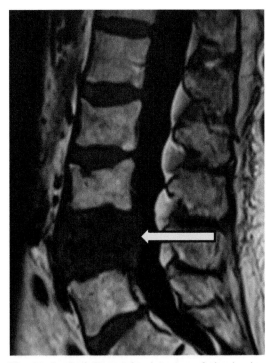

Fig. 18. Sagittal T1-weighted image of the lumbar spine in a patient with known metastatic melanoma. Note the complete replacement of normal T1 hyperintensity within the L4 vertebral body with hypointense signal (*yellow arrow*).

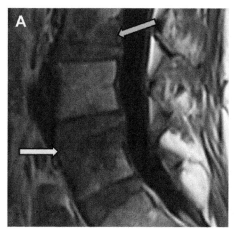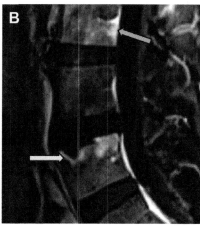

Fig. 19. (A) Sagittal T1-weighted precontrast image in a patient with known metastatic gastric carcinoma demonstrates hypointensity underlying the superior L5 endplate (*yellow arrow*). In isolation, this may be mistaken for degenerative endplate changes or developing discitis-osteomyelitis. The presence of other metastases (*blue arrow*) is a helpful clue. (B) Sagittal T1-weighted post-contrast image in the same patient demonstrates enhancing metastatic disease surrounding the site of pathologic fracture (*yellow arrow*). Aside from the presence of other metastases (*blue arrow*), the sparing of the disc space should make discitis-osteomyelitis much less likely.

also cause neck and back pain, presenting as localized spinal tenderness or radicular discomfort that radiates from the spine into an arm or leg.

Leptomeningeal carcinomatosis in systemic tumors such as melanoma and breast cancer can be caused by hematogenous spread, by direct extension, or by perineural or perivascular extension.[57] Central nervous system tumors such as ependymoma, glioblastoma, or germinoma can also seed the CSF. Contrast-enhanced MR imaging will reveal nodular or diffuse enhancement of the nerve roots on postcontrast T1-weighted images (Fig. 20). Abnormal neuroimaging is more likely in patients with solid tumors (72%–80%) versus hematologic malignancies (48%–62%).[58]

DEGENERATIVE
Acute Disc Herniation

An acute disc herniation can cause acute LBP ± radicular pain. Although the typical acute disc herniation may not require emergent imaging evaluation, if there are persistent symptoms and intervention is being considered, imaging may be warranted.[3] Some disc herniations are large enough to cause acute cauda equina syndrome, including saddle anesthesia and dysfunction of bowel and bladder.[59] This type of presentation is more likely when superimposed on preexisting spinal canal stenosis (Fig. 21). Routine MR axial and sagittal T1, T2, and STIR sequences enable adequate evaluation of thecal sac and foraminal narrowing, as well as any underlying signal abnormality in compressed segments of the spinal cord.

Rarely, there can be intradural disc herniations, which comprise only 0.26% to 0.30% of all disc herniations. These occur more often in the lumbar region (92%)[60,61] and usually in the setting of adhesions between the ventral dura and the posterior longitudinal ligament or annulus fibrosus.[62,63] Such herniations may resemble intradural extramedullary tumors such as a schwannoma or a neurofibroma but can be differentiated by their

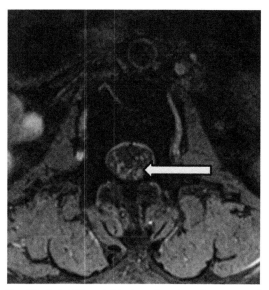

Fig. 20. Axial T1-weighted postcontrast fat-saturated image demonstrates diffuse enhancement of the cauda equina nerve roots (*yellow arrow*) in a patient with known widespread metastatic disease. Findings were consistent with leptomeningeal carcinomatosis.

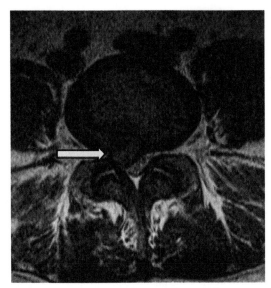

Fig. 21. Axial T2-weighted image shows a disc protrusion (*yellow arrow*) causing complete effacement of the right subarticular recess, displacement of the transiting nerve roots, and moderate narrowing of the spinal canal. The acquired stenosis is superimposed on mild congenital narrowing of the spinal canal.

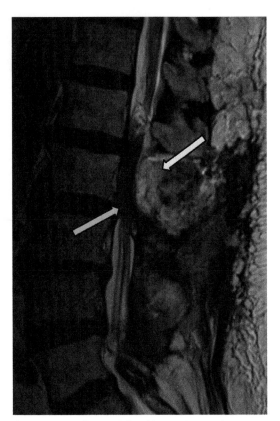

Fig. 22. Sagittal T2-weighted image in a patient status post L2 laminectomy, who presented with low back pain and cauda equina syndrome. There is a heterogeneously T2 hyperintense hematoma (*yellow arrow*) compressing the thecal sac and nerve roots at the operative site (*blue arrow*).

enhancement pattern. Although the tumors will enhance uniformly, a disc herniation will peripherally enhance due to associated granulation tissue and neovascularization.[64] Cauda equina syndrome is more frequent in the presence of intradural disc herniation.[62,65]

IATROGENIC

Iatrogenic sources of acute LBP dovetail with many of the other categories in this section. A postoperative or postprocedural hematoma causing cauda equina syndrome may compress adjacent structures (**Fig. 22**). Spinal cord infarction can result from direct spinal cord trauma, from embolization of a spinal vascular malformation, or from aortic surgery. Malposition of hardware or graft displacement can lead to compression of the thecal sac or the cord itself. Infection is also a potential source of acute back pain.

CONGENITAL

Although most congenital abnormalities of the spine are identified in childhood or adolescence, some disorders can manifest in adulthood as secondary sources of acute LBP. One such example is sickle cell disease (SCD), where acute bone infarctions and infection are well-known complications.[66] Although bone infarctions are most commonly seen in the appendicular skeleton, it is

estimated that 43% to 70% of patients with SCD suffer spine involvement.[67] Classically, the vertebral bodies of a patient with SCD are "H-shaped," with central height loss secondary to central compression deformity of the end plates. There may be patchy sclerosis due to prior infarcts. On MR imaging, the marrow will often be T1 hypointense due to a combination of prior bone infarcts, red marrow hyperplasia, and iron deposition from prior transfusions. Acute bone infarctions may show a serpentine rim of enhancement on postcontrast T1-weighted images.

Connective tissue disorders such as Marfan, Ehlers-Danlos, Loey-Dietz, and Stickler syndromes can render a patient more vulnerable to traumatic LBP resulting from hypermobility of the spine.[68-71] Beyond the imaging manifestations of trauma, look for dural ectasia and scoliosis as generic manifestations of possible underlying connective tissue disorders. One might also detect aortic dilation in the imaging field of view in these patients with connective tissue disease.

AUTOIMMUNE

When reviewing the imaging of relatively young patients presenting with acute LBP from relatively minor trauma, one may notice findings that suggest underlying HLA-B27 arthropathies, such as ankylosing spondylitis (AS). AS presents at a mean age of 26 years and affects men more than women.[72] MR imaging may show inflammatory changes at the costovertebral joints, enthesitis along the spinous processes (**Fig. 23**), and sacroiliitis. The classic "bamboo spine" due to vertebral body fusion by marginal syndesmophytes and osteoporosis predisposes to vertebral fractures, even from minor trauma (**Fig. 24**). One study estimated that patients with AS have a prevalence of osteoporosis of 25%.[73] A population-based cohort study estimated spine fracture prevalence in AS to be 10%.[74]

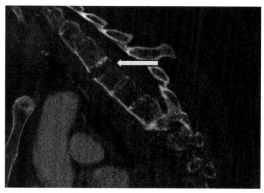

Fig. 24. Sagittal CT reformation of the thoracic spine in a patient with AS status after trauma. The patient sustained a 2-column fracture of the thoracic spine (*yellow arrow*). Note the thickening and increased density of the anterior longitudinal ligament, as well as the osteopenia of the vertebral bodies.

TRAUMA
Fractures

Traumatic spinal fracture is an obvious source of acute LBP. Major trauma from motor vehicle collisions are the most common mechanism, accounting for about 40% of all spinal injuries.[75] Of these, approximately 15% are injuries of the lumbosacral spine.[76] Minor trauma can also cause spinal fractures when the underlying bone is weakened due to decreased bone mineral density as in osteoporosis or when there are altered biomechanics with decreased mobility in conditions such as diffuse idiopathic skeletal hyperostosis or ankylosing spondylitis.

Multidetector CT is the primary modality for fracture assessment as radiographs tend to underestimate the number, extent, and stability of fractures.[77] MR imaging is reserved for cases of suspected ligamentous or spinal cord injury and in patients with neurologic deficits.

Pathologic fractures, occurring usually when most of the vertebral body has been infiltrated by tumor,[54,55] can be difficult to differentiate from benign fractures (**Table 3**). Pathologic fractures are associated with hypercellularity and, as a result, they are more likely to show diffusion restriction (bright on DWI and dark on ADC).[78] Low ADC values are often used as a proxy for hypercellularity in brain, spine, and head and neck tumors.[79] Benign fractures have preserved marrow signal on routine MR imaging sequences and typically demonstrate edema, which is bright on DWI as well as on ADC, representing "T2 shine-through."[80] Thus, benign fractures can be "white" and "wet" (white = bright on ADC, wet = edematous and possibly associated with fluid cleft) and pathologic fractures "dark" and "dry" (dark = dark on ADC, dry = less edematous and no fluid cleft). The fracture lines themselves are usually dark on T1- and T2-weighted images.

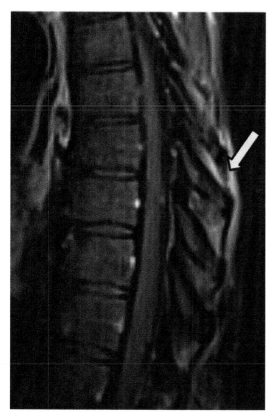

Fig. 23. Sagittal T1-weighted postcontrast fat-saturated image of the thoracic spine in a 37-year-old man with back pain and history of ankylosing spondylitis. Enthesitis along the spinous processes is noted (*yellow arrow*).

Table 3
Differentiating imaging features of benign and pathologic fractures

Benign Fracture	Pathologic Fracture
Normal marrow, bright on ADC	Patchy or diffuse replacement of normal marrow, may involve posterior elements, ADC hypointensity
Posterior bone fragment retropulsion	Bowing of the posterior cortex
Other benign compression fractures	Other spinal metastases
Fluid cleft	Typically no fluid cleft
Minimal to no abnormal extraosseous soft tissue	Epidural or paraspinal soft tissue spread
Linear horizontal T1/T2 hypointense fracture line	Bone destruction

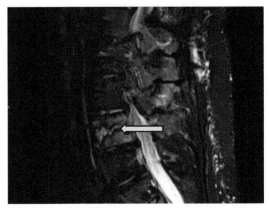

Fig. 25. Sagittal STIR image of the lumbar spine demonstrates an osteoporotic fracture with fluid cleft (*yellow arrow*). Fluid clefts are only rarely seen in pathologic fractures.

In pathologic fractures, the marrow replacement often extends into the pedicles and other posterior elements by the time a pathologic fracture takes place, and abnormal marrow signal in these regions is seen more often than in osteoporotic fractures.[81] However, other studies have suggested that this pedicle signal abnormality is not specific enough to differentiate pathologic from benign fracture.[82] Convex bowing of the posterior cortex of the vertebral body also favors a pathologic cause. Expansion of the fractured vertebral body and associated epidural mass are seen with pathologic fractures. Multiple vertebral metastases should raise the index of suspicion for pathologic fracture.[9] Enhancement is not specific,[78,83] but enhancement relative to adjacent normal vertebral bodies can be used to suggest benign versus pathologic fracture.[83–85] Other findings that favor a benign vertebral fracture include retropulsion of a bone fragment, the presence of compression fractures at other vertebral levels, and a vertebral fluid cleft (**Fig. 25**), which is rarely seen in pathologic fractures.[86]

ENVIRONMENTAL

Although there may be no direct imaging correlate of environmental conditions, it is worth briefly reviewing a few lifestyle factors that can predispose a patient to back pain. Perhaps unsurprisingly, occupations with manual labor activities such as heavy lifting, pushing, pulling, and prolonged periods of standing and walking have been shown to be predictors of future LBP.[87–91] Some studies have also established a link between smoking and increased prevalence of LBP.[92,93] Elevated body mass index has also been associated with increased prevalence of LBP.[94] Although these do not directly relate to imaging of acute LBP, they are factors that can be borne in mind while evaluating for its causes.

SUMMARY

After reviewing the multitude of causes of acute LBP, it bears repeating that because most cases are musculofascial in origin and without the "red flags," immediate imaging assessment is not warranted. When evaluating the imaging study of a patient presenting with acute LBP, develop the differential diagnoses in the context of the clinical history (ie, history of cancer, immunocompromised, etc.) as well as the imaging features. It is as important to exclude causes as it is to include potential causes in order to render a meaningful interpretation.

REFERENCES

1. Hoy D, Bain C, Williams G, et al. A systematic review of the global prevalence of low back pain. Arthritis Rheum 2012;64(6):2028–37.
2. Waterman BR, Belmont PJ, Schoenfeld AJ. Low back pain in the United States: incidence and risk factors for presentation in the emergency setting. Spine J 2012;12(1):63–70.

3. Patel ND, Broderick DF, Burns J, et al. ACR appropriateness criteria low back pain. J Am Coll Radiol 2016;13(9):1069–78.

4. Modic MT, Obuchowski NA, Ross JS, et al. Acute low back pain and radiculopathy: MR imaging findings and their prognostic role and effect on outcome. Radiology 2005;237(2):597–604.

5. Srinivas SV, Deyo RA, Berger ZD. Application of "less is more" to low back pain. Arch Intern Med 2012;172:1016–20.

6. Krings T, Geibprasert S. Spinal dural arteriovenous fistulas. AJNR Am J Neuroradiol 2009;30(4):639–48.

7. Dziedzic T, Kunert P, Krych P, et al. Management and neurological outcome of spontaneous spinal epidural hematoma. J Clin Neurosci 2015;22:726–9.

8. Zhong W, Chen H, You C, et al. Spontaneous spinal epidural hematoma. J Clin Neurosci 2011;18:1490–4.

9. Bhat KJ, Kapoor S, Watali YZ, et al. Spontaneous epidural hematoma of spine associated with clopidogrel: a case study and review of the literature. Asian J Neurosurg 2015;10:54.

10. Foo D, Rossier AB. Preoperative neurological status in predicting surgical outcome of spinal epidural hematomas. Surg Neurol 1981;15:389–401.

11. Holtas S, Heiling M, Lonntoft M. Spontaneous spinal epidural hematoma: findings at MR imaging and clinical correlation. Radiology 1996;199(2):409–13.

12. Fukui MB, Swarnkar AS, Williams RL. Acute spontaneous spinal epidural hematomas. AJNR Am J Neuroradiol 1999;20(7):1365–72.

13. Tawk C, El Hajj Moussa M, Zgheib R, et al. Spontaneous epidural hematoma of the spine associated with oral anticoagulants: 3 case studies. Int J Surg Case Rep 2015;13:8–11.

14. Mull M, Thron A. Spinal infarcts. In: von Kummer R, Back T, editors. Magnetic Resonance Imaging in Ischemic Stroke. Berlin: Springer; 2006. p. 251–67.

15. Weidauer S, Nichtweiß M, Hattingen E, et al. Spinal cord ischemia: aetiology, clinical syndromes and imaging features. Neuroradiology 2014;57(3):241–57.

16. Gravereaux EC, Faries PL, Burks JA, et al. Risk of spinal cord ischemia after endograft repair of thoracic aortic aneurysms. J Vasc Surg 2001;34(6):997–1003.

17. Mikulis DJ, Ogilvy CS, McKee A, et al. Spinal cord infarction and fibrocartilagenous emboli. AJNR Am J Neuroradiol 1992;13(1):155–60.

18. Lyders EM, Morris PP. A case of spinal cord infarction following lumbar transforaminal epidural steroid injection: MR imaging and angiographic findings. AJNR Am J Neuroradiol 2009;30(9):1691–3.

19. Nogueira RG, Ferreira R, Grant PE, et al. Restricted diffusion in spinal cord infarction demonstrated by magnetic resonance line scan diffusion imaging. Stroke 2012;43:532–5.

20. Kumral E, Polat F, Güllüoglu H, et al. Spinal ischaemic stroke: clinical and radiological findings and short-term outcome. Eur J Neurol 2011;18(2):232–9.

21. Vargas MI, Gariani J, Sztajzel R, et al. Spinal cord ischemia: practical imaging tips, pearls, and pitfalls. AJNR Am J Neuroradiol 2015;36(5):825–30.

22. Yuh WT, Marsh EE, Wang AK, et al. MR imaging of spinal cord and vertebral body infarction. AJNR Am J Neuroradiol 1992;13(1):145–54.

23. Koenig E, Thron A, Schrader V, et al. Spinal arteriovenous malformations and fistulae: clinical, neuroradiological and neurophysiological findings. J Neurol 1989;236(5):260–6.

24. Gueguen B, Merland JJ, Riche MC, et al. Vascular malformations of the spinal cord: intrathecal perimedullary arteriovenous fistulas fed by medullary arteries. Neurology 1987;37(6):969–79.

25. Mourier KL, Gobin YP, George B, et al. Intradural perimedullary arteriovenous fistulae: results of surgical and endovascular treatment in a series of 35 cases. Neurosurgery 1993;32(6):885–91 [discussion: 891].

26. Hong T, Park JE, Ling F, et al. Comparison of 3 different types of spinal arteriovenous shunts below the conus in clinical presentation, radiologic findings, and outcomes. AJNR Am J Neuroradiol 2017;38(2):403–9.

27. Singh R, Lucke-Wold B, Gyure K, et al. A review of vascular abnormalities of the spine. Ann Vasc Med Res 2016;3(4):1045.

28. Gross BA, Du H. Spinal glomus (type II) arteriovenous malformations: a pooled analysis of hemorrhage risk and results of intervention. Neurosurgery 2013;72(1):25–32 [discussion: 32].

29. Mylona E, Samarkos M, Kakalou E, et al. Pyogenic vertebral osteomyelitis: a systematic review of clinical characteristics [review]. Semin Arthritis Rheum 2009;39(1):10–7.

30. Early SD, Kay RM, Tolo VT. Childhood diskitis. J Am Acad Orthop Surg 2003;11(6):413–20.

31. Tins BJ, Cassar-Pullicino VN, Lalam RK. Magnetic resonance imaging of spinal infection. Top Magn Reson Imaging 2007;18(3):213–22.

32. Yoon SH, Chung SK, Kim KJ, et al. Pyogenic vertebral osteomyelitis: identification of microorganism and laboratory markers used to predict clinical outcome. Eur Spine J 2010;19:575–82.

33. Resnik D. Osteomyelitis, septic arthritis and soft tissue infection: axial skeleton. In: Resnick D, editor. Diagnosis of Bone and Joint Disorders. 4th edition. Philadelphia: Saunders; 2002.

34. Ledbetter LN, Salzman KL, Shah LM. Imaging psoas sign in lumbar spinal infections: evaluation of diagnostic accuracy and comparison with established imaging characteristics. AJNR Am J Neuroradiol 2016;37(4):736–41.

35. Hong SH, Choi JY, Lee JW, et al. MR imaging assessment of the spine: infection or an imitation? Radiographics 2009;29(2):599–612.

36. Ledermann HP, Schweitzer ME, Morrison WB, et al. MR imaging findings in spinal infections: rules or myths? Radiology 2003;228(2):506–14.

37. Modic MT, Steinberg PM, Ross JS, et al. Degenerative disk disease: assessment of changes in vertebral body marrow with MR imaging. Radiology 1988;166(1):193–9.

38. Tali ET. Spinal infections. Eur J Radiol 2004;50(2): 120–33.

39. Eguchi Y, Ohtori S, Yamashita M, et al. Diffusion magnetic resonance imaging to differentiate degenerative from infectious endplate abnormalities in the lumbar spine. Spine (Phila Pa 1976) 2011;36(3): E198–202.

40. Patel KB, Poplawski MM, Pawha PS, et al. Diffusion-weighted MRI "claw sign" improves differentiation of infectious from degenerative modic type 1 signal changes of the spine. AJNR Am J Neuroradiol 2014;35(8):1647–52.

41. Ledbetter LN, Salzman KL, Sanders RK, et al. Spinal neuroarthropathy: pathophysiology, clinical and imaging features, and differential diagnosis. Radiographics 2016;36(3):783–99.

42. Narvaez J, Nolla JM, Narvaez JA, et al. Spontaneous pyogenic facet joint infection. Semin Arthritis Rheum 2006;35:272–83.

43. Tali ET, Oner AY, Koc AM. Pyogenic spinal infections. Neuroimaging Clin N Am 2015;25(2):193–208.

44. Lehman VT, Murthy NS, Diehn FE, et al. The posterior ligamentous complex inflammatory syndrome: spread of fluid and inflammation in the retrodural space of Okada. Clin Radiol 2015;70(5):528–35.

45. Moritani T, Kim J, Capizzano AA, et al. Pyogenic and non-pyogenic spinal infections: emphasis on diffusion-weighted imaging for the detection of abscesses and pus collections. Br J Radiol 2014; 87(1041):20140011.

46. Meltzer CC, Fukui MB, Kanal E, et al. MR imaging of the meninges. Part I. Normal anatomic features and nonneoplastic disease. Radiology 1996;201(2): 297–308.

47. Gilbert MR, Grossman SA. Incidence and nature of neurologic problems in patients with solid tumors. Am J Med 1986;81:951–4.

48. Clouston PD, DeAngelis LM, Posner JB. The spectrum of neurological disease in patients with systemic cancer. Ann Neurol 1992;31:268–73.

49. Kassamali RH, Ganeshan A, Hoey ET, et al. Pain management in spinal metastases: the role of percutaneous vertebral augmentation. Ann Oncol 2011; 22(Issue 4):782–6.

50. Rodallec MH, Feydy A, Larousserie F, et al. Diagnostic imaging of solitary tumors of the spine: what to do and say. Radiographics 2008;28(4):1019–41.

51. Toma CD, Dominkus M, Nedelcu T, et al. Metastatic bone disease: a 36-year single centre trend-analysis of patients admitted to a tertiary orthopaedic surgical department. J Surg Oncol 2007;96(5):404–10.

52. Klimo P, Schmidt MH. Surgical management of spine metastases. Oncologist 2004;9:188–96.

53. Gokaslan ZL, York JE, Walsh GL, et al. Transthoracic vertebrectomy for metastatic spinal tumors. J Neurosurg 1998;89(4):599–609.

54. Jacobs WB, Perrin RG. Evaluation and treatment of spinal metastases: an overview. Neurosurg Focus 2001;11(6):e10.

55. Carroll KW, Feller JF, Tirman PF. Useful internal standards for distinguishing infiltrative marrow pathology from hematopoietic marrow at MRI. J Magn Reson Imaging 1997;7(2):394–8.

56. Newton HB. Neurologic complications of systemic cancer [review]. Am Fam Physician 1999;59(4): 878–86 [Erratum appears in Am Fam Physician 1999;59(9):2435].

57. Grossman SA, Krabak MJ. Leptomeningeal carcinomatosis. Cancer Treat Rev 1999;25(2):103–19.

58. Clarke JL, Perez HR, Jacks LM, et al. Leptomeningeal metastases in the MRI era. Neurology 2010; 74(18):1449–54.

59. Fraser S, Roberts L, Murphy E. Cauda equina syndrome: a literature review of its definition and clinical presentation. Arch Phys Med Rehabil 2009;90(11): 1964–8.

60. Aydin MV, Ozel S, Sen O, et al. Intradural disc mimicking: a spinal tumor lesion. Spinal Cord 2004;42(1):52–4.

61. Epstein NE, Syrquin MS, Epstein JA, et al. Intradural disc herniations in the cervical, thoracic, and lumbar spine: report of three cases and review of the literature. J Spinal Disord 1990;3(4):396–403.

62. Lee JS, Suh KT. Intradural disc herniation at L5-S1 mimicking an intradural extramedullary spinal tumor: a case report. J Korean Med Sci 2006;21(4):778–80.

63. Koc RK, Akdemir H, Oktem IS, et al. Intradural lumbar disc herniation: report of two cases. Neurosurg Rev 2001;24(1):44–7.

64. Kobayashi K, Imagama S, Matsubara Y, et al. Intradural disc herniation: radiographic findings and surgical results with a literature review. Clin Neurol Neurosurg 2014;125:47–51.

65. Yildizhan A, Paşaoğlu A, Okten T, et al. Intradural disc herniations pathogenesis, clinical picture, diagnosis and treatment. Acta Neurochir (Wien) 1991; 110(3–4):160–5.

66. Lonergan GJ, Cline DB, Abbondanzo SL. Sickle cell anemia. Radiographics 2001;21(4):971–94.

67. Kosaraju V, Harwani A, Partovi S, et al. Imaging of musculoskeletal manifestations in sickle cell disease patients. Br J Radiol 2017;90(1073):20160130.

68. Dietz H. Marfan syndrome. In: Adam MP, Ardinger HH, Pagon RA, et al, editors. GeneReviews®. Seattle (WA):

University of Washington, Seattle; 2017. Available at: https://www.ncbi.nlm.nih.gov/books/NBK1335. Accessed November 19, 2018.

69. Villeirs GM, Van Tongerloo AJ, Verstraete KL, et al. Widening of the spinal canal and dural ectasia in Marfan's syndrome: assessment by CT. Neuroradiology 1999;41(11):850–4.

70. Loeys BL, Dietz HC. Loeys-Dietz syndrome. In: Adam MP, Ardinger HH, Pagon RA, et al, editors. GeneReviews®. Seattle (WA): University of Washington, Seattle; 2018. Available at: https://www.ncbi.nlm.nih.gov/books/NBK1133. Accessed November 19, 2018.

71. Rose PS, Ahn NU, Levy HP, et al. Thoracolumbar spinal abnormalities in Stickler syndrome. Spine (Phila Pa 1976) 2001;26(4):403–9.

72. Braun J, Sieper J. Ankylosing spondylitis. Lancet 2007;369(9570):1379–90.

73. Ghozlani I, Ghazi M, Nouijai A, et al. Prevalence and risk factors of osteoporosis and vertebral fractures in patients with ankylosing spondylitis. Bone 2009; 44(5):772–6.

74. Cooper C, Carbone L, Michet CJ, et al. Fracture risk in patients with ankylosing spondylitis: a population based study. J Rheumatol 1994;21(10):1877–82.

75. Parizel PM, van der Zijden T, Gaudino S, et al. Trauma of the spine and spinal cord: imaging strategies. Eur Spine J 2010;19(suppl 1):8–17.

76. Sekhon LH, Fehlings MG. Epidemiology, demographics, and pathophysiology of acute spinal cord injury. Spine 2001;26(24 suppl):S2–12.

77. Campbell SE, Phillips CD, Dubovsky E, et al. The value of CT in determining potential instability of simple wedge-compression fractures of the lumbar spine. AJNR Am J Neuroradiol 1995;16(7):1385–92.

78. Baur A, Huber A, Ertl-Wagner B, et al. Diagnostic value of increased diffusion weighting of a steady-state free precession sequence for differentiating acute benign osteoporotic fractures from pathologic vertebral compression fractures. AJNR Am J Neuroradiol 2001;22(2):366–72.

79. Chen L, Liu M, Bao J, et al. The correlation between apparent diffusion coefficient and tumor cellularity in patients: a meta-analysis. PLoS One 2013;8(11): e79008.

80. Baur A, Dietrich O, Reiser M. Diffusion-weighted imaging of bone marrow: current status. Eur Radiol 2003;13(7):1699–708.

81. Jung HS, Jee WH, McCauley TR, et al. Discrimination of metastatic from acute osteoporotic compression spinal fractures with MR imaging. Radiographics 2003;23(1):179–87.

82. Ishiyama M, Fuwa S, Numaguchi Y, et al. Pedicle involvement on MR imaging is common in osteoporotic compression fractures. AJNR Am J Neuroradiol 2010;31(4):668–73.

83. Rupp RE, Ebraheim NA, Coombs RJ. Magnetic resonance imaging differentiation of compression spine fractures or vertebral lesions caused by osteoporosis or tumor. Spine (Phila Pa 1976) 1995; 20(23):2499–503 [discussion: 2504].

84. Cuénod CA, Laredo JD, Chevret S, et al. Acute vertebral collapse due to osteoporosis or malignancy: appearance on unenhanced and gadolinium-enhanced MR images. Radiology 1996; 199:541–9.

85. Shih TT, Huang KM, Li YW. Solitary vertebral collapse: distinction between benign and malignant causes using MR patterns. J Magn Reson Imaging 1999;9:635–42.

86. Baur A, Stäbler A, Arbogast S, et al. Acute osteoporotic and neoplastic vertebral compression fractures: fluid sign at MR imaging. Radiology 2002; 225:730–5.

87. Sitthipornvorakul E, Janwantanakul P, Purepong N, et al. The association between physical activity and neck and low back pain: a systematic review. Eur Spine J 2011;20:677–89.

88. Macfarlane GJ, Thomas E, Papageorgiou AC, et al. Employment and physical work activities as predictors of future low back pain. Spine 1997; 22:1143–9.

89. Harkness EF, Macfarlane GJ, Nahit ES, et al. Risk factors for new onset low back pain amongst cohorts of newly employed workers. Rheumatology (Oxford) 2003;42:959–68.

90. Vingård E, Alfredsson L, Hagberg M, et al. To what extent do current and past physical and psychosocial occupational factors explain care-seeking for low back pain in a working population? Results from the Musculoskeletal Intervention Center-Norrtälje Study. Spine 2000;25:493–500.

91. Thorbjörnsson CB, Alfredsson L, Fredrikkson K, et al. Psychosocial and physical risk factors associated with low back pain: a 24-year follow-up among women and men in a broad range of occupations. Occup Environ Med 1998;55:84–90.

92. Leboeuf-Yde C. Smoking and low back pain. A systematic literature review of 41 journal articles reporting 47 epidemiologic studies. Spine 1999;24: 1463–70.

93. Leboeuf-Yde C, Kyvik KO, Bruun NH. Low back pain and lifestyle. Part I. Smoking: information from a population based sample of 29,424 twins. Spine 1998;23:2207–14.

94. Leboeuf-Yde C. Bodyweight and low back pain: a systematic literature review of 56 journal articles reporting on 65 epidemiologic studies. Spine 2000;25: 226–37.

Postoperative Spine
What the Surgeon Wants to Know

Laura Eisenmenger, MD[a], Aaron J. Clark, MD, PhD[b], Vinil N. Shah, MD[c],*

KEYWORDS

• Postoperative spine • Spine surgery • Fusion • Hardware • Imaging • Complications

KEY POINTS

• Imaging plays a critical role in assessment of the postsurgical spine, which is often challenging to interpret.
• An accurate and useful imaging interpretation requires the radiologist to be familiar with the preoperative spinal pathologic condition, the surgical procedure performed, the expected imaging appearance of postsurgical changes, and the common postoperative complications.
• Optimal imaging protocol and type of imaging modality to be used depend on the clinical question, surgical procedure, and length of time since surgery.
• Both early and late complications may occur following spinal surgery, some of which may require urgent intervention.
• The radiologist should be familiar with advanced MR imaging techniques (diffusion tensor imaging, FIESTA [fast imaging employing steady-state acquisition], MR neurography) that can be helpful to arrive at a concise and relevant differential diagnosis.

INTRODUCTION

Imaging plays a critical role in the assessment of the postoperative spine. Accurate and clinically relevant interpretation of postoperative imaging requires a strong understanding of the preoperative spinal pathologic condition, the surgical procedure performed, and the expected imaging appearance of postoperative changes. This article reviews common surgical approaches to the degenerative spine, the most appropriate imaging modalities to use, how to optimize imaging protocols, and how to interpret those images. The reader will therefore possess the tools required to effectively assess postoperative spine imaging, to identify early and late complications, and to provide the surgeon with relevant information to guide patient management.

SURGICAL PROCEDURES

Spine surgeries can be divided into 3 major categories: decompressive surgeries, stabilization/fusion surgeries, and lesion excision surgeries. This article focuses on decompressive and stabilization/fusion surgical techniques.

Decompressive Procedures

Decompressive procedures include 3 main techniques: laminotomy, laminectomy, and laminectomy with facetectomy, with the common goal of relieving spinal cord or neural root compression due to herniated disc material or other structural causes.[1–3] Varying degrees of discectomy are often involved in all of the above decompressive procedures.

Disclosure Statement: A.J. Clark is a consultant for NuVasive. No relevant disclosures for L. Eisenmenger or V. Shah.
[a] University of Wisconsin School of Medicine and Public Health, 600 Highland Avenue, Madison, WI 53792, USA; [b] University of California, San Francisco, 400 Parnassus Avenue, Third Floor, San Francisco, CA 94143, USA; [c] University of California, San Francisco, 505 Parnassus Avenue, L352, San Francisco, CA 94143, USA
* Corresponding author.
E-mail address: Vinil.Shah@ucsf.edu

Radiol Clin N Am 57 (2019) 415–438
https://doi.org/10.1016/j.rcl.2018.10.003

Laminotomy removes only part of the lamina of the vertebral arch typically with partial resection of the inferior cephalic lamina. Partial resection of the superior caudal lamina is also sometimes performed with or without a microdiscectomy.[2,3] Unlike a laminotomy, a *laminectomy* involves complete removal of the lamina, and this may be either unilateral or bilateral. Although unilateral laminectomy involves removal of only one lamina, bilateral (or total) laminectomy involves excision of both laminae and the spinous process. Laminectomy is often performed in cases when removal of larger disc material is necessary.[2,3] Laminectomy is also used to treat central canal or lateral recess stenosis caused by ligamentous and facet capsule hypertrophy. The addition of *complete or partial facetectomy* to a laminectomy is primarily done when there is nerve root compression necessitating access to the neural foramen; however, overexcision of the facet joint can lead to instability and iatrogenic spondylolisthesis, so it is paramount to leave as much of the facet joint as possible.[2,3]

Stabilization/Fusion Procedures

In certain clinical settings, patients with axial back pain require a lumbar fusion. Spinal stabilization and fusion procedures are used to stabilize the spine, maintain or improve alignment, or replace removed osseous or soft tissue structures of the spine. This can be done for a wide variety of reasons, including recurrent disc disease, spondylolisthesis with stenosis, adult spinal deformity, trauma, or infection, or in the setting of spinal masses. Vertical foraminal stenosis may require interbody grafting in conjunction with fusion to reconstruct foraminal height. Lumbar fusion for patients with mechanical back pain and one- or 2-level degenerative disc disease is more controversial but may be indicated in select patients who have failed conservative management.[4] Adult spinal deformity defined as sagittal plane imbalance may require osteotomies and long segment fusion to restore harmony between the pelvic incidence and lumbar lordosis. The instrumentation used to achieve stabilization and/or fusion can be tailored as an indication for surgery and the patient's individual anatomy.[1,2,5–8] Because of this variation, the radiologist should be familiar with the general types of hardware that may be used but also be prepared for individual hardware constructs on a patient-by-patient basis.

SURGICAL HARDWARE
Rods, Plates, and Screws

The most common hardware used in posterior spinal fusion is rods in combination with either lateral mass screws in the cervical spine or transpedicular screws in the thoracic and lumbar spine. Rod constructs allow the surgeon to make short or long segment fusions of multiple vertebral body levels with secure fixation to the spinal column provided by the attachment to the screws and possibly cross bars.[2,5,9] The screws traverse the lateral mass or pedicle, depending on the spinal level, entering the lateral aspect of the vertebral body anteriorly. Although exact screw length and placement vary according to surgeon preference and patient factors, the screws should not extend into the neural foramen or spinal canal, and they should not protrude anterior to the ventral aspect of the vertebral body cortex. Although bicortical purchase of the anterior sacral cortex in lumbosacral fixation for the treatment of lumbosacral instability adds additional biomechanical benefit to the lumbosacral construct, anterior sacral penetration of the screw and drilling the anterior sacral cortex carry additional risk of neurovascular injury.[10–13] Anterior spine fusion often involves an anterior plate along the anterior aspects of the vertebral bodies in combination with screws extending into the vertebral bodies. The main advantage of hardware-based stabilization/fusion using rods, plates, and screws is that it provides immediate postoperative fixation and alignment. In addition, hardware also has improved fusion rates.[2,5–9,14]

Interbody Spacers

Interbody spacers are solid or open structures placed in the intervertebral disc space after discectomy to promote fusion, maintain alignment, and provide spinal column support. Spacers can be composed of titanium, carbon fiber, or polyetheretherketone and are often filled with bone graft material to further promote osseous fusion between vertebral body levels. Spacers can also be used to replace a resected vertebra in corpectomy cases with the spacer taking the form of an expandable cage filled with bone graft or cement. In most cases of corpectomy, rods and/or plates with screws are placed for added stability.[5,14] Most spacers contain radiopaque markers for better evaluation of their position on imaging. Although placement of the spacer may be different depending on the patient and product being used, a general rule is that a posterior marker located approximately 2 mm anterior to the posterior cortex of the adjacent vertebral body indicates good position.[2,5,14]

Bone graft material may represent autograft (eg, bone harvested from the iliac crest) or donor allograft. Bone graft substitutes, such as recombinant human bone morphogenic protein (rh-BMP), are also used in the spine to improve fusion rates; however, use of BMP has become less common due to known complications (discussed later in the complications section).

Motion Preservation Devices

Disc arthroplasty and disc stabilization devices may be used in cases without spinal cord or neural foraminal narrowing and do not have the goal of spinal fusion. The goals of disc arthroplasty are to preserve physiologic range of motion and reduce the incidence of adjacent-level disease. Although the indication for lumbar arthroplasty is axial back pain, radiculopathy and possibly myelopathy (in the setting of anterior cord compression at the level of the disc space) are indications for cervical arthroplasty. There should be no dynamic contribution to the myelopathy if disc arthroplasty is being considered. In general, the procedure involves removal of the native disc and replacement with an artificial disc that contains core material, such as polyethylene between 2 metal plates that are attached to the adjacent vertebral bodies. Disc arthroplasty is designed to allow motion and provide cushioning similar to a healthy disc.[5,9] *Dynamic stabilization* devices, in contrast, are used in cases of more extensive spine degeneration to alter the load-bearing and motion of the spine to limit strain on adjacent discs and facet joints thereby reducing progressive degeneration. Stabilization devices may be used in isolation or with additional fusion hardware.[3,5,14]

SURGICAL APPROACHES FOR FUSION

Although decompressive procedures are most often performed from a posterior midline approach to provide optimal access to the posterior elements, spinal canal, and the intervertebral disc, approaches for stabilization/fusion procedures vary widely and are often categorized based on the direction from which the spine is approached (anterior, posterior, lateral, caudal) as well as the degree of invasiveness.[2,5-7]

A posterior approach is used when decompression is required in addition to stabilization/fusion. Posterior interbody fusion includes both bilateral laminectomy and discectomy with fixation hardware and interbody spacer placement providing immediate support to the spine before osseous fusion.[2,5-7] Transforaminal interbody fusion is a variant using a posterolateral approach, leaving the midline structures intact and causing less disruption of the spinal canal; however, because of the lateral approach, a facetectomy is required to access the intervertebral disc space.[2,5] When there is severe disc height loss without the possibility of inserting a spacer, complete posterolateral fusion is performed with bone graft material placed between the transverse processes often with the addition of fixation hardware.

An anterior approach is used when decompression is not necessary; for example in cases where the patient's pain is thought to be arising from the disc and not from neural compression. Anterior interbody fusion removes the intervertebral disc and replaces it with an interbody cage spacer. Anterior plates with interlocking screws are usually used for additional stability. Performing an anterior interbody fusion in the cervical spine requires an anterolateral approach through the soft tissues of the neck near the carotid arteries, jugular veins, and cervical portions of the 9th to 12th cranial nerves. In the lumbar spine, an anterior abdominal incision or a retroperitoneal approach from the flanks is used with close proximity to the aortoiliac bifurcation and visceral organs.[2,5-7] In stand-alone interbody fusion, the interbody cage spacer is directly attached to the adjacent vertebral bodies using screws, eliminating the need for any additional surgical hardware, but similar surgical approaches are used.[5]

CLINICAL SITUATIONS REQUIRING POSTOPERATIVE IMAGING

Indications, timing, and modality of postoperative imaging vary among spine surgeons. As a general rule, patients who experience stabilization or improvement of symptoms after noninstrumented simple decompressive spinal surgery (ie, laminectomy, microdiscectomy, foraminotomy) do not need postoperative imaging. Patients who undergo instrumented fusions should be imaged at certain time points for 1 year following surgery to assess hardware positioning and progression of fusion. One example of a standard protocol is standing anteroposterior (AP) and lateral plain radiographs focused on the instrumented spinal region at 6 weeks and 3, 6, and 12 months after the operation. The same protocol is applied for instrumented nonfusion operations, such as cervical disc replacement. Patients undergoing long segment instrumented fusions for spinal deformity correction should be followed with imaging for 2 years or more.[15]

Concern for postoperative complication should prompt imaging at different time points. New pain or neurologic deficit immediately after surgery warrants urgent imaging. If a patient has had a decompression, MR imaging can elucidate new compressive pathologic conditions, such as a hematoma. In patients who have undergone instrumentation placement and there is concern for malposition, a computed tomography (CT) scan should be obtained to assess the hardware. In the early postoperative period, fever, chills, leukocytosis, wound drainage, or dehiscence should prompt an MR imaging with and without contrast to evaluate for infection. However, note that imaging in the immediate/recent postoperative period can be difficult to interpret because postoperative changes themselves can disrupt the myofascial planes and be associated with enhancement. Patients with a reported intraoperative dural tear may experience positional headaches, wound fluctuance, or serous drainage, and MR imaging of the operated spinal segment should be evaluated. MR imaging brain of these spinal dural tear patients may reveal findings of intracranial hypotension, and rarely, there may be parenchymal or subarachnoid hemorrhage hypothesized to be from changes in cerebrospinal fluid (CSF) pressures and tearing of bridging veins.[16,17] Patients with persistent radicular symptoms that have not resolved after several months may have residual stenosis, which should be evaluated with an MR imaging scan. CT/CT myelogram may be helpful to delineate any osseous component to the nerve impingement. Note, however, that stabilization of symptoms in patients with long-standing neurologic deficits before surgery may be the expected outcome and is not an indication for repeat studies. Recurrence of radicular symptoms after an initial positive surgical result may suggest recurrent disc herniation, epidural fibrosis, or arachnoiditis. In patients who have undergone interbody grafting, recurrent vertical foraminal stenosis due to graft subsidence is a consideration. MR imaging with and without contrast and/or CT scan can elucidate the cause of recurrent radicular pain. Recurrence of axial back pain after a fusion may be caused by pseudarthrosis often with hardware loosening or fracture and adjacent level degeneration. A CT scan at 1 year would be expected to show solid fusion after a successful arthrodesis. Upright radiographs with flexion and extension can provide functional information of abnormal motion at the fused levels. Loss of correction after long segment fusion for spinal deformity is typically noted on standing 36-inch radiographs. Causes can range from pseudarthrosis, hardware failure, or proximal junctional kyphosis/failure.

POSTOPERATIVE IMAGING MODALITIES

When evaluating the postsurgical spine, the indication for the study will most often guide the imaging modality, but the surgical procedure will heavily impact the technique or sequences used.

Radiographs, CT, and MR imaging play important roles in postoperative imaging and can provide complementary information. The radiologist should know how to optimize the imaging obtained from each modality in order to answer the specific clinical question.

Radiography

Radiographs play a key role in immediate postoperative imaging as well as in monitoring the bones and hardware over longer periods of time. Baseline radiographs are helpful for assessing implant position after surgery, and future studies evaluate any changes from this baseline should there be any concern for complications.[18] Follow-up radiographs can assess changes in bony alignment, component position, implant fractures, and changes in the bone-implant interface.[19,20] AP, lateral, and oblique images can provide static information, whereas dynamic imaging (flexion and extension) can provide information regarding instability. Upright lateral radiographs also give functional information on axial loading.

Computed Tomography

CT with multiplanar reconstruction is the modality of choice for assessing bony detail and evaluating instrumentation; however, because of higher cost and radiation dose than radiographs, CT should be used for more targeted examinations with specific indications rather than for serial monitoring. In addition to evaluating degenerative disease, CT in the postsurgical spine provides better evaluation of fusion progression than dynamic radiography and is also more accurate in detection of hardware failure.[21] Development of pseudarthrosis and other osseous complications of spine surgery can also be better detected with CT. MR imaging has widely replaced CT myelography for the evaluation of the intrathecal contents. Despite this, CT myelography continues to play an important role in patients who have contraindications to MR imaging and when MR artifacts due to surgical hardware obscure important anatomic detail, such as the spinal canal and nerve roots.[22] CT after intravenous contrast enhancement can also provide reliable differentiation between postoperative extradural fibrosis (scarring) and recurrent disc herniation[23–26] as well as detect postoperative collections.

The major challenge of using CT in postoperative evaluation is the beam-hardening artifact caused by the metallic prosthesis. Beam hardening can not only limit evaluation of the hardware itself but also cause difficulty in soft tissue interpretation in the spinal canal.[27] Although beam

Table 1	
Tips for improving computed tomography imaging quality of the postoperative spine	
During image acquisition	Use high-peak voltage (kilovolts peak)
	Use high tube current (milliampere-seconds)
	Use narrow collimation
	Acquire thin sections
During image reconstruction	Use thick sections
	Use lower-kernel values

Box 1
Tips for reducing metal artifact in postoperative spine MR imaging
Position the patient with the long axis of metallic hardware parallel to B0
Use fast-spin echo sequences
Use inversion recovery for fat suppression
Swap phase and frequency encoding direction
Use vie-angle tilting
Increase the bandwidth
Decrease the voxel size

hardening is less with the newer titanium implants compared with stainless steel,[5] the radiologist should always try to improve the image quality. In addition to positioning the x-ray beam perpendicular to the orthopedic implant, there are several other imaging parameters that can be adjusted (**Table 1**).[9]

MR Imaging

Because of its superior evaluation of soft tissue structures, MR imaging is often the preferred imaging modality in the evaluation of the postoperative spine.[28] Evaluation of spinal cord and nerve roots abnormalities, the bone marrow, neuroforaminal and spinal canal narrowing, soft tissue inflammation, infection, and hemorrhage are much more accurate with MR imaging than CT or radiography.[29,30] Tissue enhancement is better evaluated on MR imaging than on CT,[31] allowing easier discrimination between normal postoperative changes, such as epidural fibrosis, and complications, such as discitis-osteomyelitis or recurrent disc herniation.

In the past, MR imaging use was limited because of extensive artifacts caused by magnetic field inhomogeneity. Although artifacts still exist, the change to the use of titanium in spinal hardware instead of stainless steel has largely reduced these artifacts. In addition, multiple specialized pulse sequences have been developed, also leading to significant improvement in postoperative spine imaging.[32–34] Several imaging techniques can reduce metallic susceptibility artifact (**Box 1**).[35–38]

Routine imaging of the postoperative spine includes T1- and T2-weighted imaging in sagittal and axial planes as well as postcontrast T1-weighted images. Precontrast T1- and T2-weighted images offer complementary information. Sagittal and axial T2-weighted images can depict the contour of the thecal sac as well as evaluate the spinal cord and nerve roots. T1-weighted images are useful for assessing the osseous structures with axial images being particularly useful in evaluating for the areas of bone that have been altered or removed as well as changes to the normal epidural fat. Postgadolinium contrast-enhanced, fat-saturated T1-weighted images can not only assist in evaluating for complications but also differentiate between expected scar tissue and recurrent disc herniation or other complications that may require additional surgery.[39,40]

Other Modalities

Other imaging modalities can be used to focus on very specific questions of the postoperative spine. Ultrasound can be used for assessing and guiding aspiration of superficial postoperative collections, hematomas, and abscesses.[41] Radionuclide scans can be used to detect pseudarthrosis or infection, attempting to differentiate those complications from normal postoperative changes[42]; however, radionuclide scans may remain positive for 1 year or more in the region of the operative bed and instrumentation. More recently, PET has been shown to be useful for evaluating infection around metal implants[43] and may also play a role in evaluating for altered mechanical stresses and other causes of inflammation.

EXPECTED POSTSURGICAL CHANGES

There is considerable imaging overlap between expected early postoperative findings and surgical complications (**Figs. 1–3**). For this reason, postoperative MR imaging in the first 6 weeks can be challenging to interpret and is not routinely obtained. Following a posterior approach for spinal surgeries, such as laminectomies, MR imaging often demonstrates disruption of the margins of the paraspinal muscles as well as edema of the adjacent soft tissues. Paraspinal soft tissue and facet joint enhancement can persist up to 6 months

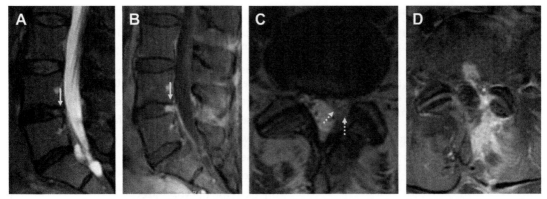

Fig. 1. Expected postdiscectomy changes. MR imaging performed within weeks of an L4-L5 discectomy shows edema and enhancement within the posterior annulus (*arrows* in *A* and *B*) at the site of curettage. (*C*) Axial T2-weighted (T2W) image shows mildly hyperintense granulation tissue within the left lateral epidural space, consistent with peridural fibrosis (*dashed arrows*). (*D*) Axial postcontrast image shows prominent avidly enhancing granulation tissue along the instrumentation tract, within the left lateral epidural space, as well as within the posterior annulus. Peridural fibrosis surrounds the traversing left L5 nerve roots in the lateral recess (*asterisk*).

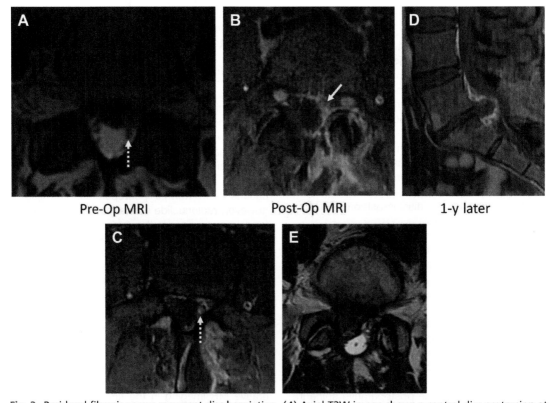

Pre-Op MRI   Post-Op MRI   1-y later

Fig. 2. Peridural fibrosis versus recurrent disc herniation. (*A*) Axial T2W image shows a central disc protrusion at L5-S1 contacting and mildly posteriorly displacing the traversing left S1 nerve root (*dashed arrow*). (*B, C*) Expected postdiscectomy changes including left lateral peridural fibrosis (*solid arrow* in *B*) and enhancement of the left S1 nerve root (*dashed arrow* in *C*) just inferior to image in (*B*). (*D, E*) One year later, right S1 radiculopathy prompted a repeat MR imaging, which shows a recurrent disc herniation at L5-S1. Note the large right central and subarticular disc extrusion compressing the right S1 nerve root. This disc extrusion is predominantly low in signal on T2 (*E*) and demonstrates thin peripheral enhancement on the postcontrast sagittal image (*D*). The patient underwent repeat discectomy.

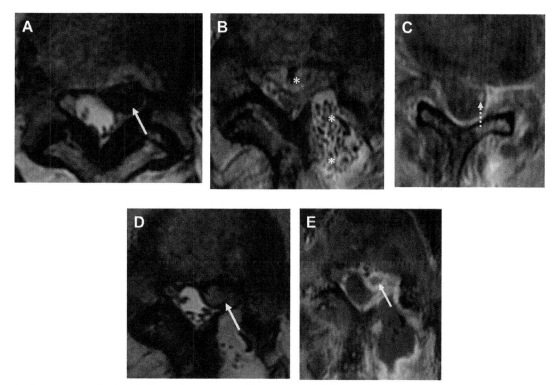

Fig. 3. Recurrent disc herniation. (*A*) A 77-year-old woman with left L5 radiculopathy secondary to a left lateral recess disc extrusion at L4-5 (*solid arrow*) that compresses the traversing left L5 nerve root. Note on the axial T2W image that the disc extrusion is low in signal. The patient underwent left L4-5 laminectomy and microdiscectomy. (*B, C*) Postoperative imaging was obtained on day 5 due to persistent low back and left lower-extremity lateral pain. Axial T2W image (*B*) shows effacement of the thecal sac from injected gelatin-thrombin matrix (*asterisks*) within the ventral epidural space and left laminectomy bed that was injected during the surgery to control local bleeding. This hemostatic matrix is recognized by its characteristic speckled T2 hypointensity in a background of surrounding T2 hyperintensity. Axial postcontrast image (*C*) just inferior to the image in (*B*) demonstrates enhancement of the previously compressed left L5 nerve root (an expected postoperative finding). The patient's postoperative pain was managed conservatively. (*D, E*) Repeat MR imaging obtained due to worsening left lower-extremity pain 6 weeks later. Axial T2W image (*D*) shows a recurrent subarticular zone disc herniation at L4-5 (*solid arrow*) impinging on the traversing left L5 nerve root. Note that this recurrent disc herniation shows elevated T2 signal. The previously seen gelatin-thrombin matrix has expectedly decreased in volume. Axial postcontrast image (*E*) shows peripheral enhancement surrounding the recurrent disc herniation (*solid arrow*).

after surgery. T1-weighted axial images often best evaluate the osseous changes. STIR (short T1 inversion recovery) and T2-weighted images will show endplate marrow edema related to the discectomy. The dural sac may protrude toward the laminectomy defect.[2]

Following discectomy, increased T2 signal and enhancement within the disc space extending to the posterior annulus at the site of curettage are expected findings and should decrease in intensity after 3 months (see **Fig. 1**).[44] Decrease in disc height compared with preoperative images at 3 months is also an expected finding.[44] On post-contrast imaging, thin linear disc enhancement, paralleling the endplates and converging onto the surgical site in the posterior annulus, is an expected finding in the first few months after discectomy, can be seen up to 6 months, and may be associated with adjacent vertebral end-plate enhancement.[41–44] Postdiscectomy changes may mimic reherniation. The intraoperative disruption of the epidural soft tissues and annulus fibrosus result in edema in the epidural space. Postoperative edema may mildly efface the thecal sac, similar in appearance to a recurrent disc. These changes within the anterior epidural space gradually involute 2 to 6 months after surgery.[45–47] Recurrent disc herniations may occur after surgery, but they may not be symptomatic or the cause of persistent or recurrent pain. One study of asymptomatic patients showed residual or recurrent disc herniation in 24% of patients at the operated level within 6 weeks of surgery. In 16% of subjects, there was mild to moderate mass effect on the dural sac, and 5% had severe compression of the dural sac. These herniated disc fragments can regress spontaneously over time.[2,48,49] Therefore, caution must be used in interpreting MR imaging within the first few months after surgery.

Solitary, asymptomatic, nerve root enhancement, ipsilateral to the site of discectomy, typically of the nerve root previously compressed by the disc herniation, can be seen at 3 to 6 weeks post-operatively and usually resolves by 6 months.[39] Nerve root enhancement is likely secondary to breakdown of the blood-nerve barrier, related to compression from disc herniation and/or surgical manipulation. The enhancement likely represents a postsurgical aseptic reaction and does not cause symptoms.[2,9,48,49] Although nerve root enhancement in the first few months after surgery is often asymptomatic, nerve root enhancement after 6 months shows a good correlation with clinical symptoms in patients with residual or recurrent sciatica.[50]

Postinstrumentation

Baseline radiographs of spine hardware should include description of the type of hardware used and its exact location within the spine. Special attention should be given to lateral mass/pedicle screws; optimal pedicle screw placement is parallel to the vertebral endplate traversing the central portion of the lateral mass or pedicle[2,9] (**Fig. 4**). Equally important is evaluation for complications such as fracture or malalignment of the operated or adjacent level or implant malpositioning.[2,9,49,51] Because these conditions may require more urgent surgical revision, they should be promptly reported to the surgeon. Although evaluation of soft tissues is limited on radiography, it is important to remember that there can be soft tissue swelling along the surgical trajectory. For example, prevertebral soft tissue swelling is expected acutely after ACDF, and this abates on subsequent radiographs in uncomplicated cases.

EARLY COMPLICATIONS
Postoperative Fluid Collections

Postoperative fluid collections in the operative bed are commonly seen in the immediate postsurgical setting and can be difficult to differentiate from pseudomeningocele, postoperative hematoma, or infected collection. Pseudomeningoceles are postoperative fluid collections that are continuous with the thecal sac resulting from a tear in the dura during the surgery (**Figs. 5–7**). Acute

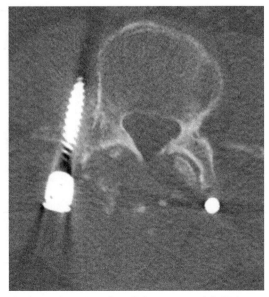

Fig. 4. Malpositioned pedicle screw. Axial CT image shows a malpositioned right pedicle screw, which is entirely extrapedicular and extends through a fractured right transverse process into the right psoas muscle.

pseudomeningoceles can be complex on MR imaging depending on the amount of protein or blood with possible fluid-fluid levels.[52] With the evolution of the blood products over time, the pseudomeningocele will follow CSF signal on all sequences. The key imaging finding that distinguishes pseudomeningoceles from other postoperative collections is identification of direct communication with the thecal sac or adjacent CSF flow artifact, best seen on T2-weighted or on high-resolution balanced steady state gradient echo sequences such as fast imaging employing steady-state acquisition (FIESTA) or CISS (constructive interference steady state) sequences (see **Figs. 5** and **6**). However, the direct communication can be challenging to visualize in the postoperative spine with distortion of the tissue planes. In certain cases, CT myelogram may be needed to identify the site of communication. Pseudomeningoceles and other sterile postoperative collections may demonstrate thin peripheral enhancement on postcontrast imaging (see **Fig. 5**). Clinically, pseudomeningoceles are often asymptomatic but may cause back pain, may present as a palpable mass (see **Fig. 7**), or may be associated with postural headaches in the setting of CSF hypotension.

Hematoma and seroma are common postsurgical collections. Pure seroma typically follows CSF on all MR imaging sequences, whereas hematomas have variable signal depending on the

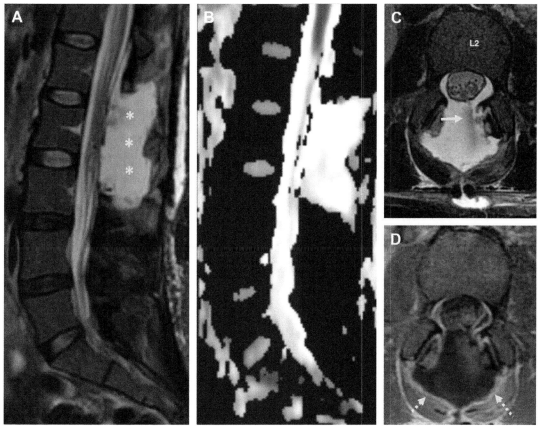

Fig. 5. Postoperative pseudomeningocele confirmed on imaging by presence of a CSF flow jet. (A) Sagittal T2W MR imaging obtained in a patient with worsening postoperative back and buttock pain and new onset postural headaches shows a postoperative fluid collection (*asterisks*) in the L1-L3 laminectomy bed resulting in mild mass effect on the dorsal thecal sac. (B) Sagittal apparent diffusion coefficient image shows facilitated diffusion within the collection, suggesting noninfectious process. (C) Axial T2W image shows a CSF flow jet (*arrow*) extending dorsal to the small dural defect confirming the collection to be a pseudomeningocele. (D) Axial T1 postcontrast image shows thin peripheral enhancement (*dashed arrows*) of the collection.

age of the blood products. Small postoperative epidural hematomas, particularly in the lumbar spine, are usually asymptomatic. However, large hematomas or those that result in mass effect may need to be urgently evacuated to prevent permanent neurologic injury (Figs. 8 and 9). New neurologic symptoms in the immediate postoperative period, such as myelopathy or weakness, should prompt urgent imaging to look for an epidural hematoma. MR imaging is the study of choice, even in the presence of hardware, because CT is relatively insensitive for diagnosing epidural hematoma (see Fig. 9). However, CT may still be obtained as the first imaging study in this scenario due to ease of obtaining that study in a rapid time frame. If MR imaging is nondiagnostic due to presence of extensive hardware, then a CT myelogram may be considered. However, note that acute severe neurologic deficit localizing to the spinal cord level may require emergent surgical exploration without waiting for imaging studies.

Sterile fluid collections evolve slowly over time and usually resolve by 6 weeks; however, their appearance can be mistaken for infection because peripheral enhancement can occur. Diffusion-weighted imaging (DWI) can be helpful to confirm infection in the paraspinal, epidural, or disc space because purulent material demonstrates reduced diffusion. Although echo planar DWI images may be distorted in the presence of hardware, making evaluation of the contents of the spinal canal difficult, they may still be helpful for assessment of paraspinal collections (Fig. 10). One important pitfall with DWI to keep in mind is that hemorrhagic postoperative collections may also demonstrate reduced diffusion (see Fig. 9). Therefore, the images need to be interpreted in the appropriate clinical context.

Timing in relation to the surgery can help in diagnosis with seromas and hematomas occurring

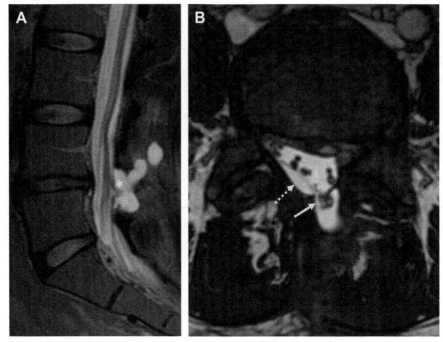

Fig. 6. Postoperative pseudomeningocele confirmed on FIESTA imaging in a patient with left foot numbness after recent discectomy. (*A*) Sagittal T2W image shows a small postoperative collection in the left L4 laminotomy bed with suggestion of posterior dural tenting into the collection (*asterisk*). (*B*) Axial FIESTA image confirms a left dorsal dural defect at L4-5 with nerve roots herniating through the dural defect into an adjacent pseudomeningocele (*solid arrow*). Also noted is a small postoperative subdural collection (*dashed arrow*) in the right dorsolateral canal ventrally displacing the adjacent cauda equina nerve roots.

immediately or days after surgery and abscesses usually taking more time to form, typically multiple days to weeks. Clinical presentation of fever and elevated inflammatory markers, such as elevated white blood cell count and rising serum C-reactive protein, suggest infection; however, aspiration may be needed for definitive answer in some cases.

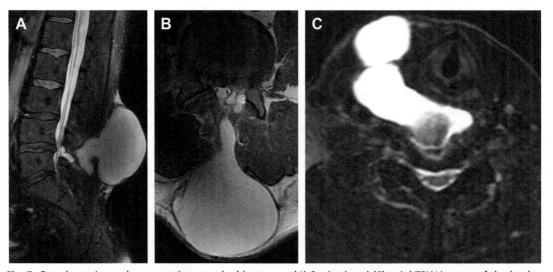

Fig. 7. Pseudomeningoceles presenting as palpable masses. (*A*) Sagittal and (*B*) axial T2W images of the lumbar spine demonstrate a large postoperative pseudomeningocele presenting as a palpable back mass. (*C*) Axial T2W image in a patient after ACDF shows a large pseudomeningocele tracking through the interbody spacer into the right anterior neck. The dural defect was repaired surgically in both cases.

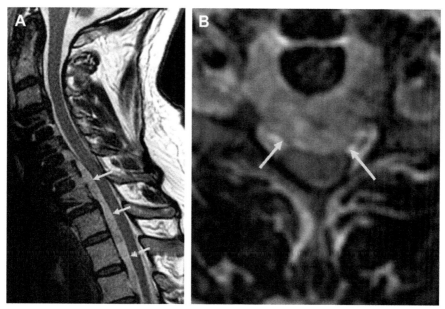

Fig. 8. Postoperative epidural hematoma after ACDF. (*A*) Sagittal and (*B*) axial T2W images obtained in a patient with progressive bilateral lower-extremity weakness immediately following ACDF show a longitudinally extensive ventral epidural hematoma (*arrows*) spanning C6-T2. This collection results in severe spinal canal stenosis and mass effect upon and posterior displacement of the cervical spinal cord. The patient underwent an emergent surgical evacuation of the hematoma.

Operative Injury (Vascular, Neural, Dural)

In the cervical spine, injuries during posterior approach are mainly neurologic, including dural, nerve root, or cord injury. An anterior approach is associated with risks of injuring the vascular and soft tissue structures, such as the carotid arteries, recurrent laryngeal nerve, esophagus, trachea, or lungs (**Fig. 11**). Similarly, in the thoracolumbar spine, vascular injuries are more common with anterior surgeries, and neural injury is more common with posterior surgeries[53] (**Figs. 12** and **13**).

Incidental dural tears can be a complication of lumbar spine surgery with an incidence of 12.5% to 16%, and in general, depend on the type and

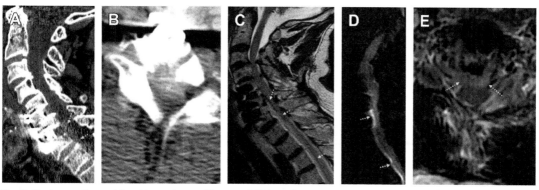

Fig. 9. Postoperative epidural hematoma. CT versus MR imaging. Noncontrast CT sagittal (*A*) and axial (*B*) images obtained after C5-7 ACDF due to perioperative lower-extremity paralysis and T2 sensory level show subtly increased density within the ventral epidural space at C6-7 (*dashed arrows* and *asterisk*), which raised the concern for an epidural hematoma and for which an urgent MR imaging was performed. (*C*) Sagittal T2W MR image performed on a 1.5-T MR image clearly shows a longitudinally extensive ventral epidural collection (*dashed arrows*) extending from C6 to the upper thoracic spine confirming the presence of a postoperative epidural hematoma. (*D*) Sagittal DWI shows reduced diffusion within the collection (*dashed arrows*) confirming the presence of blood products. (*E*) Axial T2W image shows effacement of the ventral CSF space by the collection (*dashed arrows*) and dorsal displacement of the spinal cord at the C6-7 level. This collection was urgently evacuated surgically.

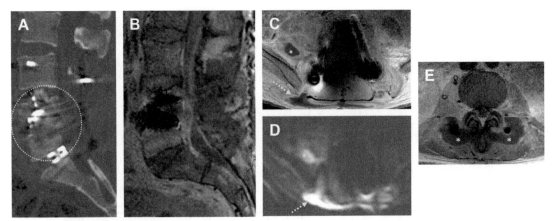

Fig. 10. Postsurgical infection after fusion. (*A*) Sagittal reformat from a CT scan obtained in a patient with worsening back pain after prior L3-S1 posterior spinal and interbody fusion shows endplate destructive changes at L4-5 (*dashed circle*). (*B*) Sagittal postcontrast T1-weighted (T1W) MR image confirms L4-5 discitis osteomyelitis with ventral epidural abscess and resultant severe canal narrowing. Axial postcontrast image (*C*) shows right psoas (*asterisk*) and right iliac bone graft harvest site (*dashed arrow*) rim enhancing collections with reduced diffusion (*D*) consistent with abscess. (*E*) Axial T1W postcontrast image more cranially shows a larger paraspinal abscess (*asterisks*) surrounding the L2-L4 interconnecting rods and posterior screws.

complexity of the surgery.[54,55] Previous surgery and older age are predisposing factors for incidental durotomy.[54] When dural injury occurs, in most cases it is detected intraoperatively, and primary repair is usually performed. If a defect goes undetected or is not properly closed, the patient may present with a spectrum of findings from postural headache to diplopia due to VI cranial nerve paresis and photophobia. As stated above, fluid-sensitive MR imaging sequences can be helpful to identify the site of the dural tear.

Graft/Hardware Malposition

Hardware malposition or displacement may cause symptoms in the immediate postoperative period. Pedicle screw malpositioning (see **Fig. 4**) can lead to nerve root irritation or cord compression secondary to excessive medial screw placement violating the medial cortex. Significant vascular injury in the cervical spine may also be encountered if a screw violates the foramen transversarium injuring the vertebral artery.[56] Poor pedicle screw placement can also lead to long-term

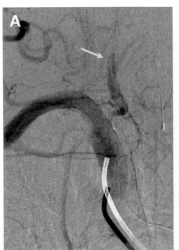
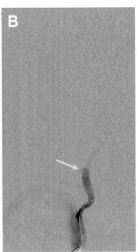
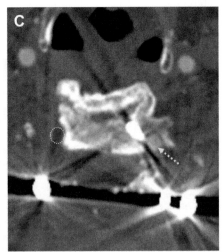

Fig. 11. Vertebral artery injury during a cervical fusion. (*A*, *B*) Bleeding in the region of the right vertebral artery after a C6-7 pedicle subtraction osteotomy during an extensive C2-thoracic spine posterior spinal fusion surgery prompted a postoperative angiogram. Angiographic images after catheterization of the right subclavian artery (*A*) and right vertebral artery (*B*) show a right vertebral artery stump (*arrows*) occluded at the C7 level. (*C*) CT angiogram a few days later shows a persistently occluded right vertebral artery (*circle*), while the dominant left vertebral artery is patent (*dashed arrow*).

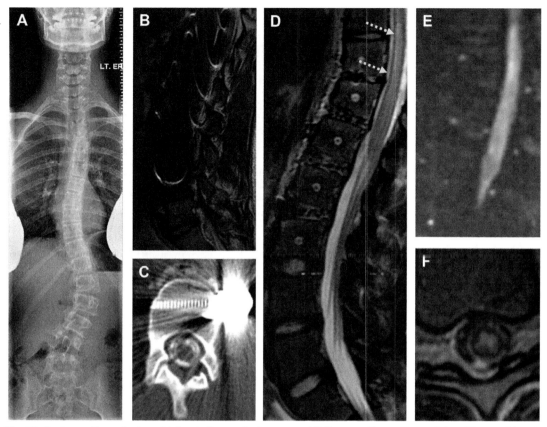

Fig. 12. Postoperative spinal cord infarct after scoliosis surgery. (A) Preoperative radiograph in a 15-year old male adolescent shows spinal scoliosis. (B) Postoperative MR imaging obtained for acute lower-extremity paralysis following a lateral spinal fusion is nondiagnostic due to extensive metallic susceptibility artifact from the spinal hardware. (C) CT myelogram obtained on the same day shows the spinal canal to be patent and no evidence of epidural hematoma. (D–F) MR imaging obtained after hardware removal but with no improvement in symptoms shows abnormal long segment T2 signal abnormality of the lower spinal cord and conus (dashed arrows in D), predominantly within the central gray matter (F) and with associated reduced diffusion (E). This is consistent with a spinal cord infarct and was presumed to be a watershed injury related to intraoperative hypotension, although the exact mechanism remains unclear.

hardware failure if there is poor osseous purchase. In anterior plate and screw fixation, the screws may be proud and impinge upon prevertebral soft tissues or may overpenetrate the posterior cortex and impinge on the cord. Another complication that can occur at or close to the time of surgery is intervertebral graft displacement, which can cause nerve root or cord compression if retropulsion occurs (Fig. 14). Migration of a ventral fixation plate in the cervical spine can cause dysphagia or even an esophageal injury.

Retained Foreign Body

Detection of metallic foreign bodies after spinal surgery is usually quite simple because surgical sponges contain a radiopaque barium sulfate filament that is easily seen on CT and plain films (Fig. 15). However, as this filament is not magnetic or paramagnetic, it will not be easily seen on follow-up MR imaging.[2] Therefore, intraoperative counts are critical, and the radiologist should be alerted to any possible retained foreign bodies. On MR imaging, a sponge can have varying T1- and T2-weighted properties with the actual sponge material being hypointense on both, but blood products within the sponge can give a component of hyperintensity. With time, a peripheral rim of low T2-weighted signal and enhancement form, related to a peripheral inflammatory foreign body reaction.[2] The imaging appearance could be confused with a postoperative collection, abscess formation, or even a mass. Correlation with additional imaging and surgical history is critical to correct diagnosis.

Intracranial Hemorrhage Following Spine Surgery

Although rare, intracranial hemorrhage (ICH) can occur following lumbar spinal surgery (Fig. 16).

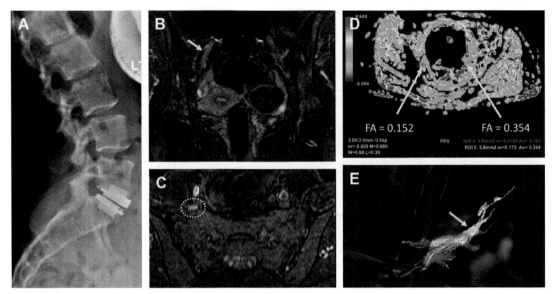

Fig. 13. Right sciatic neuropathy following disc arthroplasty. (A) Postoperative lateral radiograph demonstrates an L5-S1 disc arthroplasty. (B, C) Coronal T2 IDEAL (Iterative decomposition of water and fat with echo asymmetry and least-squares estimation) images from an MR neurogram obtained postoperatively demonstrate abnormally increased signal and caliber of right L5 ventral ramus and lumbosacral trunk (arrow and circle), presumably from a traction injury. Origin of the nerve signal abnormality at the L5 foraminal level suggests relation to the operative site. (D) Postprocessed diffusion tensor imaging images demonstrate abnormally decreased fractional anisotropy of the right lumbosacral trunk compared with the left (arrows), likely due to axonal degeneration as a sequela of the injury. (E) Tractography shows an intact but thickened right lumbosacral trunk (arrow).

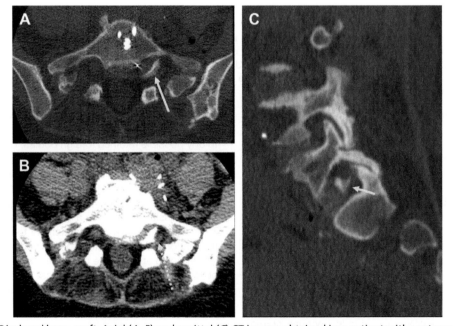

Fig. 14. Displaced bone graft. Axial (A, B) and sagittal (C) CT images obtained in a patient with postoperative left L5 radiculopathy after L3-S1 anterior interbody fusion shows migration of bone graft material (solid arrows) into the left L5-S1 neural foramen, compressing the extraforaminal left L5 nerve (dashed arrow). Actifuse, a synthetic bone graft material, was used during the surgery. During the second surgery of posterior spinal fusion and decompression, the previously placed bone graft was noted to be loose.

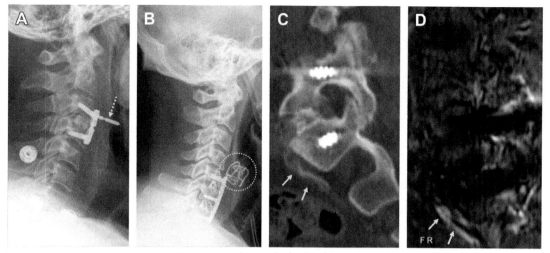

Fig. 15. Retained surgical material. (*A*) Lateral radiograph obtained in patient with postoperative dysphagia after a C3-4 ACDF shows a retained C3 screw post (*dashed arrow*). This was surgically removed. (*B*) Lateral radiograph shows a retained sponge as indicated by a radiopaque marker (*circle*) in patient after C5-7 ACDF. (*C*) Sagittal CT image in a patient who underwent an anterior and posterior lumbar fusion shows a retained sponge (*arrows*) anterior to the S1 vertebral body. (*D*) Sagittal T2 fat-saturated MR image in same patient as (*C*) shows fluid signal (*arrows*) within the retained sponge.

This complication may be asymptomatic or present with headache or focal neurologic symptoms.[17] ICH is associated with CSF leakage and use of drains postoperatively. Not all postoperative spines with lumbar drains will develop ICH, but those patients with continued and worsening neurologic symptoms, usually within the first 24 hours after spinal surgery, may warrant cranial imaging to evaluate for ICH.[16]

LATE COMPLICATIONS
Infection

Postoperative infection may be a result of the initial surgery or may occur later in recovery and is a common indication for imaging. Infection can occur in the soft tissues surrounding the operative site or involve the adjacent osseous structures, epidural space, or intradural space (see **Fig. 10**; **Figs. 17** and **18**). Osteomyelitis is often accompanied

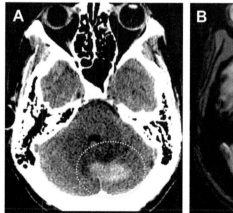
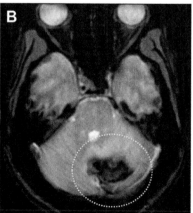
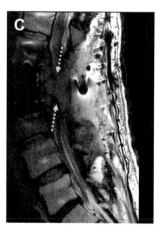

Fig. 16. ICH following spine surgery. (*A*) A 41-year-old man with metastatic testicular cancer after L2 corpectomy and cage placement for a paraspinal mass resection. The surgery was complicated by a ventral dural tear and CSF leak that was repaired intraoperatively. Altered mental status in the perioperative period prompted a noncontrast head CT scan. Axial CT image shows hyperdensity in the left posterior cerebellum (*circle*) consistent with acute intraparenchymal hemorrhage. (*B*) Iron-sensitive axial MR imaging sequence shows susceptibility artifact in the left cerebellum (*circle*) due to the presence of acute blood products. (*C*) Sagittal T2W from a postoperative spine MR imaging shows changes related to L2 corpectomy and cage placement with an associated large ventral dural defect at L2 (*dashed arrows*) consistent with a pseudomeningocele.

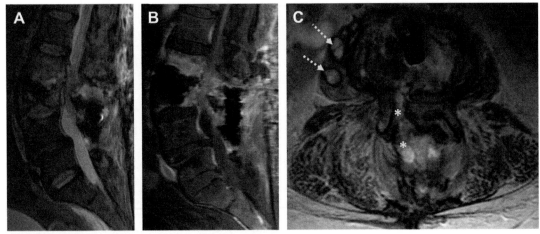

Fig. 17. Postoperative infection after posterior decompression. (*A*) Sagittal T2W and (*B*) postcontrast T1 fat-saturated images obtained in patient with worsening back pain 6 months after an L2-3 laminectomy show findings consistent with discitis osteomyelitis and ventral epidural abscess with resultant severe spinal canal stenosis and obliteration of the cauda equina nerve roots. (*C*) Axial T2W image shows small abscesses within the right psoas muscle (*dashed arrows*) and within the laminectomy bed (*asterisks*).

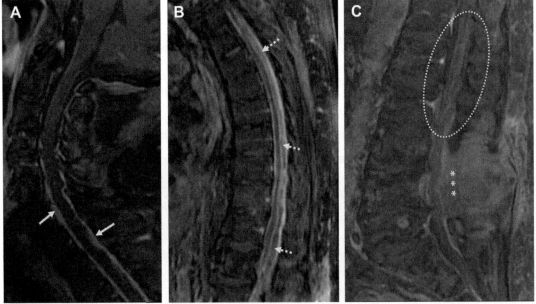

Fig. 18. Postoperative subdural Staphylococcal empyema with cord involvement and meningoradiculitis. (*A, B*) Sagittal postcontrast T1W fat-saturated images obtained in patient with worsening back pain and progressive lower-extremity weakness after recent lumbar laminectomies. These images show diffuse dural enhancement (*arrows* in *A*) and a longitudinally extensive subdural abscess (*dashed arrows* in *B*) with mass effect upon and ventral displacement of the cord. (*C*) Sagittal postcontrast T1W fat-saturated image of the lumbar spine shows expected enhancing postoperative granulation tissue in the L4 and L5 laminectomy bed (*asterisks*). However, also present is abnormal enhancement of the cauda equina nerve roots and pial surface of the cord (*dashed oval*) consistent with meningitis from Staphylococcal infection. This abscess was urgently evacuated surgically and confirmed to be in the subdural space. Subdural abscesses of the spine are uncommon but can be associated with infections of the dura. Prior surgery is a risk factor. The spinal subdural space has no barriers to prevent spread of infection. Therefore, spinal subdural empyemas can rapidly expand to involve multiple spinal levels and may produce extensive cord injury and profound neurologic deficit within 48 to 72 hours. Immediate surgery with complete exposure and drainage of the abscess is therefore needed and was performed in this case.

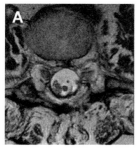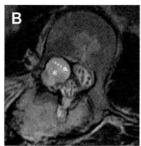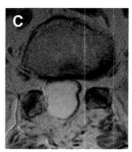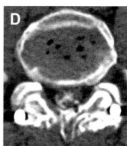

Fig. 19. Postoperative arachnoiditis in different patients. (*A*) Axial T2W image shows thickened and clumped cauda equina nerve roots. (*B*) Axial T2W image shows an intradural cyst (*asterisk*) and thick adhesions (*dashed arrow*) within the subarachnoid space. (*C*) Axial T2W image shows an "empty" thecal sac sign with peripheralization of the cauda equina nerve roots along the margins of the thecal sac. (*D*) Noncontrast axial CT image shows subarachnoid space calcifications along the cauda equina nerve roots consistent with arachnoiditis ossificans, representing sequela of end-stage adhesive arachnoiditis.

by a component of discitis or synovitis. Although bone destruction can be seen at later stages on radiographs and CT, MR imaging is more sensitive for detecting infection in the early stages.[56] The affected spinal level will demonstrate edema (low signal intensity on T1-weighted images and high signal intensity on T2-weighted images) and enhancement of the endplates and/or facet bone with additional edema and enhancement of the disc space or joint capsule, respectively.[57] In the postoperative state, this can be confusing with expected bone changes from the surgical procedure; however, adjacent soft tissue myositis, abscess, or epidural abscess assists in the diagnosis of infection. DWI can also be helpful in confirming disc or paraspinal abscess and may help guide site of biopsy. Image-guided aspiration can be used to isolate the microorganisms.

Infection can also lead to bone destruction and resorption around the implant, leading to hardware loosening, which will be further discussed later.

Failed Back Surgery Syndrome

Continued low back and/or radicular pain after lumbar surgery may be due to arachnoiditis, epidural fibrosis, recurrent disc herniation, instability, or stenosis.

Arachnoiditis

Inflammation of the cauda equina nerve roots, or arachnoiditis, can be caused by the spine surgery itself, the presence of intradural blood after surgery, perioperative spinal infection, or myelographic contrast media. Both CT myelography and MR imaging can be used for diagnosis. CT myelography is often used in cases of extensive hardware whereby metallic artifact can limit the diagnostic quality of the MR images. Imaging patterns included thickened or "clumped" nerve

roots, an "empty" thecal sac caused by adhesion of the nerve roots to the peripheral dura, or an intrathecal soft tissue "mass," representing a large group of matted roots[58] (**Fig. 19**). Nerve root thickening and adhesion often persist even after appropriate treatment. Arachnoiditis ossificans, sequela of end-stage adhesive arachnoiditis, can occur rarely and cause neurologic decline.[59]

Peridural Fibrosis and Recurrent Disc Herniation

Recurrent disc herniation has similar symptoms to primary disc herniation; however, other causes of pain must be excluded especially in postoperative spine cases. MR imaging is the modality of choice to identify recurrent disc herniation from other soft tissue disease processes,[53] including peridural fibrosis/scarring. Recurrent disc herniation often has smooth margins and no significant or only mild peripheral early contrast enhancement, whereas peridural fibrosis has irregular margins with early homogenous enhancement[60] (see **Figs. 1–3**). If imaging is delayed (>10 minutes) after the administration of contrast, recurrent disc may enhance diffusely.[61] On noncontrast imaging, peridural fibrosis is isointense or hypointense on T1 and hyperintense on T2 relative to the annulus of the adjacent postoperative disc[62] (see **Fig. 1**). Recurrent disc herniations are usually isointense or hypointense in signal intensity on all sequences to the adjacent posterior annulus and typically hypointense on T2 relative to peridural fibrosis (see **Fig. 2**). Free disc fragments, on the other hand, may be hyperintense on T1 and isointense on T2 relative to peridural fibrosis. In general, however, recurrent disc may have variable signal intensity relative to peridural fibrosis and may be hypointense or hyperintense on T2-weighted images (see **Fig. 3**). Peridural fibrosis can surround

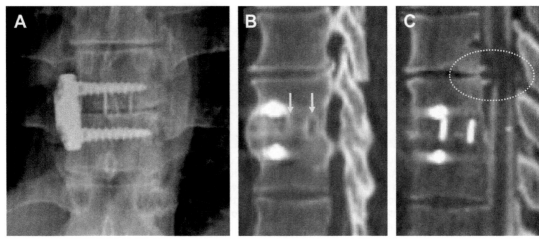

Fig. 20. Normal progression of interbody fusion. (*A*) AP radiograph shows right lateral interbody fusion at T9-10. (*B*) Nine months after surgery, sagittal CT reconstruction shows mature osseous fusion and bony bridging across the disc space (*solid arrows*). (*C*) Worsening leg pain 3 years later prompted a CT myelogram, which shows adjacent segment degeneration above the level of the fusion with resultant high-grade partial myelographic block (*dashed oval*).

or displace the adjacent nerve root, which may be increased in caliber (see **Fig. 1**). In patients with failed back surgery, identification of peridural fibrosis alone is not an indication for operation, often yielding poor reoperative results. Patients with extensive scar have been shown to experience recurrent radicular pain more often than patients with less extensive epidural scarring.[63]

Pseudarthrosis

Pseudoarthrosis, or fibrous union, results from failure to obtain bony union after fusion surgery and occurs at sites of continued mobility. Appropriately fused segments will show mature bridging bone on CT (**Fig. 20**) and radiographs and no motion on flexion-extension radiographs. Pseudoarthrosis can be seen on radiographs as a lucent line and on CT as the lack of bone bridging with or without adjacent sclerosis (**Box 2, Fig. 21**). In asymptomatic patients, intervention can be deferred and the patient followed[64]; however, pseudoarthrosis itself can result in pain as well as cause increased stress on the hardware leading to hardware failure due to persistent motion.[64]

Radiologic fusion occurs with development of bridging trabecular bone and is typically seen 6 to 9 months after surgery. Posterolateral fusions take longer than interbody fusions (9–12 months vs 3–9 months).[65] Fusions in the cervical spine occur faster than the thoracic or lumbar spine. With interbody fusion, trabecular fusion initially develops outside the interbody cage spacer and should completely bridge the intervertebral disc

space by 6 to 9 months. Increased radiotracer uptake on bone scan beyond 12 months after surgery is suggestive of pseudoarthrosis.[65] Risk factors for pseudoarthrosis include chronic illness, smoking, long-term use of nonsteroidal anti-inflammatory drugs, and revision surgery for prior nonunion.[66]

Bone Morphogenic Protein Complications

Bone graft substitutes, such as BMP, have been commonly used in spinal fusion surgeries to hasten healing and to decrease rate of pseudoarthrosis associated with autografts.[67] BMP may cause an intense symptomatic local inflammatory reaction in the first 2 weeks; its use during anterior cervical discectomy and fusion (ACDF) surgeries may

---

Box 2
Radiographic criteria for fusion

No motion or less than 3° of intersegment position change on flexion and extension views

Lack of a lucent area around the implant

Minimal loss of disc height

No fracture of the implant, bone graft, or vertebrae

No sclerotic change in the bone graft or adjacent vertebrae

Visible osseous formation in or around the cage

Data from Ray CD. Threaded fusion cages for lumbar interbody fusions. An economic comparison with 360 degrees fusions. Spine (Phila Pa 1976) 1997;22(6):681–5.

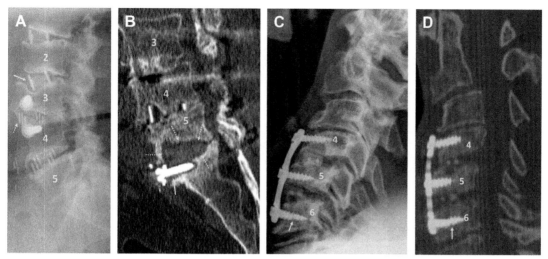

Fig. 21. Pseudoarthrosis due to subsidence and failed fusion. (*A*) Back pain in patient after prior discectomy and inter-body fusion at the L1-L5 levels. Lateral radiograph of the lumbar spine shows subsidence of the L2-3 intervertebral graft (*solid arrow*) into the superior endplate of the L3 vertebral body. Similar findings involving the L3-4 intervertebral graft subsiding into the inferior endplate of L3 are noted (*dashed arrow*). (*B*) Another patient with L3-S1 interbody fusion shows a lucent halo surrounding the L5-S1 graft (*dashed arrows*) as well as abnormal lucency surrounding an S1 screw. Findings are consistent with failed fusion and hardware loosening. (*C, D*) Patient with prior C4-6 ACDF and recurrent neck pain. Subsidence of C4-5 intervertebral bone graft into the C5 vertebral body seen on lateral radiograph (*C*) and sagittal CT image (*D*). At C5-6, there is immature osseous fusion with lucency surrounding the graft. Also noted is lucency surrounding the C6 screws, consistent with loosening, as well as a right C6 screw fracture (*solid arrow* in *C* and *D*).

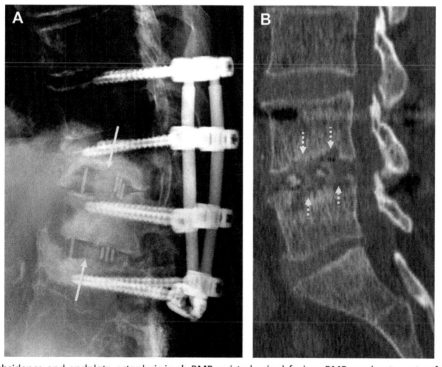

Fig. 22. Subsidence and endplate osteolysis in rh-BMP-assisted spinal fusion. BMP accelerates rate of interbody spinal fusion but can produce a marked inflammatory response that manifests as subsidence, endplate resorption, cage migration, and prevertebral swelling. (*A*) Subsidence of lower thoracic intervertebral cages into the adjacent endplates (*solid arrows*) in patient 3 months after rh-BMP-assisted spinal fusion. (*B*) Another patient with L4-5 endplate osteolysis (*dashed arrows*) 4 months after BMP-assisted fusion. These findings are commonly seen at level of BMP-assisted spinal fusion in the absence of infection.

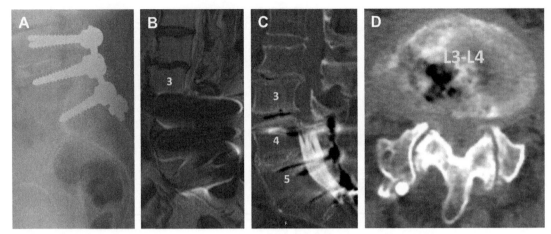

Fig. 23. Spinal canal stenosis from adjacent segment degeneration. (*A*) Lateral radiograph shows prior instrumented posterior spinal fusion from L4-S1. There is endplate sclerosis and disc space narrowing at L3-4, the level above the fusion. Fusion hardware obscures visualization of the spinal canal at L3-4 on the (*B*) sagittal T2W image. (*C*) Sagittal and (*D*) axial images from a CT myelogram demonstrate a complete myelographic block at L3-4 due to adjacent segment disease with no passage of injected contrast above the level of the severe canal stenosis. The patient underwent a decompression and extension of fusion.

result in prominent prevertebral edema and soft tissue swelling associated with dysphagia.[68,69] BMP also promotes higher rates of bone resorption than that associated with autografts.[65,66] BMP-induced osteolysis is maximal from 6 weeks to 6 months and usually decreases by 9 to 12 months, during which time bone formation occurs. Complications of osteolysis include graft migration, endplate resorption, and cage subsidence with resultant disc space narrowing

(**Fig. 22**). BMP is also associated with heterotopic bone formation in the spinal canal and neural foramen, particularly in patients who have undergone a transforaminal lumbar interbody fusion. Heterotopic bone formation in the neural foramen can be symptomatic and present as new radiculopathy after surgery. Although the use of BMP has decreased recently, in part due to known adverse reactions associated with its use, radiologists should be aware of BMP-related complications.

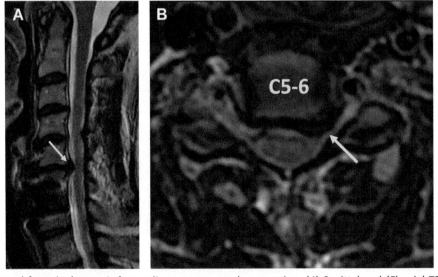

Fig. 24. Neural foraminal stenosis from adjacent segment degeneration. (*A*) Sagittal and (*B*) axial T2W images demonstrate prior C6-7 ACDF and show a left posterolateral disc extrusion at C5-6 (*arrows*) effacing the left ventral CSF space and narrowing the adjacent neural foramen accounting for the patient's left C6 radiculopathy.

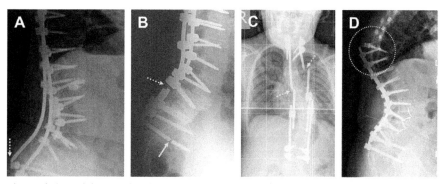

Fig. 25. Hardware failure. (A) Lateral radiograph in a patient with extensive prior thoracolumbar fusion shows disconnection of the distal aspect of the left posterior rod from the adjacent iliac bolt (*dashed arrow*). (B) Fractured rods (*dashed arrow*) and fractured iliac bolt (*solid arrow*) in another patient. (C, D) Fractured posterior fusion rods (*dashed arrows* in C) with posterior retraction of the left T10 pedicle screw, extrusion of left rod through skin, and separation of the right T10 pedicle screw from the right posterior rod (*circle* in D).

Adjacent Segment Degeneration

Because of altered biomechanics caused by spinal surgeries, degenerative changes can be accelerated at levels above and below the level of spinal fusion (**Figs. 23** and **24**). The fusion shifts the weight-bearing load away from the fused segments to the adjacent vertebrae and reduces overall flexibility and motion of the spine.[2,9] Adjacent segment degeneration is more common in the lumbar spine and most often observed cranial to the surgical level, because the superior spine is leveraged against the fused segment.[9] This complication is reported in 10.2% of patients with posterior fusion and instrumentation[70] and is reported even more frequently in long-term follow-up. Adjacent segment degeneration is a radiographic finding as compared with symptomatic adjacent segment disease. Adjacent segment degeneration is seen at a rate of 5.9% per year, whereas adjacent segment disease occurs at a rate of 1.8% per year.[71] The latter is associated with laminectomy adjacent to a fusion and sagittal imbalance. There is no strong correlation of adjacent segment degeneration with clinical outcomes.

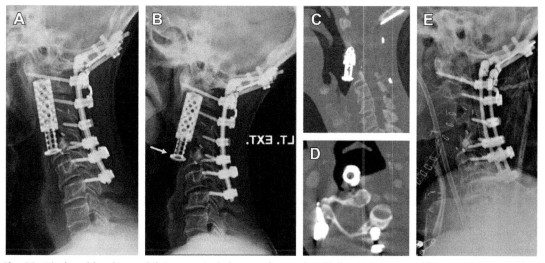

Fig. 26. Displaced hardware. (A) Postsurgical changes from prior C2-4 corpectomies with expandable vertebral bone cage placement as well as occiput to C6 posterior instrumented fusion. Hardware is intact. (B) Several months after surgery, new dysphagia with inability to swallow any solid food prompted repeat imaging. Lateral radiograph shows anterior migration of the inferior aspect of the expandable vertebral bone cage (*solid arrow*), which erodes through the posterior pharynx. (C) Sagittal and (D) axial CT images confirm the radiographic findings. The expandable cage has pierced the posterior pharyngeal wall and entered the oropharynx. (E) The patient underwent surgical removal of the displaced cage and repair of the posterior pharyngeal defect. Postsurgical lateral radiograph confirms removal of the cage.

Hardware Failure

In addition to complications related to the initial hardware placement, hardware failure can occur many years after the original surgery. Implant loosening can be caused by osseous resorption surrounding the hardware, most commonly involving screws, anchoring rods, or plates. Loosening is diagnosed on both radiographs and CT as lucency of greater than 2 mm around the fusion device. This loosening allows for hardware movement, which causes worsening resorption and increased mobility, eventually leading to screw pullout or fractures[72] (Fig. 25). Interbody spacer subsidence is another common complication seen in fusion cases, more frequently occurring with stand-alone interbody fusion[73–75] (see Fig. 21). Although some degree of spacer migration into the adjacent vertebrae is expected and may even facilitate fusion, subsidence (defined as >3 mm of migration) leads to loss of disc height and may cause recurrent radicular symptoms.[73–75] Chronic metal fatigue from repetitive stress can also lead to implant fractures. If fractured hardware allows increased motion, it may lead to or be the result of pseudarthrosis[18] or cause chronic tissue irritation, bursa formation, and even pressure sores with tissue necrosis. Hardware loosening, subsidence, or fracture may lead to additional revision surgeries or the need for hardware removal (Fig. 26).

SUMMARY

Postoperative spine imaging is commonly obtained both for confirmation of expected postsurgical changes and also to assess for complications. Interpretation of these images can be challenging, but by making an accurate diagnosis, the radiologist can substantially influence patient management. The radiologist should know how to best use the imaging modalities available, be aware of the commonly used surgical techniques and hardware, recognize expected postoperative changes, and accurately identify the complications that can occur at different time points after surgery. In this way, the radiologist can provide the most clinically useful images and relevant report for the surgeon to best assist in patient care.

REFERENCES

1. Bittane RM, de Moura AB, Lien RJ. The postoperative spine: what the spine surgeon needs to know. Neuroimaging Clin N Am 2014;24(2):295–303.
2. Van Goethem JW, Parizel PM, Jinkins JR. Review article: MRI of the postoperative lumbar spine. Neuroradiology 2002;44(9):723–39.
3. Eliyas JK, Karahalios D. Surgery for degenerative lumbar spine disease. Dis Mon 2011;57(10): 592–606.
4. Eck JC, Sharan A, Ghogawala Z, et al. Guideline update for the performance of fusion procedures for degenerative disease of the lumbar spine. Part 7: lumbar fusion for intractable low-back pain without stenosis or spondylolisthesis. J Neurosurg Spine 2014;21(1):42–7.
5. Rutherford EE, Tarplett LJ, Davies EM, et al. Lumbar spine fusion and stabilization: hardware, techniques, and imaging appearances. Radiographics 2007;27(6):1737–49.
6. Slone RM, MacMillan M, Montgomery WJ. Spinal fixation. Part 1. Principles, basic hardware, and fixation techniques for the cervical spine. Radiographics 1993;13(2):341–56.
7. Slone RM, MacMillan M, Montgomery WJ, et al. Spinal fixation. Part 2. Fixation techniques and hardware for the thoracic and lumbosacral spine. Radiographics 1993;13(3):521–43.
8. Slone RM, McEnery KW, Bridwell KH, et al. Fixation techniques and instrumentation used in the thoracic, lumbar, and lumbosacral spine. Radiol Clin North Am 1995;33(2):233–65.
9. Thakkar RS, Malloy JPt, Thakkar SC, et al. Imaging the postoperative spine. Radiol Clin North Am 2012;50(4):731–47.
10. Lehman RA Jr, Kuklo TR, Belmont PJ Jr, et al. Advantage of pedicle screw fixation directed into the apex of the sacral promontory over bicortical fixation: a biomechanical analysis. Spine (Phila Pa 1976) 2002;27(8):806–11.
11. Leong JC, Lu WW, Zheng Y, et al. Comparison of the strengths of lumbosacral fixation achieved with techniques using one and two triangulated sacral screws. Spine (Phila Pa 1976) 1998;23(21):2289–94.
12. Mirkovic S, Abitbol JJ, Steinman J, et al. Anatomic consideration for sacral screw placement. Spine (Phila Pa 1976) 1991;16(6 Suppl):S289–94.
13. Zindrick MR, Wiltse LL, Widell EH, et al. A biomechanical study of intrapeduncular screw fixation in the lumbosacral spine. Clin Orthop Relat Res 1986;203:99–112.
14. Murtagh RD, Quencer RM, Castellvi AE, et al. New techniques in lumbar spinal instrumentation: what the radiologist needs to know. Radiology 2011; 260(2):317–30.
15. Daniels AH, Bess S, Line B, et al. Peak timing for complications after adult spinal deformity surgery. World Neurosurg 2018;115:e509–15.
16. Kaloostian PE, Kim JE, Bydon A, et al. Intracranial hemorrhage after spine surgery. J Neurosurg Spine 2013;19(3):370–80.
17. Khalatbari MR, Khalatbari I, Moharamzad Y. Intracranial hemorrhage following lumbar spine surgery. Eur Spine J 2012;21(10):2091–6.

18. Venu V, Vertinsky AT, Malfair D, et al. Plain radiograph assessment of spinal hardware. Semin Musculoskelet Radiol 2011;15(2):151–62.

19. Berquist TH. Imaging of the postoperative spine. Radiol Clin North Am 2006;44(3):407–18.

20. Lonstein JE, Denis F, Perra JH, et al. Complications associated with pedicle screws. J Bone Joint Surg Am 1999;81(11):1519–28.

21. Williams AL, Gornet MF, Burkus JK. CT evaluation of lumbar interbody fusion: current concepts. AJNR Am J Neuroradiol 2005;26(8):2057–66.

22. Harreld JH, McMenamy JM, Toomay SM, et al. Myelography: a primer. Curr Probl Diagn Radiol 2011; 40(4):149–57.

23. Kleffer SA, Wltwer GA, Cacayorln ED, et al. Recurrent post-discectomy pain. CT–surgical correlation. Acta Radiol Suppl 1986;369:719–22.

24. Teplick JG, Haskin ME. Intravenous contrast-enhanced CT of the postoperative lumbar spine: improved identification of recurrent disk herniation, scar, arachnoiditis, and diskitis. AJR Am J Roentgenol 1984;143(4):845–55.

25. Cecchini A, Garbagna P, Martelli A, et al. Computerized tomography in surgically treated lumbar disk hernia. Multicenter study. Radiol Med 1988;75(6): 565–76 [in Italian].

26. Braun IF, Hoffman JC Jr, Davis PC, et al. Contrast enhancement in CT differentiation between recurrent disk herniation and postoperative scar: prospective study. AJR Am J Roentgenol 1985;145(4):785–90.

27. Mall JC, Kaiser JA. The usual appearance of the postoperative lumbar spine. Radiographics 1987; 7(2):245–69.

28. Grane P. The postoperative lumbar spine. A radiological investigation of the lumbar spine after discectomy using MR imaging and CT. Acta Radiol Suppl 1998;414:1–23.

29. Masaryk TJ, Modic MT, Geisinger MA, et al. Cervical myelopathy: a comparison of magnetic resonance and myelography. J Comput Assist Tomogr 1986; 10(2):184–94.

30. Modic MT, Masaryk T, Boumphrey F, et al. Lumbar herniated disk disease and canal stenosis: prospective evaluation by surface coil MR, CT, and myelography. AJR Am J Roentgenol 1986;147(4):757–65.

31. Bundschuh CV, Stein L, Slusser JH, et al. Distinguishing between scar and recurrent herniated disk in postoperative patients: value of contrast-enhanced CT and MR imaging. AJNR Am J Neuroradiol 1990;11(5):949–58.

32. Petersilge CA, Lewin JS, Duerk JL, et al. Optimizing imaging parameters for MR evaluation of the spine with titanium pedicle screws. AJR Am J Roentgenol 1996;166(5):1213–8.

33. Rudisch A, Kremser C, Peer S, et al. Metallic artifacts in magnetic resonance imaging of patients with spinal fusion. A comparison of implant materials and imaging sequences. Spine (Phila Pa 1976) 1998;23(6):692–9.

34. Viano AM, Gronemeyer SA, Haliloglu M, et al. Improved MR imaging for patients with metallic implants. Magn Reson Imaging 2000;18(3):287–95.

35. Lee MJ, Kim S, Lee SA, et al. Overcoming artifacts from metallic orthopedic implants at high-field-strength MR imaging and multi-detector CT. Radiographics 2007;27(3):791–803.

36. Suh JS, Jeong EK, Shin KH, et al. Minimizing artifacts caused by metallic implants at MR imaging: experimental and clinical studies. AJR Am J Roentgenol 1998;171(5):1207–13.

37. Vandevenne JE, Vanhoenacker FM, Parizel PM, et al. Reductlon of metal artefacts ln musculoskeletal MR imaging. JBR-BTR. 2007;90(5):345–9.

38. Frazzini VI, Kagetsu NJ, Johnson CE, et al. Internally stabilized spine: optimal choice of frequency-encoding gradient direction during MR imaging minimizes susceptibility artifact from titanium vertebral body screws. Radiology 1997;204(1):268–72.

39. Jinkins JR, Van Goethem JW. The postsurgical lumbosacral spine. Magnetic resonance imaging evaluation following intervertebral disk surgery, surgical decompression, intervertebral bony fusion, and spinal instrumentation. Radiol Clin North Am 2001;39(1):1–29.

40. Suk KS, Lee HM, Moon SH, et al. Recurrent lumbar disc herniation: results of operative management. Spine (Phila Pa 1976) 2001;26(6):672–6.

41. Slone RM, MacMillan M, Montgomery WJ. Spinal fixation. Part 3. Complications of spinal instrumentation. Radiographics 1993;13(4):797–816.

42. Gates GF. SPECT bone scanning of the spine. Semin Nucl Med 1998;28(1):78–94.

43. Guhlmann A, Brecht-Krauss D, Suger G, et al. Chronic osteomyelitis: detection with FDG PET and correlation with histopathologic findings. Radiology 1998;206(3):749–54.

44. Balagura S, Neumann JF. Magnetic resonance imaging of the postoperative intervertebral disk: the first eight months–clinical and legal implications. J Spinal Disord 1993;6(3):212–7.

45. Annertz M, Jonsson B, Stromqvist B, et al. Serial MRI in the early postoperative period after lumbar discectomy. Neuroradiology 1995;37(3):177–82.

46. Boden SD, Davis DO, Dina TS, et al. Contrast-enhanced MR imaging performed after successful lumbar disk surgery: prospective study. Radiology 1992;182(1):59–64.

47. Ross JS, Masaryk TJ, Modic MT, et al. Lumbar spine: postoperative assessment with surface-coil MR imaging. Radiology 1987;164(3):851–60.

48. Dina TS, Boden SD, Davis DO. Lumbar spine after surgery for herniated disk: imaging findings in the early postoperative period. AJR Am J Roentgenol 1995;164(3):665–71.

49. Herrera Herrera I, Moreno de la Presa R, Gonzalez Gutierrez R, et al. Evaluation of the postoperative lumbar spine. Radiologia 2013;55(1):12–23.

50. Lee YS, Choi ES, Song CJ. Symptomatic nerve root changes on contrast-enhanced MR imaging after surgery for lumbar disk herniation. AJNR Am J Neuroradiol 2009;30(5):1062–7.

51. Hayashi D, Roemer FW, Mian A, et al. Imaging features of postoperative complications after spinal surgery and instrumentation. AJR Am J Roentgenol 2012;199(1):W123–9.

52. Ross JS. Magnetic resonance imaging of the postoperative spine. Semin Musculoskelet Radiol 2000; 4(3):281–91.

53. Lee JK, Amorosa L, Cho SK, et al. Recurrent lumbar disk herniation. J Am Acad Orthop Surg 2010;18(6): 327–37.

54. Smorgick Y, Baker KC, Herkowitz H, et al. Predisposing factors for dural tear in patients undergoing lumbar spine surgery. J Neurosurg Spine 2015; 22(5):483–6.

55. Sin AH, Caldito G, Smith D, et al. Predictive factors for dural tear and cerebrospinal fluid leakage in patients undergoing lumbar surgery. J Neurosurg Spine 2006;5(3):224–7.

56. Young PM, Berquist TH, Bancroft LW, et al. Complications of spinal instrumentation. Radiographics 2007;27(3):775–89.

57. Van Goethem JW, Parizel PM, van den Hauwe L, et al. The value of MRI in the diagnosis of postoperative spondylodiscitis. Neuroradiology 2000;42(8):580–5.

58. Ross JS, Masaryk TJ, Modic MT, et al. MR imaging of lumbar arachnoiditis. AJR Am J Roentgenol 1987;149(5):1025–32.

59. Liu LD, Zhao S, Liu WG, et al. Arachnoiditis ossificans after spinal surgery. Orthopedics 2015;38(5): e437–42.

60. Babar S, Saifuddin A. MRI of the post-discectomy lumbar spine. Clin Radiol 2002;57(11):969–81.

61. Hueftle MG, Modic MT, Ross JS, et al. Lumbar spine: postoperative MR imaging with Gd-DTPA. Radiology 1988;167(3):817–24.

62. Bundschuh CV, Modic MT, Ross JS, et al. Epidural fibrosis and recurrent disk herniation in the lumbar spine: MR imaging assessment. AJR Am J Roentgenol 1988;150(4):923–32.

63. Ross JS, Obuchowski N, Zepp R. The postoperative lumbar spine: evaluation of epidural scar over a 1-year period. AJNR Am J Neuroradiol 1998;19(1): 183–6.

64. Emami A, Deviren V, Berven S, et al. Outcome and complications of long fusions to the sacrum in adult spine deformity: luque-galveston, combined iliac and sacral screws, and sacral fixation. Spine (Phila Pa 1976) 2002;27(7):776–86.

65. Zampolin R, Erdfarb A, Miller T. Imaging of lumbar spine fusion. Neuroimaging Clin N Am 2014;24(2): 269–86.

66. Suda K, Ito M, Abumi K, et al. Radiological risk factors of pseudoarthrosis and/or instrument breakage after PLF with the pedicle screw system in isthmic spondylolisthesis. J Spinal Disord Tech 2006;19(8): 541–6.

67. Hsu WK, Wang JC. The use of bone morphogenetic protein in spine fusion. Spine J 2008;8(3):419–25.

68. Carragee EJ, Hurwitz EL, Weiner BK. A critical review of recombinant human bone morphogenetic protein-2 trials in spinal surgery: emerging safety concerns and lessons learned. Spine J 2011;11(6): 471–91.

69. Sethi A, Craig J, Bartol S, et al. Radiographic and CT evaluation of recombinant human bone morphogenetic protein-2-assisted spinal interbody fusion. AJR Am J Roentgenol 2011;197(1):W128–33.

70. Cho KJ, Suk SI, Park SR, et al. Complications in posterior fusion and instrumentation for degenerative lumbar scoliosis. Spine (Phila Pa 1976) 2007; 32(20):2232–7.

71. Zhang C, Berven SH, Fortin M, et al. Adjacent segment degeneration versus disease after lumbar spine fusion for degenerative pathology: a systematic review with meta-analysis of the literature. Clin Spine Surg 2016;29(1):21–9.

72. Tehranzadeh J, Ton JD, Rosen CD. Advances in spinal fusion. Semin Ultrasound CT MR 2005;26(2): 103–13.

73. Barsa P, Suchomel P. Factors affecting sagittal malalignment due to cage subsidence in standalone cage assisted anterior cervical fusion. Eur Spine J 2007;16(9):1395–400.

74. Bartels RH, Donk RD, Feuth T. Subsidence of stand-alone cervical carbon fiber cages. Neurosurgery 2006;58(3):502–8 [discussion: 502–8].

75. Gercek E, Arlet V, Delisle J, et al. Subsidence of stand-alone cervical cages in anterior interbody fusion: warning. Eur Spine J 2003;12(5):513–6.

Spontaneous Intracranial Hypotension
Imaging in Diagnosis and Treatment

Timothy J. Amrhein, MD*, Peter G. Kranz, MD

KEYWORDS

- Spontaneous intracranial hypotension • CSF Leak • CSF to venous fistula • Epidural blood patch
- Myelogram

KEY POINTS

- Spontaneous intracranial hypotension (SIH) is a potentially debilitating condition resulting from low cerebrospinal fluid (CSF) volume secondary to a spontaneous spinal CSF leak or CSF to venous fistula (CVF).
- There are 3 causes of SIH: (1) CSF leak due to a nerve root sleeve diverticulum, (2) CSF leak due to an osteophyte spur, and (3) CVF.
- Multiple spinal imaging modalities are available to assess for the underlying pathologic condition in SIH, including computed tomographic (CT) myelography, dynamic myelography, dynamic (ultra-fast) CT myelography, MR imaging, and MR myelography with intrathecal gadolinium.
- Each imaging modality has strengths and weaknesses related to spatial, temporal, and contrast resolution. The optimal diagnostic test depends on the underlying pathologic condition (slow CSF leak, fast CSF leak, or CVF).
- Treatment options for SIH include conservative measures, surgery, and blood patching. Imaging guidance plays an integral role in targeted patching.

INTRODUCTION

Spontaneous intracranial hypotension (SIH) is an often-misdiagnosed condition resulting from cerebrospinal fluid (CSF) hypovolemia.[1] This CSF hypovolemia is, by definition, noniatrogenic (ie, not secondary to a lumbar puncture or surgery) and typically occurs due to a spinal CSF leak. The reported incidence of SIH is approximately 5 in 100,000, but is likely considerably higher due to lack of awareness among both physicians and the general population.[2] SIH can occur in anyone with reported ages ranging from 3 to 86 years; however, it most commonly occurs in the fifth or sixth decade of life. SIH patients are slightly more commonly female (1.5:1).[3]

Clinical Symptoms

Patients with SIH most characteristically report an orthostatic headache (ie, one that is worse with upright posture).[4] In addition, they can experience a myriad of variably present symptoms related to cranial nerve dysfunction, including diplopia, reduced visual acuity, nausea, vomiting, tinnitus, hearing loss, disequilibrium, paresthesias, and cognitive deficits. These symptoms, in combination with headaches, can lead to considerable disability resulting in a loss of work productivity and a markedly reduced quality of life. Although less common, some patients with SIH have nonorthostatic headaches, and some may not have headaches at all. Furthermore, there are

No conflicts of interest to disclose.
Department of Radiology, Duke University Medical Center, Box 3808, Durham, NC 27710, USA
* Corresponding author.
E-mail address: timothy.amrhein@duke.edu

Radiol Clin N Am 57 (2019) 439–451
https://doi.org/10.1016/j.rcl.2018.10.004
0033-8389/19/Published by Elsevier Inc.

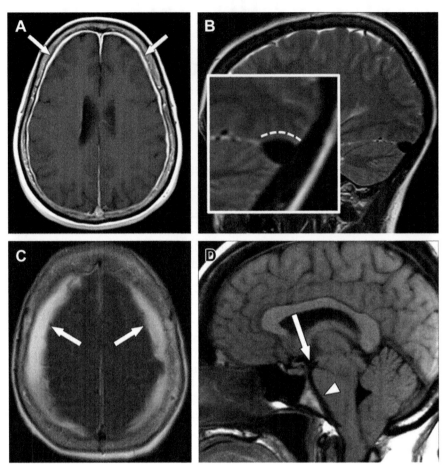

Fig. 1. Brain MR imaging signs in SIH. (*A*) Axial T1-weighted postcontrast image demonstrating diffuse smooth dural (pachymeningeal) enhancement (*arrows*). Note that the pattern of enhancement does not extend into the sulci, as would be seen with leptomeningeal enhancement. This distinction is important because diffuse *smooth* dural enhancement is not associated with meningitis or leptomeningeal carcinomatosis and should raise suspicion for SIH. (*B*) Sagittal T2-weighted image demonstrating venous distension sign. Note convex bowing of the transverse sinus at the level of the orbit (*inset; dashed line*). (*C*) Axial FLAIR image demonstrates symmetric bilateral hyperintense subdural effusions (*arrows*). (*D*) Sagittal T1-weighted image demonstrating brain sagging in SIH. Prepontine cistern is narrowed (*arrowhead*). Note that the floor of the third ventricle is downsloping (*arrow*), a finding never seen with Chairi I malformations.

alternative causes for orthostatic headaches, including postural orthostatic tachycardia syndrome and cervicogenic headache.[5,6] For this reason, symptoms alone can be an unreliable diagnostic tool and a combination of tests, including brain imaging, spinal imaging, and CSF pressure measurement, is often required to confirm the diagnosis.

Brain and Spine MR Imaging

SIH patients commonly undergo a brain MR imaging for assessment of headaches. At the time of ordering this examination, the referring physician often does not suspect SIH and, for this reason, the radiologist may be the first to suggest this

diagnosis, preventing prolonged misdiagnosis, which is all too common in this patient population.[1]

There are several brain MR imaging signs in SIH. The most important of these include (a) smooth diffuse dural (or pachymeningeal) enhancement, which is found in up to 83% of SIH patients on contrasted MR images (**Fig. 1**A); (b) the venous distension sign (75% of SIH patients) (**Fig. 1**B); (c) bilateral subdural effusions (23% of SIH patients) (**Fig. 1**C); (d) brain sagging (61% of SIH patients) (**Fig. 1**D).[7,8] It should be emphasized that a negative brain MR imaging does *not* exclude a diagnosis of SIH.[9,10]

Occasionally, a CSF leak will be incidentally visualized on spinal imaging acquired for neck or back pain associated with undiagnosed SIH,

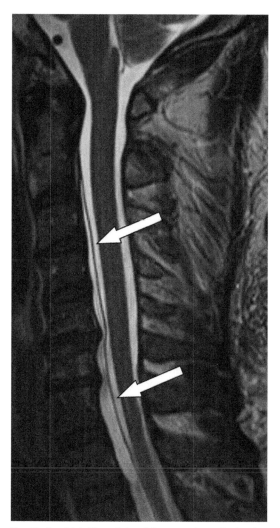

Fig. 2. Sagittal T2-weighted image of cervical spine demonstrates a ventral CSF leak. A large extradural fluid collection is identified in the ventral spinal canal. Intervening dura appears as a low signal line (*white arrows*) dividing the CSF leak from CSF within the true subarachnoid space.

most commonly on an MR imaging of the cervical or thoracic spine. In this case, one may identify an extradural fluid collection indicating the presence of a CSF leak with intervening low linear signal representing the dura (**Fig. 2**).[11] Although this finding signifies the presence of a high flow CSF leak, one cannot determine the location of the dural defect with standard MR imaging alone.

SPONTANEOUS INTRACRANIAL HYPOTENSION SUBTYPES

There are 3 general subtypes of SIH, classified by the underlying cause: (1) CSF leak due to a nerve root sleeve diverticulum, (2) CSF leak due to an osteophyte spur, and (3) CSF to venous fistula (CVF)[12] (**Fig. 3**).

Most CSF leaks in SIH occur because of a diverticulum of a spinal nerve root sleeve.[12] Although nerve root sleeve CSF leaks can occur abruptly due to traumatic tearing of the meninges surrounding the nerve root, most cases are thought to occur secondary to denuding of the overlying dura, which allows for protrusion and exposure of the more friable arachnoid. The arachnoid then tears, even in the absence of significant trauma, resulting in a CSF leak.[13–15] Nerve root sleeve diverticula can occur anywhere within the spine but are most commonly along thoracic nerve roots.[16] In contrast to diverticula, a perineural cyst is a normal dilation of the nerve root sleeve that contains all 3 intact meningeal layers and can occur in patients without CSF leaks. In patients with nerve root sleeve origin CSF leaks, the size of dural defect determines the morphology of the resultant CSF leak. Smaller dural defects cause slow-flow CSF leaks and result in a small volume of extradural CSF, whereas larger dural defects cause high-flow CSF leaks and result in a large volume of extradural CSF. These different types of leaks produce different imaging appearances.

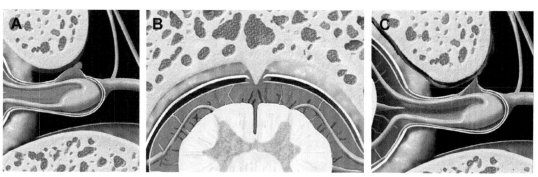

Fig. 3. Subtypes of SIH. (*A*) CSF leak due to a nerve root sleeve diverticulum. (*B*) CSF leak due to an osteophyte spur. (*C*) CSF to venous fistula. (*Courtesy of* Richard H. Wiggins, MD, Salt Lake City, UT.)

CSF leaks may also occur secondary to an osteophyte that pierces the dura and arachnoid. Typically, these spurs are associated with a disc herniation leading to a ventral dural tear.[12] However, tears of the dorsal dural surface have also been reported, arising because of ligamentum flavum calcification and facet osteophytosis.[17] Osteophytes most commonly result in high-flow, large-volume CSF leaks.

CVF have only recently been discovered but are an increasingly recognized and important cause of SIH.[18] It is hypothesized that this acquired pathologic connection between the subarachnoid space and an adjacent epidural vein allows for unregulated rapid transfer of CSF into the bloodstream resulting in CSF hypovolemia. CVFs are usually located in the neuroforamen and are associated with a nerve root sleeve diverticulum. Although CVFs can occur along with slow-flow CSF leaks from the diverticulum, more commonly they have no associated CSF leak.

Two common misconceptions about the cause of SIH are (1) that it is caused by skull base CSF leaks and (2) that multiple leaks are present. In actuality, nearly all cases of SIH occur due to pathologic condition in the spine and, in particular, skull base CSF leaks do *not* cause SIH.[19] Furthermore, in the authors' experience, patients nearly always have only one CSF leak or CVF.

The underlying cause of SIH determines the appearance of the pathologic condition on spinal imaging and helps to guide decision making regarding optimal therapy. For this reason, understanding these SIH subtypes is critical for both diagnosis and treatment.

IMAGING MODALITIES AND TECHNIQUES

Identifying the causative spinal CSF leak or CVF in a patient with SIH can be challenging. Although spinal imaging will not localize a CSF leak or CVF in all SIH patients, the chances of success can be maximized by choosing the appropriate imaging test and by paying meticulous attention to imaging technique.

The investigation begins with an initial screening spinal imaging examination, most commonly standard MR imaging, heavily T2-weighted MR imaging, or a CT myelogram. Based on the findings from this initial examination, one may then need to select a secondary problem-solving imaging modality in order to confirm the location and presence of the CSF leak or CVF.

The most important factor in choosing an imaging modality is the suspected subtype of SIH, which helps to determine the particular spatial, contrast, and temporal resolution needs. For example, in the setting of a known high-flow and high-volume CSF leak, rapid temporal resolution is paramount because one is hoping to capture the exact moment that contrast material escapes through the dural defect, confirming the origin of the leak. Conversely, CVFs can be relatively diminutive structures and will most commonly have no associated CSF leak. For this reason, spatial and contrast resolution become priorities in order to identify the often-subtle contrast opacification of an adjacent paraspinal vein, which can be only several millimeters in size.[20]

There are several different imaging modalities that can be used in an effort to identify and localize a spinal CSF leak or CVF.[11] These imaging modalities include (1) CT myelography, (2) dynamic (or ultrafast) CT myelography, (3) dynamic myelography under conventional fluoroscopy (with or without digital subtraction), and (4) MR myelography with intrathecal gadolinium. Nuclear medicine cisternography has also been used in the assessment of SIH and may allow one to identify slow-flow or intermittent CSF leaks given its ability to image over longer time periods. However, it suffers from relatively poor spatial and temporal resolution, high false negative rates, and false positives.[21,22] For this reason, this modality is not discussed further in this article.

Computed Tomographic Myelography

CT myelography is an excellent imaging modality for identifying the cause of SIH. This technique provides very good spatial resolution as well as CSF-specific contrast via injection of myelographic contrast material into the subarachnoid space. Furthermore, CT myelography allows for imaging of the entire spine as well as cross-sectional visualization allowing one to identify degenerative changes that may be the cause of a CSF leak (eg, spiculated disc osteophytes). Potential weaknesses of this technique include radiation dose and relatively poor temporal resolution.

In the authors' experience, a few modifications to the standard CT myelography technique can greatly improve the probability of diagnostic success. First, temporal resolution can be maximized by performing the lumbar puncture under CT fluoroscopy guidance with rapid subsequent scanning of the patient soon after injecting contrast. Doing so serves to eliminate any delays that may occur in transferring the patient from the conventional fluoroscopy table to the CT scanner after the myelogram. Improving temporal resolution is particularly important in the setting of a high-flow large-volume CSF leak, where delaying CT scan acquisition by 20 to 30 minutes may result in diffuse contrast opacification of the extradural CSF precluding one's ability to identify the exact origin of the leak. In addition to a CT fluoroscopy-guided lumbar puncture, a breath-hold during CT scan acquisition is critical in order to reduce motion artifact because the causative pathologic condition in SIH is frequently in the thoracic spine. Finally, reviewing thin-section images is imperative because many CSF leaks and CVFs can be subtle findings. At the authors' institution, they routinely review 0.625-mm axial images with 1-mm coronal and sagittal reformats.

CSF leaks arising from nerve root sleeve diverticula may have a variety of appearances on CT myelography depending on the size of the meningeal defect and the volume of resultant extradural CSF. Slow leaks typically result in small volumes of contrast within the foramen adjacent to an irregular nerve root sleeve, which can sometimes be quite subtle. Higher-flow leaks will manifest as a large volumes of extradural contrast centered on the nerve root of origin (**Fig. 4**).

CSF leaks caused by spiculated osteophytes are usually high flow and result in a large volume of contrast external to the subarachnoid space, which may extend multiple vertebral segments on CT myelography. Because most of these spurs are secondary to disc degenerative changes that cause defects of the ventral dura, the extradural contrast is typically centered in the ventral epidural space. An advantage of CT myelography is the ability to identify these causative disc osteophyte spurs as well as the CSF leak (**Fig. 5**).

CVF identification can be aided by the presence of a hyperdense paraspinal vein indicating pathologic egress of contrast from the subarachnoid space into the vein[20] (**Fig. 6**). These hyperdense veins may be identified anywhere in the region of the CVF, which is usually located in the neuroforamen, but are most commonly found in the form of the segmental veins located adjacent to the vertebral body. On CT myelography, the Hounsfield unit measurements within these veins are typically greater than 70 and therefore considerably higher than adjacent normal veins (~30 HU).

As previously mentioned, in the setting of a large-volume high-flow CSF leak, rapid imaging is important in order to identify the exact origin of the dural defect. Occasionally, CT myelography may not provide the temporal resolution necessary to identify the exact leak origin. Dynamic myelography or dynamic (ultrafast) CT myelography may then be required given their superior temporal resolution. However, often the gradient of contrast density within the large-volume CSF leak on CT myelography can be used to narrow down the potential locations of the dural defect, because greater contrast is typically identified closer to the origin of the leak[23] (**Fig. 7**).

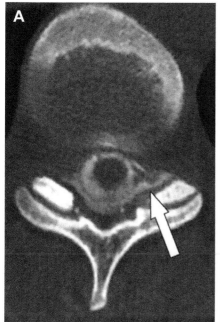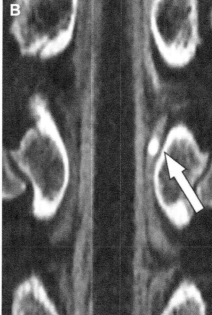

Fig. 4. High-flow CSF leak arising from a nerve root sleeve diverticulum. Axial (*A*) and coronal (*B*) CT myelogram images demonstrating a high-flow CSF leak arising from the left T10 nerve root sleeve (*arrows*). Note the subtly increased contrast density surrounding this nerve root on the coronal image.

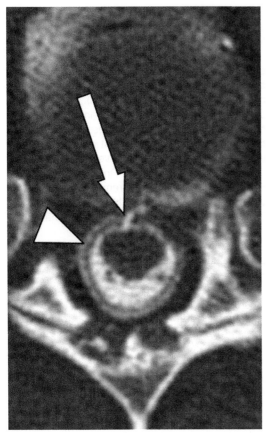

Fig. 5. Axial CT myelogram image demonstrating a spiculated disc osteophyte spur (*arrow*) piercing the dura and resulting in a CSF leak (*arrowhead*). (*Courtesy of* J. Michael Hazenfield, MD, Cincinnati, OH.)

Dynamic Myelography with or Without Digital Subtraction

Dynamic myelography refers to conventional myelography using a tilt table in conjunction with rapid image capture that is focused over an area of concern (the suspected CSF leak or CVF).[24] It affords superior temporal resolution compared with CT myelography as well as excellent spatial resolution. Potential shortcomings of this technique include the lack of cross-sectional imaging, the inability to image the entire spine at once, and the requirement for considerable patient cooperation.[11]

Dynamic myelography begins with a standard lumbar puncture under conventional fluoroscopic guidance. The patient is placed securely on a tilt table, and the table is then tilted to allow myelographic contrast to flow along the dependent surface of the thecal sac over the area of concern. Contrast migration is visualized in real time using intermittent fluoroscopy, and images are rapidly acquired in an attempt to capture the exact location of a high-flow CSF leak.[25] Because this technique is dependent on contrast flowing over the area of pathologic condition, it is important to position the patient such that the suspected pathologic condition is dependent. For example, if a ventral CSF leak is suspected, the patient should be prone. Similarly, the patient is placed in a lateral decubitus position for suspected nerve root sleeve origin CSF leaks and CVFs.

On dynamic myelography, one expects CSF leaks to manifest as a split or "Y" in the normal

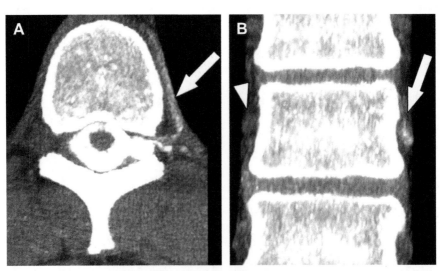

Fig. 6. Hyperdense paraspinal vein sign confirming the presence of a CVF. (*A*) Axial maximum intensity projection (MIP) image from a CT myelogram demonstrates asymmetric contrast opacification of the left paraspinal vein (*arrow*). (*B*) Coronal MIP of same patient demonstrates the hyperdense paraspinal vein (*arrowhead*). Note much lower density of normal contralateral paraspinal vein (*arrowhead*).

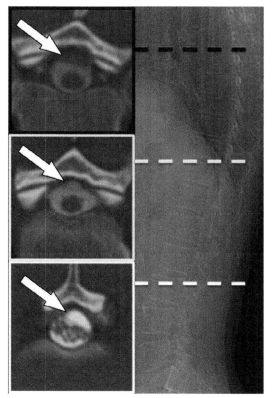

Fig. 7. Contrast gradient to help localize large-volume high-flow CSF leak on CT myelogram. Lateral scout image (*right*) and 3 magnified axial CT myelogram images (*left*) from spinal levels demarcated by respective dashed lines. Dorsal CSF leak (*arrows*) exhibits progressively decreased contrast density relative to the subarachnoid space as one extends superiorly from the lumbar spine (*white box*) to the lower thoracic spine (*yellow box*) to the upper thoracic spine (*blue box*).

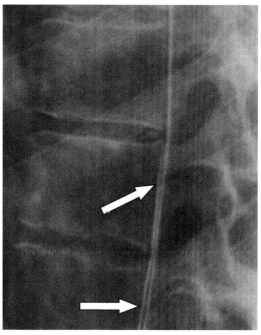

Fig. 8. High-flow ventral CSF leak. Dynamic myelogram with patient in the prone position exhibits split or "Y" of contrast column (*arrows*) beginning at the disc interspace confirming the location of the dural defect.

subarachnoid contrast column indicating the location of the dural defect (Fig. 8). This split of the contrast column typically occurs either on the ventral dural surface due to a disc osteophyte spur or laterally within the neuroforamen in the setting of a nerve root sleeve diverticulum. CSF leaks arising from nerve root sleeve diverticula tend to occur characteristically along the axilla of the nerve root (Fig. 9).

Dynamic myelography can also be very helpful in confirming the presence of a CVF, particularly if it is suspected based on prior imaging, such as an initial CT myelogram. In this scenario, the superior spatial resolution of dynamic myelography allows one to better visualize contract opacification of the often diminutive veins in a CVF. Furthermore, the tilt table and decubitus positioning allow for maximal concentrations of contrast in the region of the nerve root sleeve giving rise to the fistula. CVFs manifest as

branching contrast-opacified vessels extending from a nerve root sleeve (Fig. 10).

Digital subtraction can be applied during a dynamic myelogram allowing for removal of osseous structures via a mask. Applying digital subtraction is particularly useful near the cervicothoracic junction given attenuation from the shoulders. It may also prove useful in the presence of spinal orthopedic hardware. Furthermore, removal of background can increase the conspicuity of subtle CVFs. Digital subtraction is susceptible to artifact from patient motion and, therefore, does require either patient breath-holding or general anesthesia with suspension of respirations.

Dynamic (Ultrafast) Computed Tomographic Myelography

Dynamic (or ultrafast) CT myelography involves modifications to the aforementioned CT myelography technique in an effort to improve temporal resolution.[26] This technique is used when attempting to identify the otherwise occult origin of a known high-flow CSF leak. However, the markedly improved temporal resolution comes at the cost of a considerably higher radiation dose.[27]

Dynamic CT myelography is performed with the patient positioned such that the area of concern is dependent. The patient is also supported on foam

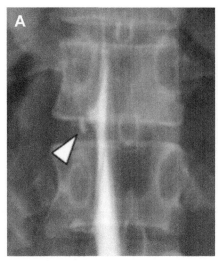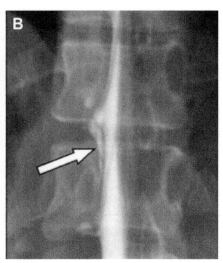

Fig. 9. CSF leak arising from a nerve root sleeve axilla. Consecutive dynamic myelogram images (patient left lateral decubitus) demonstrate progressive contrast opacification of the left T11 nerve root sleeve (*A*: *arrowhead*). Contrast spills through the dural defect near the axilla (*B*: *arrow*) confirming the origin of the leak.

pads or pillows in order to elevate the hips above the shoulders. This patient positioning allows for a downward slope toward the cervical spine mimicking a tilt table. A CT fluoroscopy-guided lumbar puncture is then performed. Subsequently, myelographic contrast is rapidly injected followed

immediately by multiple CT scans of the entire spine (or of a shorter z-axis, if a more focused area of concern can be established).

The goal of dynamic CT myelography is for one of the scans to capture the exact moment that subarachnoid contrast escapes into the extradural space, thereby localizing the dural defect. Analogous to dynamic myelography, this manifests as a split in the contrast column (**Fig. 11**).

Given the relatively increased radiation dose of dynamic CT myelography compared with the other modalities described in this article, it is typically used as a problem-solving examination reserved for selected cases with known high-flow CSF leaks in which the exact origin of the leak is unknown.

MR Myelography with Intrathecal Gadolinium

In cases in which a suspected slow-flow CSF leak remains occult on primary imaging modalities (ie, CT myelography), some investigators advocate for the use of MR myelography with intrathecal injection of gadolinium-based contrast agents. This technique combines CSF-specific contrast with the superior contrast resolution of MR imaging. Weaknesses of MR myelography with intrathecal gadolinium include its susceptibility to artifacts, relatively inferior spatial resolution compared with other imaging modalities, and poor temporal resolution (given the long image acquisition times). In addition, intrathecal injection of gadolinium is an off-label use of this contrast material and, although it is generally well tolerated, the long-term risks are unknown.

After a lumbar puncture, 0.3 to 0.5 mL of Magnevist (gadopentetate dimeglumine; 0.5 mol/L;

Fig. 10. CVF. Oblique projection image from a dynamic myelogram demonstrates contrast opacification of a CVF appearing as multiple branching vessels adjacent to the nerve root sleeve (*arrowhead*). Note also the subtle but abnormal contrast opacification of the paraspinal veins (*arrows*) both superior and inferior to the neuroforamen indicating a direct connection between the subarachnoid space and the venous system.

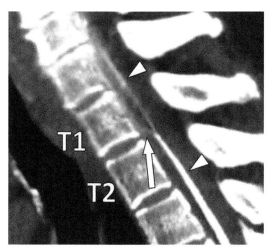

Fig. 11. Ultrafast (dynamic) CT myelography confirms the presence of a dural tear at T1/2. Contrast column within the subarachnoid space (*arrowheads*) splits at the level of the T1/2 disc interspace (*arrow*) and spills into a ventral epidural collection (not shown).

Schering, Berlin, Germany) is injected into the CSF. (Most studies on intrathecal gadolinium have used Magnevist.) Subsequently, patients are scanned with a heavily T1-weighted fat-saturated technique.

Slow flow CSF leaks appear as a T1 hyperintense halo around a nerve root sleeve or as a curvilinear hyperintensity in the ventral epidural space in the setting of a disc osteophyte spur (Fig. 12). In SIH patients with a negative CT myelogram, prior investigations have found that MR myelography with intrathecal gadolinium is successful in identifying the CSF leak in 21% to 25% of cases.[28,29]

Because of the long image acquisition times and the delay between contrast injection and the MR scan, MR myelography with intrathecal gadolinium is typically not helpful in the assessment of high-flow, large-volume CSF leaks. Although its sensitivity for the detection of CVFs is unknown, the reduced spatial resolution may make detection difficult.

SPONTANEOUS INTRACRANIAL HYPOTENSION SUBTYPES: CHOOSING THE APPROPRIATE DIAGNOSTIC IMAGING

Although there is no agreed upon consensus regarding a diagnostic imaging algorithm for assessment of spinal pathologic condition in SIH, many centers will start with either standard MR imaging, heavily T2-weighted MR imaging, or a CT myelogram of the spine. Spine MR imaging

typically will not reveal a slow-flow CSF leak or a CVF, but may confirm the presence of a high-flow high-volume CSF leak directing one toward a modality with maximal temporal resolution, such as dynamic myelography or a dynamic (ultrafast) CT myelogram. This algorithm has been shown to reduce the need for repeat myelography.[30] However, it should be noted that, if this initial MR imaging is negative, an alternative imaging modality will be needed in order to assess for a slow CSF leak or CVF.

Beginning with a CT myelogram may result in definitive identification of the causative pathologic condition precluding the need for additional imaging. Alternatively, it could reveal findings that are suggestive of the presence of (1) a slow-flow CSF leak directing the algorithm toward MR myelography with intrathecal gadolinium or conventional myelography; (2) a high-flow leak directing one toward dynamic myelography or dynamic (ultrafast) CT myelography if the origin cannot be determined on initial imaging; or (3) a CVF. Further interrogation of a potential CVF may include imaging the patient in the decubitus position with either CT myelography or dynamic myelography with or without digital subtraction.

Cases in which the patient clearly has SIH but the spinal cause cannot be identified can be challenging. Sometimes diagnostic spinal imaging will need to be repeated in order to find the CSF leak or CVF. Newer techniques such as positive pressure myelography (during which the CSF pressure is artificially elevated via infusion of saline) or dual-energy CT may prove capable of increasing the diagnostic yield but are currently investigational.

In general, the authors advocate for the use of CT myelography, with the technique modifications outlined above, as the first-line modality in assessing for a spinal CSF leak or CVF. When a high-flow or high-volume CSF leak is identified, one may then need to use dynamic myelography in an attempt to identify the exact location of the CSF leak. The addition of digital subtraction may be required if the suspected leak is in a region with considerable attenuation of the x-ray beam due to overlying structures, such as the shoulders at the cervicothoracic junction.

A CVF can be a subtle finding with any imaging modality. If a hyperdense paraspinal vein is identified on initial CT, decubitus dynamic myelography may be helpful in confirming the finding. The authors will often also perform a post dynamic myelogram CT scan through the area of concern with the patient kept in the decubitus position, because this can help improve conspicuity of the CVF.

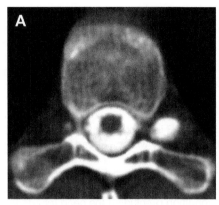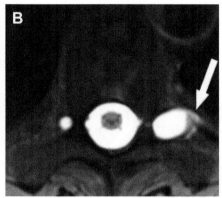

Fig. 12. Slow-flow CSF leak arising from the left T7 nerve root sleeve. (*A*) Axial CT myelogram image demonstrates a prominent left T7 nerve root sleeve without discernible CSF leak. (*B*) Axial fat-saturated T1-weighted image from an MR myelogram with intrathecal gadolinium reveals a contrast halo around the nerve root confirming the presence of a slow-flow CSF leak (*arrow*).

TREATMENT OF SPONTANEOUS INTRACRANIAL HYPOTENSION

In general, there are 3 main approaches to treating a patient with SIH: (1) conservative measures, (2) blood patching, and (3) surgery.

Conservative measures in the treatment of SIH are analogous to those for a post lumbar puncture headache and include strict bed rest, hydration, caffeine, and an abdominal binder. Many patients will be refractory to these simple measures, however, requiring further intervention. One study found that only 37% of patients received headache relief at 6 months and 63% at 2 years.[31] Prolonged bed rest, without certainty of a cure, is quite burdensome, and many patients will therefore pursue other therapies.

Epidural blood patching (EBP) is the widely accepted primary method for treatment of CSF leaks in SIH. Relative to surgery, EBP is less invasive. EBP involves acquiring sterile autologous blood from the patient's intravenous line and injecting it through a needle or catheter placed in the epidural space in order to seal a CSF leak. Some treatment centers will also inject dural sealant materials, such as fibrin glue in an effort to achieve improved patching efficacy. EBP can be targeted to the site of a known CSF leak or nontargeted. Nontargeted patches are generically injected in the dorsal epidural space irrespective of the location of a CSF leak, typically in either the lumbar spine or at the thoracolumbar junction. Nontargeted patches are presumed to work by either achieving successful spread of patching material to the unknown leak site or by creating nonspecific mass effect within the spinal canal.[32] Although nontargeted patches are sometimes performed without imaging guidance, targeted

patches require the use of either fluoroscopic or CT guidance. With imaging-guided targeted patching, one can direct the needle tip to the location of a previously identified CSF leak.

The technique for needle placements in EBP is similar to that used for other epidural injections in the spine (eg, corticosteroid delivery for treatment of pain) and most commonly involves either a transforaminal or an interlaminar approach. During an interlaminar approach, the spinal needle is advanced via a posterior approach through the ligamentum flavum into the dorsal epidural space of the spinal canal (**Fig. 13**A). Loss-of-resistance technique is used, although this can be less reliable in the cervical spine given the relatively diminutive size of the ligamentum flavum and known midline gaps. Therefore, direct visualization of the needle tip position is more important in these cases.[33,34] Once the target dorsal epidural space is reached, an extravascular needle tip location is confirmed by noting absence of blood return in the needle hub, no blood return with aspiration, and by direct visualization on imaging after injection of myelographic-safe contrast material.[35,36] This contrast epidurogram can also serve to demonstrate the locations of potential spread of patching material. Finally, patching material is injected (autologous blood with or without fibrin glue). The total volume of injected material is dependent on patient symptoms and mass effect on the thecal sac as visualized on imaging. Indications to terminate the injection include excessive pain, neurologic deficit, or if there is significant compression of the thecal sac and spinal cord.

The transforaminal approach involves advancing the spinal needle under imaging

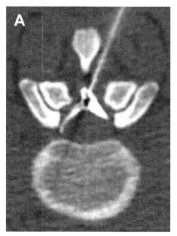 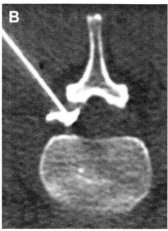 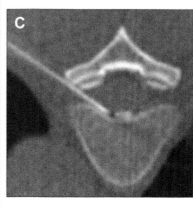

Fig. 13. Needle approaches during EBP. (*A*) CT fluoroscopy-guided interlaminar epidural needle placement. Contrast is noted surrounding the tip of the needle within the dorsal epidural space covering the entirety of the dorsal dura. (*B*) CT fluoroscopy-guided transforaminal epidural needle placement. Contrast opacifies the foraminal epidural space surrounding the nerve root. (*C*) CT fluoroscopy-guided ventral epidural needle placement. The needle is advanced through the foramen until the tip reaches the ventral epidural space of the spinal canal.

guidance into the posterior aspect of the neuroforamen (**Fig. 13**B). On reaching the target, an extravascular location is confirmed using contrast material, and the methods outlined in the description of the interlaminar approach are followed before patching material is injected.

Although the volume of patching material injected likely varies depending on practitioner, typical volumes range from 10 to 40 mL for nontargeted patches via the interlaminar approach.[37,38] Less volume is required when the injection is targeted to a known CSF leak, and generally less volumes are used in smaller spaces, such as the neuroforamen, during a transforaminal approach where one may inject approximately 1 to 5 mL. With higher volumes, caution must be exercised not to compress the spinal cord. Visualization of the degree of mass effect on imaging as well as feedback from the patient regarding symptoms is helpful in this regard.

Transforaminal and interlaminar approaches provide excellent coverage of CSF leaks located along the dorsal dural surface as well as CSF leaks and CVFs arising from nerve root sleeve diverticula. However, ventral epidural coverage of patching material, necessary for treatment of CSF leaks caused by spiculated disc osteophytes, is difficult to achieve using these approaches. In these cases, experienced operators may consider direct placement of the needle tip into the ventral epidural space of the spinal canal by traversing the neuroforamen during a transforaminal approach (**Fig. 13**C).[39] Ventral

epidural needle placement often allows for adequate spread of patching material over the ventral dura, particularly if bilateral placements are performed. There is a theoretic possibility of injuring a radiculomedullary artery in the neuroforamen during this needle placement resulting in spinal cord infarction. Therefore, every attempt should be made to pass the needle through the inferior aspect of the neuroforamen away from the typical anterosuperior vessel location.[40]

It is not uncommon that CSF leaks in SIH will require multiple patches in order to achieve a durable result.[9] Several retrospective studies have been published reporting variable success rates for EBP ranging from 30% to 90%.[37,38,41–45] Prospective research and clinical trials are needed to confirm the efficacy of patching, to compare different patching techniques (eg, targeted vs nontargeted, or use of fibrin glue vs blood alone), and to eventually establish a universally agreed upon treatment algorithm.

When CSF leaks and CVFs are refractory to both conservative measures and patching, surgery may be required (**Fig. 14**). Often a CSF leak or CVF arising from a nerve root sleeve can be successfully treated with ligation or clipping of the associated nerve root. Surgery for ventral dural tears is more challenging. Both intradural and extradural approaches have been performed, each with the goal of finding and closing the dural defect.[46,47] In the authors' experience, removing the causative osteophyte spur is important in order to prevent recurrence.

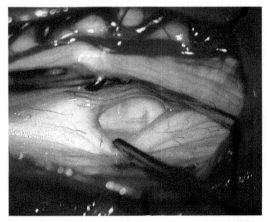

Fig. 14. Intraoperative photograph demonstrating a ventral dural tear due to a spiculated disc osteophyte spur. (*Courtesy of* Wouter Schievink, MD, Los Angeles, CA.)

SUMMARY

SIH is a debilitating and often misdiagnosed condition resulting from low CSF volume due to a spontaneous spinal CSF leak or CVF. Imaging plays a key role in diagnosis, in identification of the CSF leak or CVF, and in treatment. As such, radiologists have a central role in the care of these patients.

REFERENCES

1. Schievink WI. Misdiagnosis of spontaneous intracranial hypotension. Arch Neurol 2003;60:1713–8.
2. Schievink WI, Maya MM, Moser F, et al. Frequency of spontaneous intracranial hypotension in the emergency department. J Headache Pain 2007;8:325–8.
3. Schievink WI. Spontaneous spinal cerebrospinal fluid leaks. Cephalalgia 2008;28:1345–56.
4. Schievink WI, Deline CR. Headache secondary to intracranial hypotension. Curr Pain Headache Rep 2014;18:457.
5. Leep Hunderfund AN, Mokri B. Orthostatic headache without CSF leak. Neurology 2008;71:1902–6.
6. Becker WJ. Cervicogenic headache: evidence that the neck is a pain generator. Headache 2010;50: 699–705.
7. Kranz PG, Amrhein TJ, Choudhury KR, et al. Time-dependent changes in dural enhancement associated with spontaneous intracranial hypotension. AJR Am J Roentgenol 2016;207(6):1283–7.
8. Kranz PG, Tanpitukpongse TP, Choudhury KR, et al. Imaging signs in spontaneous intracranial hypotension: prevalence and relationship to CSF pressure. AJNR Am J Neuroradiol 2016;37:1374–8.
9. Kranz PG, Gray L, Amrhein TJ. Spontaneous intracranial hypotension: 10 myths and misperceptions. Headache 2018;58(7):948–59.
10. Lai TH, Fuh JL, Lirng JF, et al. Subdural haematoma in patients with spontaneous intracranial hypotension. Cephalalgia 2007;27:133–8.
11. Kranz PG, Luetmer PH, Diehn FE, et al. Myelographic techniques for the detection of spinal CSF leaks in spontaneous intracranial hypotension. AJR Am J Roentgenol 2016;206:8–19.
12. Schievink WI, Maya MM, Jean-Pierre S, et al. A classification system of spontaneous spinal CSF leaks. Neurology 2016;87:673–9.
13. Schievink WI, Reimer R, Folger WN. Surgical treatment of spontaneous intracranial hypotension associated with a spinal arachnoid diverticulum. Case report. J Neurosurg 1994;80:736–9.
14. Schievink WI, Jacques L. Recurrent spontaneous spinal cerebrospinal fluid leak associated with "nude nerve root" syndrome: case report. Neurosurgery 2003;53:1216–8 [discussion: 1218–9].
15. Cohen-Gadol AA, Mokri B, Piepgras DG, et al. Surgical anatomy of dural defects in spontaneous spinal cerebrospinal fluid leaks. Neurosurgery 2006;58(4 Suppl 2):ONS-238-45 [discussion: ONS-245].
16. Kranz PG, Stinnett SS, Huang KT, et al. Spinal meningeal diverticula in spontaneous intracranial hypotension: analysis of prevalence and myelographic appearance. AJNR Am J Neuroradiol 2013;34:1284–9.
17. Beck J, Ulrich CT, Fung C, et al. Diskogenic microspurs as a major cause of intractable spontaneous intracranial hypotension. Neurology 2016;87: 1220–6.
18. Schievink WI, Moser FG, Maya MM. CSF-venous fistula in spontaneous intracranial hypotension. Neurology 2014;83:472–3.
19. Schievink WI, Schwartz MS, Maya MM, et al. Lack of causal association between spontaneous intracranial hypotension and cranial cerebrospinal fluid leaks. J Neurosurg 2012;116:749–54.
20. Kranz PG, Amrhein TJ, Schievink WI, et al. The "hyperdense paraspinal vein" sign: a marker of CSF-venous fistula. AJNR Am J Neuroradiol 2016;37:1379–81.
21. Monteith TS, Kralik SF, Dillon WP, et al. The utility of radioisotope cisternography in low CSF/volume syndromes compared to myelography. Cephalalgia 2016;36:1291–5.
22. Mokri B. Radioisotope cisternography in spontaneous CSF leaks: interpretations and misinterpretations. Headache 2014;54:1358–68.
23. Yoshida H, Takai K, Taniguchi M. Leakage detection on CT myelography for targeted epidural blood patch in spontaneous cerebrospinal fluid leaks: calcified or ossified spinal lesions ventral to the thecal sac. J Neurosurg Spine 2014;21:432–41.
24. Hoxworth JM, Trentman TL, Kotsenas AL, et al. The role of digital subtraction myelography in the diagnosis and localization of spontaneous spinal CSF leaks. AJR Am J Roentgenol 2012;199:649–53.

25. Hoxworth JM, Patel AC, Bosch EP, et al. Localization of a rapid CSF leak with digital subtraction myelography. AJNR Am J Neuroradiol 2009;30:516–9.

26. Luetmer PH, Mokri B. Dynamic CT myelography: a technique for localizing high-flow spinal cerebrospinal fluid leaks. AJNR Am J Neuroradiol 2003;24:1711–4.

27. Thielen KR, Sillery JC, Morris JM, et al. Ultrafast dynamic computed tomography myelography for the precise identification of high-flow cerebrospinal fluid leaks caused by spiculated spinal osteophytes. J Neurosurg Spine 2015;22:324–31.

28. Akbar JJ, Luetmer PH, Schwartz KM, et al. The role of MR myelography with intrathecal gadolinium in localization of spinal CSF leaks in patients with spontaneous intracranial hypotension. AJNR Am J Neuroradiol 2012;33:535–40.

29. Chazen JL, Talbott JF, Lantos JE, et al. MR myelography for identification of spinal CSF leak in spontaneous intracranial hypotension. AJNR Am J Neuroradiol 2014;35:2007–12.

30. Verdoorn JT, Luetmer PH, Carr CM, et al. Predicting high-flow spinal CSF leaks in spontaneous intracranial hypotension using a spinal MRI-based algorithm: have repeat CT myelograms been reduced? AJNR Am J Neuroradiol 2016;37:185–8.

31. Kong DS, Park K, Nam DH, et al. Clinical features and long-term results of spontaneous intracranial hypotension. Neurosurgery 2005;57:91–6 [discussion: 91–6].

32. Franzini A, Messina G, Nazzi V, et al. Spontaneous intracranial hypotension syndrome: a novel speculative physiopathological hypothesis and a novel patch method in a series of 28 consecutive patients. J Neurosurg 2010;112:300–6.

33. Manchikanti L, Malla Y, Cash KA, et al. Do the gaps in the ligamentum flavum in the cervical spine translate into dural punctures? An analysis of 4,396 fluoroscopic interlaminar epidural injections. Pain Physician 2015;18:259–66.

34. Amrhein TJ, Parivash SN, Gray L, et al. Incidence of inadvertent dural puncture during CT fluoroscopy-guided interlaminar epidural corticosteroid injections in the cervical spine: an analysis of 974 cases. AJR Am J Roentgenol 2017;209:656–61.

35. Kranz PG, Amrhein TJ, Gray L. Incidence of inadvertent intravascular injection during CT fluoroscopy-guided epidural steroid injections. AJNR Am J Neuroradiol 2015;36:1000–7.

36. Furman MB, O'Brien EM, Zgleszewski TM. Incidence of intravascular penetration in transforaminal lumbosacral epidural steroid injections. Spine (Phila Pa 1976) 2000;25:2628–32.

37. Sencakova D, Mokri B, McClelland RL. The efficacy of epidural blood patch in spontaneous CSF leaks. Neurology 2001;57:1921–3.

38. Berroir S, Loisel B, Ducros A, et al. Early epidural blood patch in spontaneous intracranial hypotension. Neurology 2004;63:1950–1.

39. Amrhein TJ, Befera NT, Gray L, et al. CT fluoroscopy-guided blood patching of ventral CSF leaks by direct needle placement in the ventral epidural space using a transforaminal approach. AJNR Am J Neuroradiol 2016;37:1951–6.

40. Gregg L, Sorte DE, Gailloud P. Intraforaminal location of thoracolumbar radicular arteries providing an anterior radiculomedullary artery using flat panel catheter angiotomography. AJNR Am J Neuroradiol 2017;38:1054–60.

41. Chung SJ, Lee JH, Im JH, et al. Short- and long-term outcomes of spontaneous CSF hypovolemia. Eur Neurol 2005;54:63–7.

42. He FF, Li L, Liu MJ, et al. Targeted epidural blood patch treatment for refractory spontaneous intracranial hypotension in China. J Neurol Surg B Skull Base 2018;79:217–23.

43. Ferrante E, Arpino I, Citterio A, et al. Epidural blood patch in Trendelenburg position pre-medicated with acetazolamide to treat spontaneous intracranial hypotension. Eur J Neurol 2010;17:715–9.

44. Cho KI, Moon HS, Jeon HJ, et al. Spontaneous intracranial hypotension: efficacy of radiologic targeting vs blind blood patch. Neurology 2011;76:1139–44.

45. Wu JW, Hseu SS, Fuh JL, et al. Factors predicting response to the first epidural blood patch in spontaneous intracranial hypotension. Brain 2017;140:344–52.

46. Schievink WI, Morreale VM, Atkinson JL, et al. Surgical treatment of spontaneous spinal cerebrospinal fluid leaks. J Neurosurg 1998;88:243–6.

47. Schievink WI, Ross L, Prasad RS, et al. Vanishing calcification associated with a spontaneous ventral spinal cerebrospinal fluid leak. Cephalalgia 2016;36:1366–9.

Beyond the Spinal Canal

Prashant Raghavan, MBBS*, Jessica Record, MD, Lorenna Vidal, MD

KEYWORDS

• Spinal imaging • Extraspinal • Spinal abnormality • Incidental finding

KEY POINTS

- Incidental findings are commonly seen on cross-sectional spine imaging studies.
- Not all such findings require workup. An awareness of current recommendations for follow-up and management of these and the use of structured reporting can help minimize unnecessary interventions.
- It is important to evaluate scout views and screening images routinely so as not to miss clinically relevant incidental findings.

INTRODUCTION

The use of cross-sectional spinal imaging continues to increase,[1,2] and extraspinal findings are often incidentally identified during interpretation. Although some of these findings may in themselves cause symptoms that mimic a spinal disorder, the majority is entirely asymptomatic and incidental. It is essential that the radiologist not only identify those abnormalities that may have clinical significance but also recognize those that are clinically irrelevant and thereby prevent patients from being subjected to further unnecessary, expensive and potentially harmful interventions.[3] A comprehensive review of all such abnormalities is beyond the scope of this article. The authors' intention instead is to focus on those abnormalities that are commonly encountered and provide practical guidance for follow-up and management based on current recommendations.

A STRUCTURED APPROACH TO INCIDENTAL FINDINGS

Lee and colleagues[4] reported a prevalence of 4.3% for clinically important findings in a series of 400 lumbar spine computed tomography (CT) examinations, the most common of which were abdominal aortic aneurysms. However, although 40.5% of their patients manifested an extraspinal finding, only 14.8% required further evaluation. Barboza and colleagues[5] identified incidental findings in 230 of 1256 patients (18.3%) who underwent cervical spine CT during trauma evaluation. They noted that the likelihood of nontrauma-related incidental findings was associated with age ($P<.0001$).

Recently, several investigators have adopted a structured reporting approach to classify incidental findings. This approach uses a classification scheme first applied to CT colonography[6] (CT Colonography Reporting and Data System [C-RADS]) (Table 1). Using this approach, Quattrocchi and colleagues[7] noted a 68.6% incidence of extraspinal findings in a series of 3000 lumbar spine MR images with 17.6% demonstrating indeterminate or clinically important findings (E3 and E4) and requiring clinical correlation or further evaluation. Of the 11.3% of patients in the E3 group, the most common finding was the presence of abdominal-pelvic fluid. In the 2.5% of patients manifesting an E4 finding, the most common abnormalities included lymphadenopathy, prostate lesions, urinary bladder wall thickening, and abdominal aortic aneurysms (11/74, 14.9%). It is

Disclosure Statement: The authors have nothing to disclose.
Department of Diagnostic Radiology and Nuclear Medicine, University of Maryland School of Medicine, 655 W. Baltimore St, Baltimore, MD 21201, USA
* Corresponding author.
E-mail address: prashant.raghavan@gmail.com

Radiol Clin N Am 57 (2019) 453–467
https://doi.org/10.1016/j.rcl.2018.09.009

Table 1 Classification of incidental extracolonic findings	
Extracolonic Classification	**Clinical Significance**
E0	Limited Examination
E1	Normal examination or normal variant
E2	Clinically unimportant finding: no workup required
E3	Likely unimportant or incompletely characterized finding: referral depends on local center
E4	Potentially important finding: communicate to referring physician

Adapted from Zalis ME, Barish MA, Choi JR, et al. CT colonography reporting and data system: a consensus proposal. Radiology 2005;236(1):8; with permission.

significant that their study showed that, in the absence of structured reporting, incidental asymptomatic extraspinal findings were underrepresented in the actual radiological reports, with 85% of E3 or E4 findings not being mentioned. In another series of lumbar spine MR images (n = 3024), the investigators demonstrated an E3 finding in 22% and an E4 finding in 5%.[8] Most of the C-RADS E3 findings in their series were benign, required further workup to determine clinical relevance, and included hepatic hemangiomas, hydronephrosis, complex renal cysts, large ovarian cysts, and liver cysts. The most common C-RADS E4 findings were abdominal aortic aneurysms, renal masses, and retroperitoneal lymphadenopathy. Although lower than that reported by Quattrocchi and colleagues,[7] 40% of incidental findings in the Semaan and colleagues'[8] study were not noted in the actual radiology reports, with 38.6% of potentially important (E4) findings not being mentioned.

On the planning CT images obtained for transforaminal lumbar epidural steroid injection, Lagemann and colleagues[9] identified 10 of 400 patients with C-RADS E4 findings, most commonly vascular aneurysm or stenosis, whereas 13 demonstrated E3 findings, most of which were hepatomegaly. They also noted that in only 1 of the 22 patients with E3 or E4 findings was the abnormality communicated to the referring physician. After implementation of a checklist template to include prevertebral soft tissues and thyroid nodules, Lin and colleagues[10] demonstrated a

statistically significant decrease in missed non-fracture findings on cervical spine CT. These studies not only shed light on the frequency and types of incidental pathologies that are encountered on spine imaging but also suggest that the use of a structured approach to these may enhance diagnostic accuracy and aid the referring clinician as to what further workup, if any, is warranted.

Scout Images

Incidental findings are often evident on the scout image of a CT or localizer image of an MR imaging of the spine. Scout/localizer views may be considered the modern equivalent of the "edges of the film." These unfortunately often remain neglected during image interpretation.[11] For example, in one of the earliest studies performed addressing this subject, Johnson and colleagues[12] found that up to 23% of CT scout images contained important findings with 2% not being evident in the CT field of view. If one extrapolates this to the approximately 85 million CT studies performed annually in the United States, as many as 1.7 million patients may harbor a potentially clinically relevant finding that is demonstrated only on the scout view. It would be reasonable to surmise that this would be true of MR imaging localizer images as well. Kamath and colleagues[13] concluded that the incidental findings on localizer MR images may be more significant than the spinal problems being evaluated and can have significant impact on patient management and medicolegal implications to the radiologist. Therefore, the onus may be on the radiologist to determine the need for further management from limited images. From a medicolegal standpoint, although no current standards require the radiologist to comment on the scout images, experts believe that it constitutes a radiologist's moral as well as legal duty to interpret these so as not to miss a clinically significant finding.[13,14]

INCIDENTAL THYROID NODULES

Incidental thyroid nodules (ITN), defined as nodules detected in the absence of thyroid-related symptoms, clinical examination findings, or thyroid disease, are frequently encountered, poorly evaluated, and often overlooked entities on cross-sectional imaging of the head, neck, and spine. Youserm and colleagues[15] estimated that up to 16% of such studies may harbor an ITN[16] (**Fig. 1**). When an ITN is seen, the first step is to determine if it warrants further workup with ultrasonography, because indiscriminate workup is not cost-effective. The estimated rate of

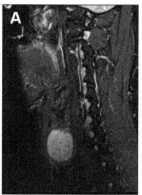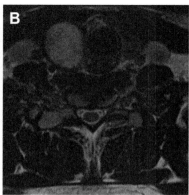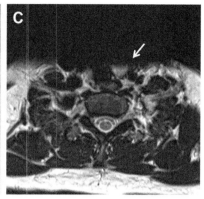

Fig. 1. Incidental thyroid nodules. Parasagittal short tau inversion recovery image (*A*) and axial T2-weighted image (*B*) demonstrate a 3 cm nodule detected incidentally in a 40-year-old patient undergoing cervical spine MR imaging for degenerative disease assessment. Given the size, this nodule requires further evaluation with ultrasound. Axial T2-weighted image (*C*) of a cervical spine MR imaging shows an incidental a 1 cm nodule in the left lobe of the thyroid (*arrow*). The saturation band partially obscures the nodule. The patient was 72 years old and no follow-up was recommended, in keeping with current guidelines.

malignancy in a patient with one or more nodules greater than 5 mm in size is only 1.6%. In addition, most small thyroid cancers are indolent and definitive pathologic diagnosis of benign nodules may require lobectomy.[16] For most patients with indolent thyroid cancer, the problems of over diagnosis and treatment, including the financial implications and treatment-associated morbidity, are not inconsiderable.[17] The current recommendations[18] are ultrasound evaluation if the nodule demonstrates suspicious CT imaging features such as local invasion and lymphadenopathy and positron emission tomography avidity (**Fig. 2**). In the absence of such features, no further workup is indicated in patients with limited life expectancy and comorbidities, unless specifically requested by the clinician. Further workup is required for nodules greater than 1 cm in patients younger than 35 years and for nodules greater than 1.5 cm in patients older than 35 years. Abnormal lymph nodes are those that are enlarged (>1.5 cm short axis diameter for jugulodigastric nodes and 1 cm for other stations), calcified, enhance avidly, or demonstrate cystic change.[18]

LYMPHADENOPATHY

Although normal and reactive lymph nodes are frequently identified on imaging studies of the spine, lymphadenopathy as a clinically significant incidental finding is only rarely present. Although Lagemann and colleagues[9] found lymphadenopathy, defined as any node larger than 1 cm in the short axis, in only 1 patient (0.3%), retroperitoneal lymphadenopathy constituted the second most common E4 finding in Semaan's series.[8] However,

if there is a clinical history of cancer, it is always prudent to scrutinize cervical, mediastinal, pelvic, and retroperitoneal nodal stations for lymphadenopathy (**Fig. 3**).

Although a universally accepted method of measuring lymph nodes is not present in the literature, there are some useful rules of thumb. Cervical nodes greater than 1.5 cm in short axis may be considered pathologically enlarged. However, size is not the only imaging feature to consider because normal-sized nodes may also be abnormal if they show necrosis, calcification, and extracapsular spread of malignancy.[19,20] In the mediastinum, the largest normal lymph nodes lie in the subcarinal and right tracheobronchial regions. In general, a mediastinal node larger than 10 mm in short axis dimension may be considered abnormal. Incidental detection of mesenteric lymph nodes is a common phenomenon on lumbar spine imaging. Normal mesenteric nodes are usually less than 5 mm in short axis, and when identified, require no further imaging.[21] With regard to abdominal lymph nodes in other locations, size thresholds for normal short axis diameters include the following: retrocrural space, 6 mm; paracardiac, 8 mm; gastrohepatic ligament, 8 mm; upper paraaortic region, 9 mm; portacaval space, 10 mm; porta hepatis, 7 mm; and lower paraaortic region, 11 mm.[22]

ABDOMEN
Liver

Incidental hepatic lesions are fairly common (**Fig. 4**). For example, in the study by Semaan and colleagues,[8] the liver was the fourth most

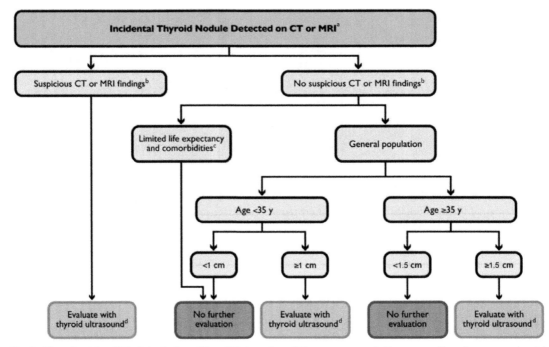

Fig. 2. Flowchart for ITNs detected on CT or MR imaging. [a] The recommendations are offered as general guidance and do not apply to all patients, such as those with clinical risk factors for thyroid cancer. [b] Suspicious CT/MR imaging features include abnormal lymph nodes and/or invasion of local tissues by the thyroid nodule. Abnormal lymph node features include calcifications, cystic components, and/or increased enhancement. Nodal enlargement is less specific for thyroid cancer metastases, but further evaluation could be considered if an ITN has ipsilateral nodes greater than 1.5 cm in short axis for jugulodigastric lymph nodes and greater than 1 cm for other lymph nodes. [c] Limited life expectancy and comorbidities that increase the risk of treatment or are more likely to cause morbidity and mortality than the thyroid cancer itself, given the nodule size. Patients with comorbidities or limited life expectancy should not have further evaluation of the ITN, unless it is warranted clinically or specifically requested by the patient or referring physician. [d] Further management of the ITN after thyroid ultrasound, including fine-needle aspiration, should be based on ultrasound findings. (*Adapted from* Hoang JK, Langer JE, Middleton WD, et al. Managing incidental thyroid nodules detected on imaging: white paper of the ACR Incidental Thyroid Findings Committee. J Am Coll Radiol 2015;12(2):146; with permission.)

common organ system associated with incidental findings with about 3.9% of studies harboring such lesions, most of which were simple cysts. Other commonly seen incidental lesions include hemangiomas, focal nodular hyperplasia, and focal perfusional changes on postcontrast studies. Current guidelines[23] state that the first step is to determine if the patient is "high risk" for having a malignant neoplasm (**Fig. 5**). Risk factors include a history of primary malignancy known to spread to the liver, cirrhosis and hepatic disease such as hepatitis, nonalcoholic steatohepatitis, sclerosing cholangitis, primary biliary cirrhosis, choledochal cysts, hemochromatosis and hereditary hepatic disease, and anabolic steroid use. Hepatic cysts have low density on CT, which can be fairly confidently determined when the cyst is greater than 1 cm in size. Perfusional changes tend to occur at characteristic locations, whereas hemangiomas

and focal nodular hyperplasia (FNH) tend to demonstrate variable imaging appearances depending on modality, sequences used, and contrast administration. In general, lesions smaller than 1 cm in size require no further workup. Those lesions that are greater than or equal to 1 cm in size, without suspicious features (sharp margins, ≤20 HU attenuation, demonstrating typical features of hemangiomas, FNH, or perfusional changes) also need no follow-up, regardless of risk level. A lesion greater than or equal to 1 cm demonstrating irregular margins, attenuation greater than or equal to 20 HU, septations, and nodularity may need evaluation by MR imaging or biopsy. Often, these lesions are incompletely characterized on the imaging study on which they were detected, such that any lesion greater than or equal to 1 cm needs further evaluation with MR imaging.

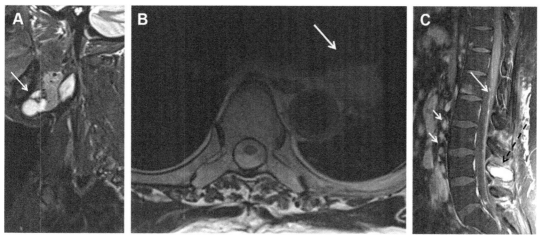

Fig. 3. Lymphadenopathy detected incidentally on spine imaging. Sagittal STIR (*A*) submandibular lymphadenopathy (*arrow*) due to lymphoma on a cervical spine MR image. Axial T2-weighted image (*B*) of a thoracic spine MR imaging shows paraesophageal lymphadenopathy (*arrow*) due to metastatic disease from chordoma, which was identified incidentally. Postcontrast sagittal T1 image with fat saturation image (*C*) reveals retroperitoneal lymph nodes (*short arrows*), biopsy proved to be sarcoidosis in a patient who also had leptomeningeal disease and osseous lesions (*long and black dashed arrows*, respectively).

Biliary Tree and Gallbladder

A dilated common bile duct was seen in 1.3% of lumbar spine MR images in Semaan's series[8] and 0.6% in the study by Quattrocchi and colleagues[7] (**Fig. 6**). Although a dilated common duct is usually consequent to prior cholecystectomy, It Is prudent to correlate with clinical findings or laboratory abnormalities to determine if the imaging findings are secondary to biliary obstruction. No further evaluation is required for a dilated common duct greater than 6 mm or greater than 10 mm after cholecystectomy, if laboratory results are normal.

Filling defects in the gallbladder may include calculi, polyps, and mass lesions. Cholelithiasis is a common finding, present in 3.7% of the study by Semaan and colleagues[8] The American College

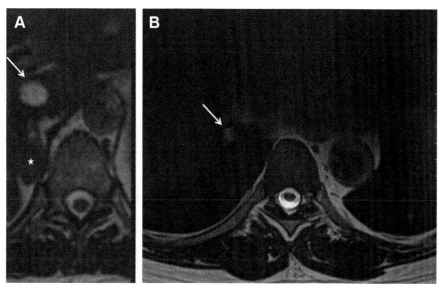

Fig. 4. (*A, B*) Incidental hepatic lesions. Axial T2-weighted images show examples of simple cysts (*arrows*). Note also an incidental adrenal adenoma (*star, A*).

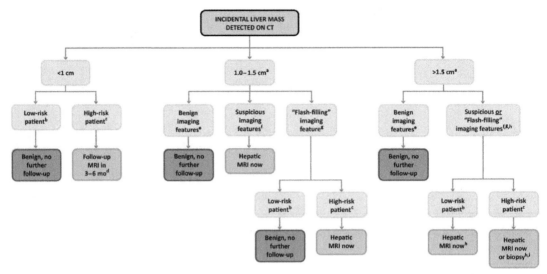

Fig. 5. Algorithm for incidental liver lesions. [a] If inadequate imaging is available to ascertain the presence of benign versus suspicious features in a ≥1 cm lesion, prompt MR imaging is advised. [b] Low-risk patient: no known primary malignancy, hepatic dysfunction, or hepatic risk factors. [c] High-risk patient: known primary malignancy with a propensity to metastasize to the liver, cirrhosis, and/or other hepatic risk factors. [d] Follow-up MR imaging in 3 to 6 months. May need more immediate follow-up in some scenarios. CT is also acceptable in a patient with cancer who is due for routine CT surveillance. [e] Benign features: sharp margin, homogeneous low attenuation (≤20 Hounsfield units [HU]) on noncontrast and/or portal venous phase imaging, and characteristic features of hemangiomas, focal nodular hyperplasia (FNH), focal fatty sparing or deposition, or perfusional changes. If pseudoenhancement is present, a benign cyst may measure greater than 20 HU; radiologists' discretion is necessary. [f] Suspicious features: ill-defined margins, heterogeneous density, mural thickening or nodularity, thick septa, and intermediate to high attenuation on portal venous phase imaging (>20 HU, in the absence of pseudoenhancement). If pre- and postcontrast CT is available, enhancement greater than 20 HU is a suspicious feature. To evaluate, prefer MR imaging. [g] "Flash-filling" feature: uniform hyperenhancement relative to hepatic parenchyma on arterial phase (including late arterial/early portal venous phase) postcontrast imaging. If additional postcontrast phases are available to characterize lesion as benign (eg, hemangioma) or suspicious (eg, hepatocellular carcinoma), the lesion should be placed in one of those respective categories and not here. [h] Incidental hepatic lesions that are greater than 1.5 cm and do not have benign features should at least undergo prompt MR imaging. Direct biopsy (without MR imaging) may be appropriate in some scenarios. Differentiation of FNH from adenoma is important, especially if larger than 3 cm and subcapsular in location; for such patients, MR imaging with hepatospecific gadoxetate disodium is advised. [i] If biopsy is pursued, core biopsy is preferred over fine-needle aspiration. (*Adapted from* Gore RM, Pickhardt PJ, Mortele KJ, et al. Management of incidental liver lesions on CT: a white paper of the ACR Incidental Findings Committee. J Am Coll Radiol 2017;14(11):1430; with permission.)

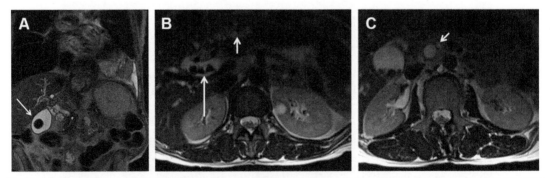

Fig. 6. (*A–C*) Incidental biliary abnormalities. Coronal localizer image (*A*) for a thoracolumbar spinal MR imaging shows a solitary gall bladder calculus (*arrow*). Axial T2-weighted images (*B, C*) reveal biliary ductal (*long arrow*, B) calculi in a patient in whom spine imaging was obtained for clinically suspected spondylodiscitis. Note the dilatation of the intrahepatic biliary radicles and the proximal pancreatic duct (*small arrows* in *B* and *C*).

of Radiology (ACR) recommends annual ultrasound follow-up of polyps between 7 to 9 mm and surgical consultation for those larger than 10 mm.[24] Follow-up is not recommended for asymptomatic gall stones, gallbladder mural calcification, polyps less than 6 mm in size, diffuse gallbladder wall thickening, or asymptomatic gallbladder distension.

Adrenal Glands

An adrenal "incidentaloma" is defined as a mass lesion greater than 1 cm in diameter, discovered serendipitously on an imaging study[25] and is relatively common (4.4% prevalence on abdominal CT) (Fig. 7). Two key questions must be addressed when an adrenal "incidentaloma" is identified: (1) is it malignant? (2) is it hormonally functional? A homogenous, smoothly marginated lesion with a mean density of less than 10 HU is highly likely to be a benign adenoma.[26] In general, larger masses are likely to be malignant (>4 cm).[27] Hamrahian and colleagues[28] found that size less than 4 cm and a mean density of less than 10 HU excluded malignancy with 100% certainty. The ACR does not recommend any workup for small incidentalomas in patients without history of malignancy.[29] Although evaluation may be limited on spine CT or MR images, worrisome features include irregular shape, inhomogeneity, high CT attenuation, diameter greater than 4 cm, and calcification. If a lesion has these imaging features, dedicated contrast-enhanced CT or MR imaging is recommended. If there is a history of malignancy, in the absence of typical benign features, or known widespread metastatic disease, PET imaging is recommended.

Kidneys

Simple renal cysts are perhaps the most commonly encountered incidental finding on lumbar spine imaging (Fig. 8). However, such renal lesions are often incompletely characterized on such examinations. Although there are accepted guidelines for the management and workup of "completely characterized" renal incidental lesions, that is, those in which imaging features allow a confident diagnosis,[30] these criteria are not tailored for the "incompletely evaluated" lesions, that is, those that are too small to characterize or are detected incidentally. Recent recommendations[30] are based on evidence that reveals a low risk of progression of many small renal masses and an improved understanding of their imaging features. As such, imaging follow-up of incompletely characterized lesions that are highly likely to be simple cysts is not recommended and follow-up of small solid lesions in selected patients may be delayed, given the indolent nature of small renal cell cancers. Incompletely characterized lesions that are homogeneously low in attenuation (≤20 HU) or homogeneously high (≥70 HU) require no additional imaging. The presence of fat is a reassuring sign of a benign angiomyolipoma[31] (see Fig. 8D). The presence of thick septations, mural nodularity, calcification, and necrosis are worrisome signs. An approach to incidental cystic and solid renal masses is presented in Figs. 9 and 10.[30]

Nephrolithiasis is frequently reported as an incidental finding on CT imaging (18.8%)[32] (Fig. 11A, B) but is rarely evident on MR imaging.

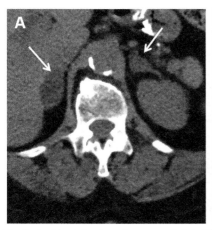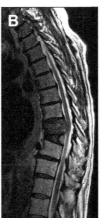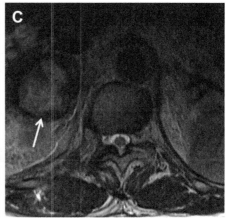

Fig. 7. Incidental adrenal masses. Axial CT (A) shows typical bilateral low-density adrenal adenomas (arrows). Sagittal T2-weighted thoracic spine MR imaging (B) obtained for a patient with lung cancer presenting with new back pain reveals metastatic lesions in the T10 and T11 vertebral bodies. A pathologic fracture of T11 is noted. Axial T2-weighed image (arrow, C) from this study shows a previously unknown right adrenal metastasis.

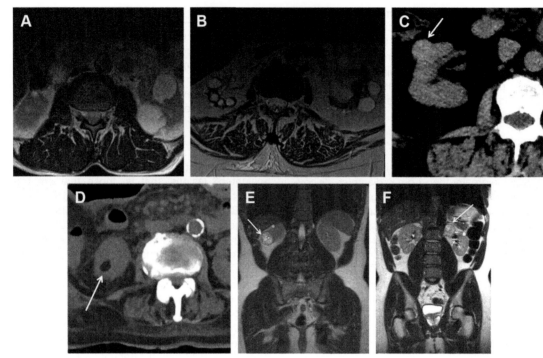

Fig. 8. Incidental renal abnormalities. Axial T2-weighted images of lumbar spine show simple cysts (*A*) and atrophic native kidneys containing multiple cysts (*B*). Axial lumbar spine CT images demonstrate a uniformly hyperdense cyst (*arrow, C*) and an angiolipoma (*arrow, D*). Coronal T2-weighted scout images (*arrows, E* and *F*) reveal heterogenous bilateral renal masses, which proved to be renal cell carcinomas.

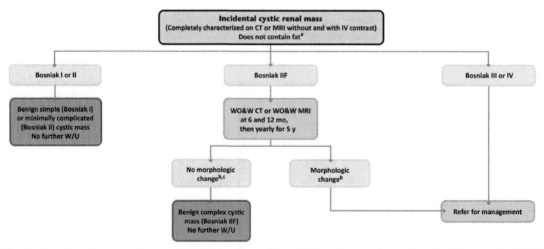

Fig. 9. Flowchart for managing a cystic renal mass on CT or MR imaging performed both without and with IV contrast. [a] If the mass contains fat attenuation (a region of interest <−10 HU). [b] Morphologic change includes increasing number of septa, thickening of the wall or septa, or development of a solid nodular component (including reclassification as Bosniak III or IV). Growth of a cystic mass without morphologic change does not indicate malignancy. [c] A Bosniak IIF cystic renal mass without change in imaging features for at least 5 years is considered stable and likely of no clinical significance. IV, intravenous; WO&W, without and with; W/U, workup. (*Adapted from* Herts BR, Sliverman SG, Hindman NM, et al. Management of the incidental renal mass on CT: a white paper of the ACR Incidental Findings Committee. J Am Coll Radiol 2018;15(2):264–73; with permission.)

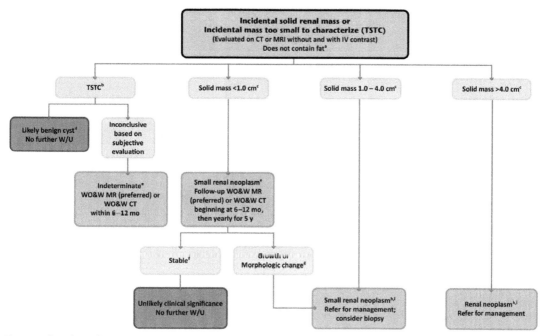

Fig. 10. Flowchart for managing a completely characterized solid renal mass or renal mass too small to characterize on CT or MR imagingl performed both without and with IV contrast. [a] Does not contain fat. [b] Too small to characterize. [c] Size = largest diameter in any plane, follows TNM version 7 staging criteria. [d] Well-circumscribed TSTC renal masses, either calcified or noncalcified but that are otherwise homogeneous and either visually much lower than the renal parenchyma on any phase or much higher than the unenhanced renal parenchyma, are probably benign cystic lesions that do not need further evaluation. [e] MR imaging is preferred for characterizing smaller renal masses (<1.5 cm) and for detecting enhancement in suspected hypovascular masses. [f] A renal mass without change in imaging features *and* with an average growth of ≤3 mm per year for at least 5 years is considered stable and likely of no clinical significance. [g] Growth is defined as ≥4 mm per year average; morphologic change is any change in heterogeneity, such as a change in contour, attenuation, or number of septa. [h] Consider biopsy, especially if hyperattenuating on unenhanced CT or hypointense on T2-weighted MR imaging, because these suggest a fat-poor angiomyolipoma. [i] If a pathologic diagnosis is desired to determine management but biopsy is technically challenging, or there is another relative contraindication to biopsy, consider MR imaging to assess the T2-weighted signal intensity. Fat-poor angiomyolipoma and papillary renal cell carcinoma may be T2 hypointense in contrast to clear cell renal cell carcinoma, which is typically heterogeneous and mildly T2 hyperintense. IV, intravenous; WO&W, without and with; W/U, workup. (*Adapted from* Herts BR, Sliverman SG, Hindman NM, et al. Management of the incidental renal mass on CT: a white paper of the ACR Incidental Findings Committee. J Am Coll Radiol 2018;15(2):267; with permission.)

Asymptomatic nephrolithiasis can, however, become symptomatic in up to 50% of patients in 5 years. Although expectant management is prudent in those who harbor small calculi without evidence of infection or obstruction, high-risk patients (ie, those with solitary kidneys, renal anatomic abnormality, etc.) may benefit from further evaluation and treatment to forestall recurrence or growth of existing calculi. Hydronephrosis[33] was found incidentally in 0.2% of lumbar spine MR images in the Quattrocchi and colleagues'[7] study (**Fig. 11C**). The cause of such hydronephrosis is often not apparent on spine imaging and further clinical and imaging evaluation is recommended.

VASCULAR FINDINGS

Aneurysms of the abdominal aorta are among the most commonly seen E4 findings on spine imaging[7–9] (**Fig. 12**). These may not necessarily be incidental given that they may also present with back pain. The ACR's Incidental Findings Committee II on Vascular Findings[34] provides follow-up guidelines on aortic ectasia and aneurysms. Complete evaluation of the blood vessels ventral to the spine may be difficult if they are obscured by saturation bands. However, when they can be confidently measured, normal diameters for the suprarenal and infrarenal abdominal aorta are 2.0 cm and 3.0 cm, respectively. Aneurysmal dilatation is

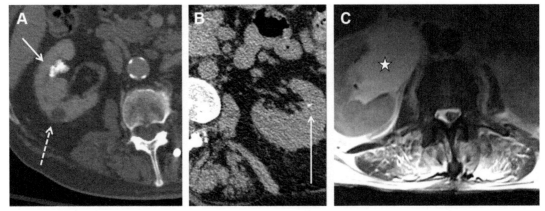

Fig. 11. Incidental staghorn calculus seen on an axial lumbar spine CT obtained for polytrauma (*arrow, A*). Note also an incidental right renal cyst (*dashed arrow*). CT lumbar spine (*B*) obtained for low back pain reveals incidental punctate nephrolithiasis (*arrow*). Axial T2-weighted image (*C*) of a lumbar spine MR imaging shows previously unknown right hydronephrosis (*star*) likely accounting for chronic flank pain.

present when the infrarenal aortic diameter exceeds 3.0 cm or when it is greater than or equal to 1.5 times the normal diameter. Abdominal aortic dilatation less than 2.5 cm generally does not require follow-up. There are recommended intervals for follow-up of aortic ectasia and aneurysms.[34] Because the rupture of smaller abdominal aortic aneurysms is less likely, longer intervals between follow-ups are recommended. Follow-up intervals may vary depending on comorbidities and the growth rate of the aneurysm. In addition to planning follow-up imaging, one should also consider surgical or endovascular referral.

Iliac artery aneurysms, defined as dilatation greater than or equal to 1.5 times the normal iliac artery diameter or greater than or equal to2.5 cm, are uncommon but can occasionally be seen on lumbar spine imaging. Iliac artery aneurysms larger than 3.0 cm in diameter should receive follow-up cross-sectional imaging in 6 months, whereas those that exceed 3.5 cm should be followed up more closely or receive treatment given the high rupture risk.[35] Other incidental vascular findings that may be observed include retropharyngeal course of the internal carotid arteries (occasionally mistaken for pathology on lateral plain radiographs or clinical

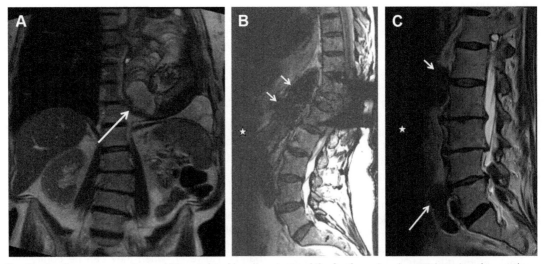

Fig. 12. Aortic aneurysms. Coronal T2-weighted localizer image (*A*) of a thoracic spine MR imaging shows a large descending aortic aneurysm (*arrow*). Sagittal T2-weighted images (*B, C*) show incidental abdominal aortic aneurysms (*short arrows*) in 2 different patients obscured partially by saturation bands (*asterisks*). Note also the iliac artery aneurysm in C (*large arrow*).

examination), aneurysms of splanchnic vessels, penetrating aortic ulcers, anatomic venous variants and thrombosis of the major cervical or abdominal veins, and vascular filter complication (**Fig. 13**).

PELVIS

Although abnormalities of the pelvic viscera are fairly frequently seen on lumbar spine imaging, adequate characterization is difficult, given the limitations of field of view and obscuration by saturation bands. However, it is helpful to be aware of some practical guidelines that may help determine the need for follow-up when these can be reasonably evaluated. Free pelvic fluid (**Fig. 14**A) is a commonly seen finding (present in 77% of the studies in the Quattrocchi's series).[7] This is usually a physiologic finding except when there is a history of abdominal/pelvic pain or trauma. Pelvic peritoneal fluid accumulation of less than 10 mL may be a normal finding in otherwise healthy men and postmenopausal women.[36] Incidental uterine findings include variant anatomy, endometrial thickening, and leiomyomas (**Fig. 14**B). The thickness of normal endometrium can be variable, depending on numerous factors, and can be difficult to measure accurately on spine imaging. It can measure up to 16 mm in the secretory phase of

menstruation in premenopausal women and is typically less than 5 mm in postmenopausal women. Incidentally seen endometrial thickness exceeding 11 mm in postmenopausal women may require biopsy.[37]

The ACR's Incidental Findings Committee II on Adnexal Findings provides useful recommendations for workup of incidental adnexal lesions.[38] Adnexal cysts are categorized as "benign-appearing" or "probably benign" depending on the morphologic features (**Fig. 15**A–C). Given that it is not likely for many of these to be well characterized on imaging studies focused on the spine, the majority would fall in the "probably benign" category, a feature described by the guidelines as "a portion of the cyst is not well imaged." The recommendations[38] are summarized in **Fig. 16**. Briefly, no follow-up is required for benign appearing adnexal cysts less than or equal to 3 cm in premenopausal women. For benign appearing adnexal cysts greater than 5 cm, ultrasound follow-up is recommended at 6 to 12 weeks. For early postmenopausal women (<5 years after last menstrual period or age 50–55 years), ultrasound follow-up is recommended for benign appearing cysts between 3 and 5 cm (in 6–12 months) and for those greater than 5 cm in size and probably benign cysts greater than 3 cm should undergo ultrasound evaluation. Prompt ultrasound evaluation

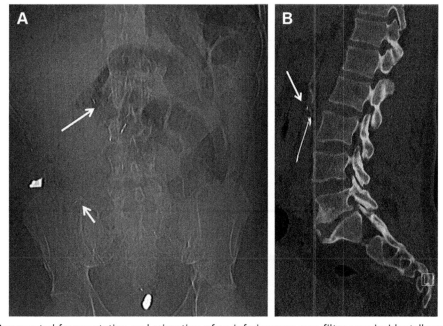

Fig. 13. Unsuspected fragmentation and migration of an inferior vena cava filter seen incidentally on a lumbar spine CT. The CT scout image (*A*) of displacement of the filter tines clearly (*long arrow*) and also migration of a tine into the right hemipelvis (*short arrow*). Parasagittal CT (*B*) clearly depicts the fractured, displaced filter (*arrow*).

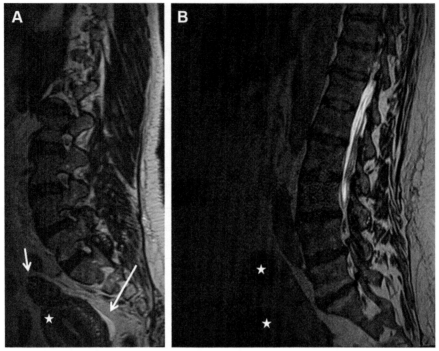

Fig. 14. Spectrum of incidental pelvic imaging findings on lumbar spine MRI. Parasagittal T2-weighted image (*A*) shows a small amount of free fluid (*long arrow*), a subserosal leiomyoma (*short arrow*), and adenomyosis (*star*). Parasagittal T2-weighted image (*B*) illustrates large intramural leiomyomas (*stars*).

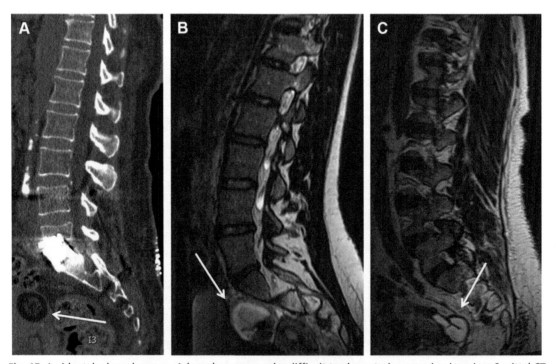

Fig. 15. Incidental adnexal masses. Adnexal masses can be difficult to characterize on spine imaging. Sagittal CT (*A*) shows a lesion in the pelvis with internal fat (*arrow*), which enabled the correct diagnosis of a dermoid cyst. Parasagittal T2-weighted image (*B*) reveals a complex adnexal cyst containing debris (*arrow*), which was determined to be a benign hemorrhagic ovarian cyst. Parasagittal T2-weighted image (*C*) shows a tubular curved lesion (*arrow*) strongly suggesting it to be a hydrosalpinx.

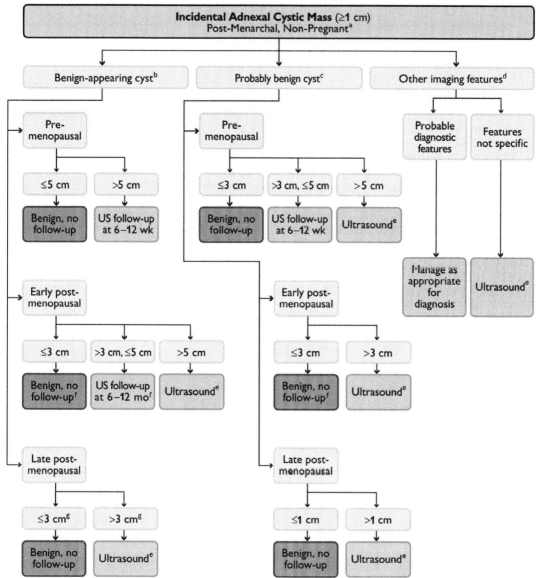

Fig. 16. Incidental adnexal cystic mass flowchart. [a] Exclusions: (1) normal findings, including hypodense ovary, crenulated enhancing wall of corpus luteum, asymmetric ovary (within 95% confidence interval for size) with normal shape; (2) unimportant findings, including calcifications without associated noncalcified mass; (3) previous characterization with ultrasound or MR imaging; and (4) documented stability in size and appearance for greater than 2 years. [b] Should have all of the following features: (1) oval or round; (2) unilocular, with uniform fluid attenuation or signal (layering hemorrhage acceptable if premenopausal); (3) regular or imperceptible wall; (4) no solid area, mural nodule; and (5) <10 cm in maximum diameter. [c] Refers to an adnexal cyst that would otherwise meet the criteria for a benign-appearing cyst except for one or more of the following specific observations: (1) angulated margins, (2) not round or oval in shape, (3) a portion of the cyst is poorly imaged (eg, a portion of the cyst may be obscured by metal streak artifact on CT of the pelvis), and (4) the image has reduced signal-to-noise ratio, usually because of technical parameters or in some cases because the study was performed without intravenous contrast. [d] Features of masses in this category include (1) solid component, (2) mural nodule, (3) septations, (4) higher than fluid attenuation, and (5) layering hemorrhage if postmenopausal. [e] This indicates that ultrasound should be performed promptly for further evaluation, rather than in follow-up. [f] A benign-appearing cyst ≤5 cm with suspected internal hemorrhage in a patient aged ≤55 years, or within 5 years of menopause, should be followed in 6 to 12 weeks because hemorrhagic cysts in early postmenopause are possible, although rare. [g] May decrease threshold from 3 cm to lower values down to 1 cm to increase sensitivity for neoplasm. (*Reproduced from* Patel MD, Ascher SM, Paspulati RM, et al. Managing incidental findings on abdominal and pelvic CT and MRI, part 1: white paper of the ACR Incidental Findings Committee II on adnexal findings. J Am Coll Radiol 2013;10(9):677; with permission.)

is recommended for benign-appearing cysts greater than 3 cm and probably benign cysts greater than 1 cm in late postmenopausal women.[38]

SUMMARY

A myriad of incidental extraspinal findings may be present on spine imaging studies, some of which may have enormous clinical implications. The authors have discussed those important entities for which established guidelines can be applied to direct follow-up and further management. The scout/screening images may contain a wealth of information, and it is important to incorporate evaluation of these images into routine practice. Look beyond the spinal canal as the findings can have significant impact on patient management and medicolegal implications to the radiologist. Using structured reporting terminology may aid the radiologist not only to more consistently identify incidental extraspinal findings but also to suggest appropriate management recommendations.

ACKNOWLEDGMENTS

The authors would like to thank Brigitte Pocta, MLA for her assistance with manuscript preparation.

REFERENCES

1. Ganduglia CM, Zezza M, Smith JD, et al. Effect of public reporting on MR imaging use for low back pain. Radiology 2015;276(1):175–83.
2. Gan G, Harkey P, Hemingway J, et al. Changing utilization patterns of cervical spine imaging in the emergency department: perspectives from two decades of national medicare claims. J Am Coll Radiol 2016;13(6):644–8.
3. Martin BI, Jarvik JG. The medicare outpatient imaging efficiency measure for low back pain ("OP-8"). Radiology 2015;276(1):1–2.
4. Lee SY, Landis MS, Ross IG, et al. Extraspinal findings at lumbar spine CT examinations: prevalence and clinical importance. Radiology 2012;263(2):502–9.
5. Barboza R, Fox JH, Shaffer LET, et al. Incidental findings in the cervical spine at CT for trauma evaluation. AJR Am J Roentgenol 2009;192(3):725–9.
6. Zalis ME, Barish MA, Choi JR, et al. CT colonography reporting and data system: a consensus proposal. Radiology 2005;236(1):3–9.
7. Quattrocchi CC, Giona A, Di Martino AC, et al. Extraspinal incidental findings at lumbar spine MRI in the general population: a large cohort study. Insights Imaging 2013;4(3):301–8.
8. Semaan HB, Bieszczad JE, Obri T, et al. Incidental extraspinal findings at lumbar spine magnetic resonance imaging: a retrospective study. Spine 2015;40(18):1436–43.
9. Lagemann GM, Aldred PW, Borhani AA, et al. Lumbar transforaminal epidural steroid injections: incidental extraspinal findings on planning imaging. AJR Am J Roentgenol 2016;207(6):1271–7.
10. Lin E, Powell DK, Kagetsu NJ. Efficacy of a checklist-style structured radiology reporting template in reducing resident misses on cervical spine computed tomography examinations. J Digit Imaging 2014;27(5):588–93.
11. Daffner RH. Reviewing CT scout images: observations of an expert witness. AJR Am J Roentgenol 2015;205(3):589–91.
12. Johnson PT, Scott WW, Gayler BW, et al. The CT scout view: does it need to be routinely reviewed as part of the CT interpretation? AJR Am J Roentgenol 2014;202(6):1256–63.
13. Kamath S, Jain N, Goyal N, et al. Incidental findings on MRI of the spine. Clin Radiol 2009;64(4):353–61.
14. Berlin L. Medicolegal-malpractice and ethical issues in radiology should CT and MRI scout images be interpreted? AJR Am J Roentgenol 2017;209(1):W43.
15. Youserm DM, Huang T, Loevner LA, et al. Clinical and economic impact of incidental thyroid lesions found with CT and MR. AJNR Am J Neuroradiol 1997;18(8):1423–8.
16. Hoang JK, Nguyen XV. Understanding the risks and harms of management of incidental thyroid nodules: a review. JAMA Otolaryngol Head Neck Surg 2017;143(7):718–24.
17. Kitahara CM, Sosa JA. The changing incidence of thyroid cancer. Nat Rev Endocrinol 2016;12(11):646–53.
18. Hoang JK, Langer JE, Middleton WD, et al. Managing incidental thyroid nodules detected on imaging: white paper of the ACR Incidental Thyroid Findings Committee. J Am Coll Radiol 2015;12(2):143–50.
19. Hoang JK, Vanka J, Ludwig BJ, et al. Evaluation of cervical lymph nodes in head and neck cancer with CT and MRI: tips, traps, and a systematic approach. AJR Am J Roentgenol 2013;200(1):W17–25.
20. Schwartz LH, Bogaerts J, Ford R, et al. Evaluation of lymph nodes with RECIST 1.1. Eur J Cancer 2009;45(2):261–7.
21. Lucey BC, Stuhlfaut JW, Soto JA. Mesenteric lymph nodes: detection and significance on MDCT. AJR Am J Roentgenol 2005;184(1):41–4.
22. Dorfman RE, Alpern MB, Gross BH, et al. Upper abdominal lymph nodes: criteria for normal size determined with CT. Radiology 1991;180(2):319–22.
23. Gore RM, Pickhardt PJ, Mortele KJ, et al. Management of incidental liver lesions on CT: a white paper

of the ACR incidental findings committee. J Am Coll Radiol 2017;14(11):1429–37.

24. Sebastian S, Araujo C, Neitlich JD, et al. Managing incidental findings on abdominal and pelvic CT and MRI, Part 4: white paper of the ACR Incidental Findings Committee II on gallbladder and biliary findings. J Am Coll Radiol 2013;10(12):953–6.

25. Young WFJ. Clinical practice. The incidentally discovered adrenal mass. N Engl J Med 2007; 356(6):601–10.

26. Grumbach MM, Biller BMK, Braunstein GD, et al. Management of the clinically inapparent adrenal mass ("incidentaloma"). Ann Intern Med 2003; 138(5):424–9.

27. Mantero F, Terzolo M, Arnaldi G, et al. A survey on adrenal incidentaloma in Italy. Study Group on Adrenal Tumors of the Italian Society of Endocrinology. J Clin Endocrinol Metab 2000,85(2):637–44.

28. Hamrahian AH, Ioachimescu AG, Remer EM, et al. Clinical utility of noncontrast computed tomography attenuation value (hounsfield units) to differentiate adrenal adenomas/hyperplasias from nonadenomas: Cleveland Clinic experience. J Clin Endocrinol Metab 2005;90(2):871–7.

29. Choyke PL. ACR Appropriateness Criteria on incidentally discovered adrenal mass. J Am Coll Radiol 2006;3(7):498–504.

30. Herts BR, Silverman SG, Hindman NM, et al. Management of the incidental renal mass on CT: a white paper of the ACR incidental findings committee. J Am Coll Radiol 2018;15(2):264–73.

31. Silverman SG, Israel GM, Herts BR, et al. Management of the incidental renal mass. Radiology 2008; 249(1):16–31.

32. Meyer HJ, Pfeil A, Schramm D, et al. Renal incidental findings on computed tomography: frequency and distribution in a large non selected cohort. Medicine (Baltimore) 2017;96(26):e7039.

33. Glowacki LS, Beecroft ML, Cook RJ, et al. The natural history of asymptomatic urolithiasis. J Urol 1992; 147(2):319–21.

34. Khosa F, Krinsky G, Macari M, et al. Managing incidental findings on abdominal and pelvic CT and MRI, Part 2: white paper of the ACR Incidental Findings Committee II on vascular findings. J Am Coll Radiol 2013;10(10):789–94.

35. Santilli SM, Wernsing SE, Lee ES. Expansion rates and outcomes for iliac artery aneurysms. J Vasc Surg 2000;31(1 Pt 1):114–21.

36. Yoshikawa T, Hayashi N, Maeda E, et al. Peritoneal fluid accumulation in healthy men and postmenopausal women: evaluation on pelvic MRI. AJR Am J Roentgenol 2013;200(6):1181–5.

37. Smith-Bindman R, Weiss E, Feldstein V. How thick is too thick? When endometrial thickness should prompt biopsy in postmenopausal women without vaginal bleeding. Ultrasound Obstet Gynecol 2004; 24(5):558–65.

38. Patel MD, Ascher SM, Paspulati RM, et al. Managing incidental findings on abdominal and pelvic CT and MRI, part 1: white paper of the ACR Incidental Findings Committee II on adnexal findings. J Am Coll Radiol 2013;10(9):675–81.

Printed and bound by CPI Group (UK) Ltd, Croydon, CR0 4YY

08/05/2025

01864741-0004